MANKIND IN THE MAKING

MANKIND IN THE MAKING

THE STORY OF HUMAN EVOLUTION

Revised Edition

WILLIAM HOWELLS

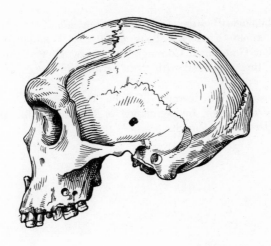

DRAWINGS BY JANIS CIRULIS

DOUBLEDAY & COMPANY, INC., GARDEN CITY, NEW YORK

Library of Congress Catalog Card Number 67–10973
Copyright © 1959, 1967 by William Howells
All Rights Reserved
Printed in the United States of America

"The Three Races" from *Cautionary Verses,* by Hilaire Belloc. Published 1941 by Alfred A. Knopf, Inc. Reprinted by permission of Alfred A. Knopf, Inc., and Gerald Duckworth and Company, Limited.

"Ethnological" from *Gaily the Troubadour,* by Arthur Guiterman. From the book *Gaily the Troubadour,* by Arthur Guiterman. Copyright, 1936, by E. P. Dutton & Co., Inc. Reprinted with their permission.

Translation into German of "The Three Races," by Dr. Gottfried Kurth, by permission of Dr. Kurth and Albert Muller Verlag, Zürich.

IN MEMORY

OF

E. A. HOOTON

CONTENTS

LIST OF ILLUSTRATIONS

LIST OF PHOTOGRAPHS, *following page 192*

NOTE TO THE READER

In the complicated story of man one has to be precise as to the animals and the ideas being talked about, and so it is absolutely necessary to use their right names and terms. I have tried to explain each one as I came to it. Unfortunately these names are seldom one syllable. In the hope of easing the reader's way I have put a glossary at the end, in which he may look for the meaning of terms that might have escaped him since their first introduction.

I have referred liberally to the writings and opinions of others, without immediately directing the reader to a footnote giving the actual source. This is unorthodox, and I apologize to those cited for the slight. I have done it simply to avoid distraction; and the anthropologists will know the sources, anyhow. I have also sometimes mentioned scientists only by name when they first appear, introducing them properly in connection with a more important matter later on. Once again, this is to avoid breaking the story's gait at that point, and I have not meant to be offhanded.

All the drawings of human skulls are, unless otherwise noted, exactly one quarter natural size. The skulls are poised in the "Frankfort Horizontal"; that is, by a horizontal passing through the lower edge of the eye socket and the upper edge of the ear opening. This has been accepted by anthropologists (first at an international convention at Frankfort) as a standard way of best showing the head in its natural position. It is important here, in comparing the features of different fossil skulls. A special effort has also been made to avoid foreshortening, or the distortion resulting when a face is viewed or photographed from a point too close.

Finally, I have added a formal classification of those main groups of vertebrates and primates which are important to man and his ancestry, simply for reference, and to show the arrangement made of these groups by zoologists.

1. EVOLUTION

A HIGH SCHOOL boy in a physics course asked his teacher about evolution. The teacher, John Thomas Scopes, described it in a few sentences. This was rash. For the place was Rhea County, Tennessee, and the time was late in April 1925, a bare month after the governor of the state had signed a new law forbidding the teaching of evolution in the public schools. And so Scopes found himself indicted, charged with having unlawfully and willfully taught a theory that man had descended from a lower order of animals, thus denying the story of divine creation.

Around the country storm clouds began to gather. William Jennings Bryan, retired presidential candidate and superlative speaker, came up from Florida to aid the prosecution and the anti-evolutionists. The famous liberals, Clarence Darrow and Dudley Field Malone, joined the defense. Through a hot July the case of Scopes, Genesis, and evolution was argued, vividly if not scientifically, by men who could hardly have been better equipped to do it before the American public.

The trial, of course, was a trial of Scopes, not of evolution. Had Scopes broken the law? Scopes had, on the testimony of a couple of schoolboys, who managed to recall a few dim vestiges of what he had told them. Scopes was sentenced to pay a fine of $100. Nevertheless, over Scopes' head the grand issues resounded so mightily that the trial became in fact the last major engagement of the two forces. The anti-evolutionists won the trial, but lost the battle and the war. For the acceptability of evolution ceased to be argued by the general public from then on.

It had been a useless war. The losers, fighting always from the purest of religious motives, defended the unity of the Bible against the unity of nature, feeling that talk of evolution was defiance of the word of God. The framers of the 1925 law in Tennessee said as much. But most of the world has come to the conclusion that it is a greater defiance to ignore the fabulous complexities of the known universe, living and inert, all obeying the same natural laws, ordained God only knows how or when. For such people, Genesis is a religious book, beautiful and commanding in its conception, but representing more the vision and outlook of three thousand years ago than the continuous revelation to be found in the knowledge of recent centuries.

There persists, however, another attitude, not actually anti-evolutionary, which probably springs from misunderstanding and unawareness of facts. One sees mention of the "Darwinian dogma" (a phrase without meaning) or of the "theory" of evolution, as though it were a hypothesis, a good guess. There is a difference between the "theory of evolution" and "evolutionary theory," for the latter means the whole body of knowledge and explanation tying the known facts together into one system. It was atomic theory, after all, which produced a new kind of explosion at Alamogordo in 1945. And evolutionary theory is not less well founded. This is the thing which is so little appreciated: the facts bearing on evolution known today, compared with those known a century ago, are as a whale to a mouse, and all these facts fall neatly into place in general evolutionary theory.

Around the time of Darwin there was little to go on. Fossils, of course, were collected in quantity, revealing animals quite different from those now living. Otherwise scholars depended on knowledge, good as it was, of the varying anatomy of living animal types. Even this was powerful evidence of close likenesses here and there; and in the late eighteenth century the great French naturalist Buffon was moved to suggest that possibly the donkey had developed from the horse by a sort of degeneration, and likewise monkeys from men. But Buffon found he had stuck his toe into very cold water. The theologians reminded him crisply of the words of Genesis, and he removed his toe to a drier situation by retracting his suggestion. After Darwin, however, Huxley, Haeckel, and the other naturalists jumped in with vigorous splashes and routed all reticence.

New realms have opened up since then. There are the fossils, no longer looked on as relics of an age destroyed in the flood. Brought back in great profusion from all over the world, they range themselves in various ascending series to make a great pattern of life's development. Constantly the gaps are filled, logically and without absurdities; and whenever time itself can be measured from radioactive minerals, existing estimates of past ages of the earth are found to have been reasonable.

Fossils will be the *dramatis personae* of a good deal of this book. But in addition to fossils we have special demonstrations of family relationships, found in the blood or the body chemistry; or in the way parts form and growth takes place; or in vestigial structures (like hair on the surface of the human body) which are pointless in their owners but have a function in near relatives. All of this supports, agrees with, explains the rest, and none of it throws a wrench in the works. Naturalists, of course, are no longer looking for proof of evolution, but only for advanced knowledge of its complex processes or for the history of certain animal lines. Yet ordinary people allow themselves to wonder audibly whether Darwin is still believed in, or if the "theory" of evolution is all it was once thought to be. The answer is a resounding "Yes."

Actually, the masses of fossilized bones and teeth, and the long shelves of biological studies, are not the true cornerstones of our understanding. The two principal foundations are the contributions of Darwin and of Mendel, and they consist respectively of a largely irresistible force and a moderately movable object. The object, which Mendel did so much to explain, is heredity. The force—Darwin's monument—is natural selection. The combination is evolution.

Heredity: A Sameness of Differences

Let us look a little further at object and force. The achievement of the followers of Mendel was the realization that inheritance is deposited in genes and chromosomes, and not in "blood" or in long, thin ancestral lines running back to William the Conqueror. (The chromosomes, found in every living cell, are strings of genes. Genes, contrariwise, are short active regions of the chromosomes, precisely localized, which in a very specific way control all the hereditary side of an animal's nature and development.) The genes constitute the estate of a human population or an animal species, the estate on which it lives from generation to generation, to which it owes its existence and nature, and which may undergo gradual modification, thus modifying the nature of the whole species.

Although its living members look and seem so much alike, every species nonetheless carries a considerable variety in its pool of heredity. Some of the variety is due to genes for marked distinctions (perhaps for color, as in our own eyes), but much of it is due to far smaller differences in genes, differences harder to see on the surface. The stock of genes, differences and all, is passed on, generation after generation, being held, like the stock of a corporation, by a whole group made up of many different individuals. New genes—mutations from existing genes—appear occasionally in the stock. Some are useful, but most of them are injurious, being failures or defects of perfectly good genes. These may have drastic effects, so changing or mutilating their possessors that they are apt to drop out of the population, although the same mutation will continue to reappear from time to time.

But the "good" mutations, those which can provide something useful, are not so dramatic, and furnish only slight steps, perhaps very small indeed. Wings, or eyes, as full-fledged organs, could never spring from a single mutation. Nevertheless, such small steps, each one useful in itself, have allowed new trends to develop, and new combinations to be made, by Darwinian selection.

In any case, with or without mutations, the bank of genes, and its creatures, the succeeding generations of animals, go on much the same, since the basic heredity of the animals is only the stirring and recombination of the same material, and there is no essential reason for change in the system itself. This has been hard to believe: that there is no inner force directing change and bringing progress. Many a writer has pleaded such a force, an *élan vital*. But the evidence is emphatically lacking. You should not try to interpret evolution as it would be if you yourself were in charge; you are not in charge, and you will not find out what has been happening, or by what rules, unless you rid yourself of all preconceptions and pay attention only to the facts.

Natural Selection

There is no evidence for an inner force, and there is no necessity for it, because Darwin discovered the outer force which provides the necessary answer. He discovered it over a hundred years ago, before the nature of Mendelian heredity was established at the start of the twentieth century. First of all, he himself, as the result of long observation and travel, appreciated the astonishing way in which living things have their forms and functions suited to the places they inhabit and the lives they lead. This is adaptation. It may be moderate in degree—color differences (as in bears, white for snow and dark for woodland) or slight differences in the teeth of closely related species. It may be profound, so that four-footed mammals gave rise by adaptive evolution to bats and to whales. These are simple, big-print examples. The archives of natural history are replete with others, and, after all, any structure is somehow a result of adaptation, just as an eye is a structure for receiving light and images.

All this beautiful joining of form and purpose was used by the creationists of the eighteenth and early nineteenth centuries as evidence of the Creator's care in His work on the fifth and sixth days of Genesis. We now know, of course, that the rise and branching of species through adaptation was a gradual process, not a sudden one. Adaptation more recently has been cited to uphold belief in a subtler kind of design, the notion of a pre-existing plan or purpose, subscribed to by many people who are otherwise willing to accept the fact of evolution. Because eyes are "for" seeing, wings "for" flying, fur "for" warmth, and nesting habits "for" the rearing of nestlings, the impulse of the imagination is to think that the plan was there all the time and that the animals evolved along a directed route to achieve it, prompted by some undetected factor in their heredity. But Darwin's explanation, natural selection, invariably turns out to be the simplest of all; it is akin to water seeking its own level. The dispute, obviously, springs from theological preferences. Still it is a curious thing that, considering the end result and the known marvels of evolution, the older explanation should be taken to reflect more credit on the Creator than the newer. I cannot help observing that the account in Genesis sounds like child's play compared to what we know actually took place.

We ourselves are thinking animals, much the highest kind of life the earth has seen. This is the main reason why we are apt to view all evolution as leading up to man, the final, perfect creature, the aim of it all. Naturally, when we look back down the trail of our history, we seem to see a plan in which the aim of evolution is progress. But when we start below and follow the trail up, we get a slightly different, more truthful view: evolution does not look ahead, its eye fixed on the distant future. Instead, it is always trying to do its best with the business at hand. In doing this—in keeping some kind of animal well adapted to the life it is living, by one device or another—it sometimes stumbles into a new avenue leading off at a tangent, into a whole new earthly career.

For example, a species of ancient air-gulping fish which was only seeking to survive by crawling on stumpy fins from one stagnant pond to another less foul, made a crucial turn and became an amphibian. It had no such plan in mind; it was not trying to be a land animal, but only trying to go on being a fish; all animals are tories. But in following the magnet of adaptation it passed through the field of a stronger magnet and veered off in a new direction. Now it could manage to live on land, though (like frogs and newts) it laid its eggs in water, passed its tadpole stage in water, and was much at home in the water as an adult.

Later some of its amphibian descendants, with no special urge to say good-by to water, nevertheless developed a better-adapted egg: a larger one, with a shell, and plenty of yolk for food, so that it could be laid in a dry, safe place and would carry the embryo right through the tadpole stage. These animals were not cursing their aqueous fate and endeavoring to be "progressive" by laying a "land egg"; they were only trying to raise a family in a more efficient way. But without any plan to do so, they had become truly equipped for land life, the first reptiles. And birds, we can be sure, did not evolve feathers because they intended to begin flying, but for some more immediately useful reason, possibly warmth. Such accidental zigzags mark the evolutionary path of many animals, and later on I think you will see how much luck we had in becoming human.

The traditional view of Darwin's argument is somewhat too dramatic and emphasizes the wrong things, but it is easy to comprehend. It goes like this. Natural selection comes about through the "struggle for existence" and the "survival of the fittest," two famous phrases, neither of which was invented by Darwin himself. Most animals multiply at a high rate, with insects and fishes being able to produce astronomical numbers of offspring, far more than could survive. Those that do survive, thus giving rise to the generation coming after them, will tend to be the most successful of their species, by being well fitted to their environment and way of life. Those that are defective, or less well suited, will tend to be selected for oblivion, and eliminated. Here is nature in the raw, a repellent idea but an appealing one to thinkers of the late nineteenth century who were inclined to apply it to human society as well as to the animal world.

But it is too simple. It does not actually reflect Darwin's own ideas, and does not stand a close inspection. The struggle within a species seldom seems so severe, and there is much co-operation and mutual protection to be seen. And the tiny new-hatched fish which are gobbled by bigger fish are usually gobbled indiscriminately, not according to special, adaptive features they might develop as adults. Biologists now know that the essential point is which animals eventually produce the most offspring, not which ones get killed off. Death is certainly a factor, but the true secret, the real distinction, is between those individual parents who are more productive and those who are less so. The distinction can be very slight and still be important.

Notice, however, that there is a booby trap in this, with a history running from Lamarck to Lysenko: the supposed "inheritance of acquired characteristics." The offspring of the successful parents do not inherit the stronger muscles, the keener sight, the better adapted coloring, or any of the myriad adaptations of those parents. Rather, they inherit the genes which tend to produce those things, and which produced them in the parents. They certainly do not inherit anything which the parents acquired or lost in life, any more than you can inherit a knowledge of French, or your mother's nice straight teeth that cost your grandparents so much to straighten. So, in the end, a selection is made among *genes;* and the heredity of the species, its

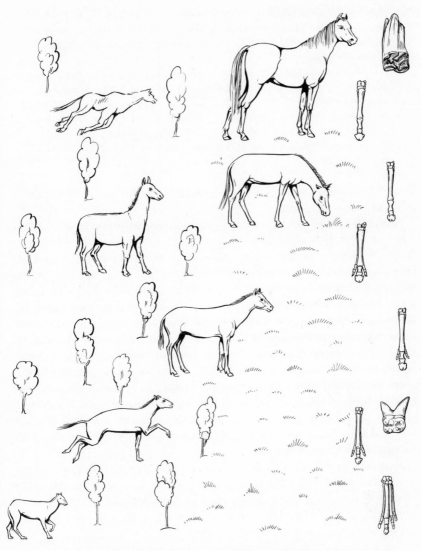

Evolution and adaptation in horses. Early small horses browsed on soft plants in the woods; they could not have chewed grass without wearing out their small teeth. Their descendants became larger, with higher-crowned, longer-lasting teeth, stronger limbs, and some reduction of toes; these horses remained in the woods and finally became extinct. Some horses developed harder tooth crowns as well, permitting grass eating and allowing horses to move into the grasslands. Some of these kept side toes (as shock absorbers?), but with the powerful, well-knit leg bones of the ancestors of modern horses, these side toes vanished. Notice that there was no single line of horse evolution, although only *Equus* survives now. Much evolution of tooth and limb was necessary before horses could take to the plains and become the kind of horse we know.

The horses shown are only a small number. They are, from the bottom up, *Hyracotherium* (*Eohippus*), *Mesophippus*, *Merychippus* (who ventured into the grasslands); *Hypohippus* (who went on being a three-toed browser), *Pliohippus* and *Equus*. Their respective footbones are shown at the side, together with molar teeth of *Eohippus*, below, and *Equus* (above). Based on Simpson and specimens.

estate, is trimmed and pruned by natural selection in the direction of advantageous adaptation.

Adaptation does not mean progress, or even evolution. It only means what it says. If a clam is perfectly suited to its mud, its food, and the temperature of the water, then it is the perfect clam (for its clamship, food, and water). Natural selection will operate purely to keep it that way. If, however, there is an avenue leading to a better state, natural selection will begin to push and pull in that direction. If they are larger, many mammals can feed more economically (consume a smaller proportion of their own weight daily) and also defend themselves better. So they show a general tendency, other things equal, to larger size. And if, in becoming larger, an appetizing herbivore can escape from carnivorous predators by becoming a powerful runner, then adaptation can mean the lengthening of legs, the growth of hoofs to take the punishment of long-distance running, and the loss of breakable side toes. Thus, over sixty or seventy million years, an eohippus becomes a horse.

So much for natural selection, the external force, that finger beckoning to the otherwise unguided heredity of an animal type. All other principles and facts of evolution may be satisfactorily related to it or explained by it, and the century following 1859 has seen Darwin triumphant.

The Genes: Safety in Numbers

As to heredity, another word or two. Evolution can be large-scale or small-scale, and the latter kind is important. Because there is always variation in a species, that species may respond quickly to slight changes and selective forces, by a shuffling and sorting of the genes it already has. Otherwise dog breeders, with their deliberate, artificial kind of selection, would never have been able to draw out the breeds we know, some of them in a relatively few years. This fact, this stock of variety, is a sort of adaptation itself, and a most important safety valve. There is such a thing as being too tightly adapted to one set of circumstances. If the species cannot virtually jump to the crack of the selection whip and adjust itself quickly to slight changes in its world, it may be able to respond only by becoming extinct, something which has happened very often. If it is fortunate, it may be able to produce a new combination of its genes to meet the new situation, and this is what much evolution consists of; it would have little chance of experiencing the right new mutations in time for its salvation.

Of course, mutations are important, as time goes on and as major amounts of change give rise to really new and different animals. The two things dovetail: the slow selective adoption of occasional new, favorable mutated genes and the constant churning and shuffling of the great mass of genetic material already present, actually the more important source of change. Sometimes the two can hardly be distinguished. Bacteria have been observed, when placed in a hostile environment (such as DDT or an antibiotic), to survive, in some cases by a variety of different mutations, in other cases by forming new combinations of genes already present. These are fine observations of evolution in operation, even though the differences between such simple creatures and higher animals makes for differences in the details of this operation. Little by little, the parts of the whole process are coming to light, either by working with cheap, quick breeders like fruit flies or by studying the nature of change in tooth, skull, and leg in the long ancestry of the horses.

One other thing, basic but often overlooked, is the fact that the species, or population of animals, undergoes its evolutionary creep together, advancing here, catching up there. It is never a case of a single individual appearing in strikingly new form and fathering a sort of secession from the old type in one generation. You could have figured this out by thinking of the nature of the stock of genes, the real object of evolution, but it should not be lost sight of.

The foregoing should convey how it is that forward evolution, or higher organization, comes about. But perhaps we should ask the question again in its plainest form: "Where do 'new' features, like feathers, or eggs, or eyes, come from?" For it once was a common objection to Darwinism that selection explains the survival of the fittest but not the arrival of the fittest; that selection eliminates but does not create. The answer today is clearer: as G. G. Simpson, the veteran paleontologist, has constantly stressed, selection *does* create. The genes and chromosomes are a rich store of possibilities and a flexible mechanism. Selection, working at many points, acts to create the most favorable combinations of existing genes, within which new, favorable mutations, even though slight in single contribution, will be cumulatively effective in a given direction of adaptation. Furthermore, many "new" things are not new, but are developments of features which are already "preadaptive." This signifies organs, whether or not they were useful before, which in changed circumstances can be called on to work for a new and more important need.[1] There is every evidence that such organs go on being useful and adapted during the transition, and need not be called out of service for remodeling. Examples of all this come later.

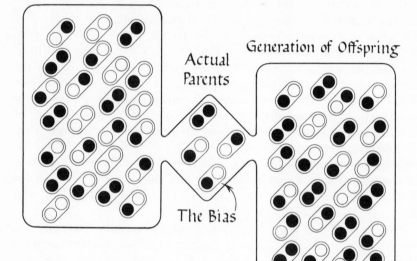

Generation of Parents

Actual Parents

Generation of Offspring

The Bias

$$24 \begin{cases} 6 \times \\ 12 \times \\ 6 \times \end{cases}$$

$$24 \begin{cases} 8 \times \\ 14 \times \\ 2 \times \end{cases}$$

Total: 24 × ●, 24 × ○

Total: 30 × ●, 18 × ○

---

[1] Preadaptation, an important idea to evolutionists, is not always defined the same way. It refers, as above, to a trait or mutation which may or may not be beneficial in the existing state of adaptation, but which proves useful in a new state or environment. It does not mean something intended by nature to fit an animal for something different or new; nor does it mean, of course, that an individual animal inherits the normal adaptations of its species ready-made.

Patterns of Adaptation

I hope I have shown why we have evolution, how it gets from here to there, and have even suggested why the little eohippus is not with us any more. But what about the whole tree of life, growing outward in so many directions? How did that come into being? You might think from natural selection that evolution travels, like light, in straight lines. It does, but seldom; it makes other figures much more often; it branches and bushes; it makes parallel lines, when two remotely related animals follow the same adaptive bent; it travels almost in circles, when reptiles go back to the sea and imitate sharks, as did the ichthyosaurs, and when mammals, long after, do the same thing again, as did the dolphins. Evolution pokes and pries, looking for opportunities going to waste. (Of course, it must have something to fill these op-

Opposite:
How natural selection changes the proportions of genes. Suppose the parent generation consists of 24 individuals. Suppose the number of black and white genes is equal in the population. With two genes to an individual, a most likely distribution is 6 with two black (homozygous), 6 with two white (also homozygous), and 12 with one of each (heterozygous).

Now suppose that only a small part becomes the parents of the next generation (a principle of Darwinism). If these number 4, the most truly representative group would be 1 with two black, 1 with two white, and 2 with a black and a white. But suppose selection favors whatever it is that black genes cause, *very slightly,* i.e., just enough to *bias* the parent group by one gene, let us say by replacing the two-white-gene individual by another having a black and a white.

Then the next generation will be expected to have a distinct majority of black genes (a ratio of 5 to 3 instead of even). If it is the same size as the previous generation, the most likely distribution of genes in the offspring, by the laws of chance, would be the one shown. The increase of black can be seen.

This imaginary example is exaggerated in several ways. (It supposes a very small number of actual parents; it takes no account of "sampling errors," assuming that only the most likely combinations will occur; it deals with only one pair of genes, not the whole animal.) It is meant simply to show how selection may have a marked and rapid effect. Notice how the complexion of the second generation has changed without a new gene having appeared, and without a long lapse of time.

portunities with when the time comes: the air with its juicy insects was going to waste until there was something which could become a bird or a bat.)

Sometimes it stands still. Sometimes it pushes forward with force and speed, especially when a major transition is taking place and a critical point being passed. Probably this was the case when animals came out on land and had to make certain choices for good and all. Probably this was the case when our own forebears stood up, for better or worse, on their hind legs. These times were important points in evolution, but they are difficult to study now, for the very reason that they were short periods and left few fossils. The times were not comfortable ones for the animals involved, since they were, in a way, having their old adaptation pulled out from under them like a rug, and were far from adapted to the radically new conditions around them. Land and sea, for example, are very different places. That the critical points were passed at all was usually due to preadaptation, that lucky existence already of something which came in handier than its possessors had any right to expect. One fine example was certainly the primitive lungs and limbs of the fishes who dared the land.

All this exploring, stopping, and rushing, in the pursuit of profitable adaptation, has resulted in the great family tree of the animals. It has a certain orderliness, as its classifiers have found, most of all in one main pattern, that of grades of organization. We will see this particularly in our own line of vertebrates. In its history, somehow a general upward step will be taken (by "upward" I invariably mean toward myself), such as that of animals coming out to make use of the land. This is followed by an adaptive radiation, meaning that this new grade of animal at once begins to explore the different niches in the environment. Adaptation leads to a general branching into many family lines, which become more and more different from one another as time goes on. Eventually, an accumulation of improvements gives rise to another new grade of animal, which can take advantage of a new set of niches or else commandeer them from lowlier competitors, who are apt reluctantly to become extinct.

Of course, niches may not be as simple as we name them. For instance, and thinking only of food, to flying insects air is air, but to birds it is air with insects in it. Furthermore, and generally speaking, bats and birds keep out of each other's way by using night and day respectively, so that the same niche is really two. At all events, once there appears such a distinct grade of animal as birds, there follows a typical adaptive radiation. And the birds, with owls, ducks, sparrows, and ostriches, have shown this on a major scale, together with a minor closeness of adaptation to the minutiae of environment that has made them one of the great objects of natural science.

Generalized and Specialized

There is a useful distinction to keep in mind in viewing this pattern. Animals, or parts of animals, may be generalized or specialized. The distinction is not really clear-cut, since the same animal may be generalized in some ways, specialized or extreme in others. But it has some meaning for man, when we come to him, since, although he is certainly specialized in some ways, he never during his long history got caught in a blind alley which would have cut him off from progress to the point he has reached.

Consider illustrations. A giraffe is quite simply specialized in height. Parasites are specialized for living on, or in, another animal and cannot exist by themselves. An anteater has let his teeth go and has emphasized claws, snout, and tongue for tearing away the ants' protection and licking them up. Specialization often runs in straight lines toward extreme forms, toward a higher degree of adaptation for the same object. That is to say, if it is successful in the first place, then more and more of the same medicine may be better and better. The steady development of size and tusks in the elephants, and then of highly peculiar teeth, is one of the clearest pages in the annals of paleontology.

The advantages of specialization are clear. The disadvantages lie in limitation of change, since specialization is something of a one-way street: a species is most unlikely to go back over the same ground, becoming less rather than more adapted to the same life. Can we imagine the happy dolphin growing back his ancestral limbs? In the limitation of change lies both a danger of extinction and a degree of improbability of evolving into a generally higher form of life, though of course this has bothered the heads of few of our dumb friends, present or past. The limitation is particularly obvious when specialization takes place, as it often does, through loss, as in the modern horse, who has narrowed the number of digits down to one on each foot. "The Moving Finger writes; and, having writ, moves on." Marked specialization is a disguised strait jacket, a surrender to environment for the sake of a close and comfortable adjustment to a narrow way of life. Of course, the rewards are great, or most animals would not be specialized.

A generalized animal, on the other hand, is one which has kept the initiative and departed less from the general form of its forebears. A truly generalized animal is apt to remain a primitive one, of course, but in the sense I am considering here, a progressive animal may undergo fundamental changes (developing the lungs of land-dwelling vertebrates or the warm blood of mammals) which still allow great variations to develop on the same pattern. Thus such changes are not specializations of the limiting variety. They are not so much meek adjustments to the environment as conquests of it, blows for freedom rather than for slavery.

Now of course neither kind of animal is necessarily inferior. There is the constant tendency for generalized forms to become specialized, and most higher animals are specialized to a clear degree. And both kinds run the hazard of extinction. Specialized types may find themselves caught in a change of their surroundings which they lack the capacity to overcome, and paleontology is the graveyard of specialized species. But it is also the graveyard of generalized ancestors who were eliminated by their own, more specialized and more successful descendants. The little eohippus, for instance, could not have survived, competing with his own ever horsier offspring, let alone fighting off the growing, specializing progeny of his carnivore contemporaries.

In any case, as I said before, the distinctions are not clear-cut. A generalized animal may be primitive or progressive, and a progressive animal may be both generalized and specialized at the same time. This is what applies to us ourselves, for man has preserved a nice balance. Springing from generalized but highly progressive relatives, he became decidedly specialized from the waist down, and this, we shall see—a specialized development—was what suddenly made him human. But his humanity is really above the waist, and here the pattern was more generalized.

Look at his brain. It is not simple, but it is not specialized, being only the most advanced, the best, of mammal brains. It is enormously developed as to size and refinement—so much so that it has been able to perform new kinds of function, like speaking in language—but as far as we can say at the moment this is a matter of size, since we are merely the biggest-brained members of a big-brained tribe, that of the apes and monkeys. Consider also the brain's connections with the rest of human anatomy. Man has long met his needs by doing things internally, in his head, rather than externally, through adaptation of his body parts. And, fortunately, whatever the course by which he attained his big brain and high mental powers, once he had done so he found himself unburdened by physical specializations like hoofs or a trunk. So he was able, because of his generalized nature, to turn his hand to the most complicated of pursuits.

In his limbs we can find the best contrast of the general and the special which man affords. His foot is a really specialized organ. From the grasping foot of his more typical relatives it has been made over into a unique arched platform. It is solid and strong: it is able to apply a powerful force at the ball, and it is thus the only foot which can take

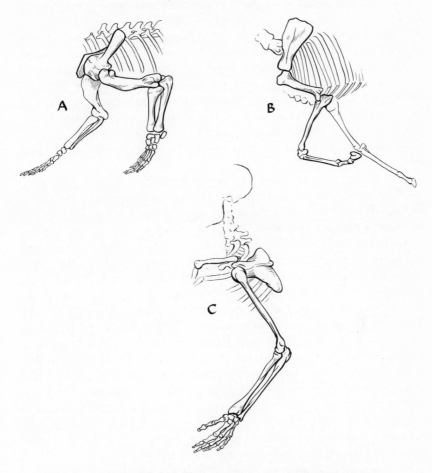

Skeletons of forelimbs, showing adaptation to the different uses.
A. the proto-mammalian pattern, in a mammal-like reptile.
B. a horse, highly modified by lengthening of the lower part, and loss of separate forearm bones and of side toes.
C. man, with a general retention of the basic pattern. Partly following Gregory.

a human step. Clearly it will never go back to being the hand-like affair which is the proper primate appendage (weird as it may look to us). In all truth, our foot is our most human characteristic.

Our hand, on the contrary, is quite generalized. It recalls the fundamental vertebrate plan and has lost virtually nothing from its most primitive mammal ancestor. This is equally true of the wrist and arm. Instead of cutting down on the varied possibilities inherent in the original pattern, we have enormously increased them. Gently evolution has modified and refined the whole limb for flexibility of movement and delicacy of grasp, through such features as the rotation of the two bones of the forearm and the ability to oppose the thumb to the fingers; until altogether the hand has become the unfettered genie of the brain. It is the best possible illustration of the blessings of keeping a generalized form, broadening and refining it, rather than accepting its distortion so as to obtain a special reward. Such hands are a feature of the whole order of Primates, which is a generalized order, anyhow. But man's hand is among the most generalized of them all.

How at last can we view the whole pattern of forces, principles, grades, specializations, as they are manifest in a typical evolutionary history? If you like mental diagrams, suppose you have a large, empty house of a number of stories, with stairs going up the center. Let the several floors represent the main grades of organization—the forward evolutionary steps—and the corridors and rooms stand for the paths of special adaptation and the environmental niches to which they lead.

Suppose our first land ancestors move into the ground floor. From the hallway there takes place an adaptive radiation throughout that floor, the occupants quite unconscious of higher floors and proud of the rooms they come to occupy. Then one family clambers up to a new floor, and a new scurry for rooms takes place. Far from the stairs, in the distant rooms (which may represent extreme redecorations like flying, swimming, or burrowing), happy recluses settle, never to see a stair again. But back at the middle certain less adventurous occupants, who have been eyeing the staircase all the time, go up to still another floor and give rise to another radiation, occupying a set of rooms having a plan rather similar to the floors below.

Man, of course, has got up into a little belfry all his own. It appears that his ancestors never got far from the stairs; his generalized nature shows it and the record proves it. And his later forebears have been rather obscure animals, leaving most of the stage to others. During recent eons, as a little ape-like person, he looked about and saw the herbivores becoming alert and speedy runners and the carnivores developing fangs and claws and a furious killing power. He had no such gaudy accomplishments, but as he came to stand on his legs he could use his hands for whatever it amused him to do, and at last he found this to be a niche of a fabulously rewarding kind. He seems at the same time to have been accustoming himself to living in families or small groups, with strong ties, for he never was a solitary animal. There was little about him then to attract attention or command respect, but this lusterless past paid off at tremendous odds in the end.

2. VERTEBRATES

IF YOU HAVE a backbone you are a vertebrate. You, dear reader, are a mammal, best of the vertebrates, but you could be a bird, a snake (reptile), a frog (amphibian), or a fish and still qualify.

This jointed backbone, the vertebral column, is the basic part of the skeleton of the vertebrate animals, together with a skull and a rib cage; and most vertebrates have two pairs of limbs. The skeleton is constructed, like the body as a whole, on a plan of bilateral symmetry, so that the two sides of the body mirror one another. And the skeleton is mainly or wholly internal. This makes it a better support than the external skeleton of lobsters or beetles, and it also allows more complicated and advantageous arrangements of the muscles. For these reasons it makes possible both large size and high activity, and only among the vertebrates have there appeared giant animals: elephants, giraffes, or the tyrannosaurs. It is true that some invertebrates have become large, like the giant clam, or the octopus, or the giant squid, when they were supported externally by a reef or water; but when vertebrates also took advantage of such support they reached bigger sizes still. Witness the colossal brontosaurs of the Mesozoic swamps and some of our modern whales, the largest creatures ever to exist.

Another trait of vertebrates, important to large size, is their internal fueling system—the combination of what we look on as our respiratory and circulatory systems. The whole thing is centralized: oxygen is supplied to the blood at centralized, specialized points (lungs or gills) and then carried by the blood, along with nutritive substances from food, over a centralized network of vessels, under pressure supplied by a special muscle, the heart. This is where insects fall down badly, since they must meet their oxygen needs by having air penetrate through small channels, opening directly to the surface of the body. This device will not work beyond a certain depth, and so the body cannot be very thick or large. Next time you dream of a tiger beetle as large as you are, do not take fright. It is not real.

The vertebrates are only one of a dozen grand divisions, or basic body plans, of animal life. Some of the invertebrates may be fantastically numerous, like the one-celled animals. And in numbers of species the arthropods (joint-legged creatures such as crabs, centipedes) lead all others, since the group includes the insects. But we put the vertebrates at the top, because they have produced men, as well as rank on rank of the other most highly organized animals of the world. Their body features are not all unique: insects have bilateral symmetry, and a head with sense organs and a mouth, as we have. And invertebrates may even have fairly good eyes. But the vertebrate combination of traits eventually allowed such size, freedom of motion, and nervous development as to put the vertebrates quite off by themselves.

The Rise of the Fishes

The first vertebrates did not look like much, suggesting a small stripped-down fish. However, the potential—the peculiarly happy combination—was there. After a very long time the fishes themselves became enormously successful, and from the fish stock stemmed the land animals, in a sequence of upward steps which at last made possible the rise of the mammals and man. The ground plan, it is true, called for a good deal of working over, and each stage of improvement needed the preceding stage as a platform to build on. We began as fishes and we ended as men, but in between we went through some profound revolutions. Amphibians got out of the water, without really conquering the land. The reptiles conquered the land, but not the weather. The mammals conquered the weather and, counting their other achievements as well, needed no further basic revolutions to produce humanity, but only some fortunate arrangements and developments of what by then had come into existence.

To begin with beginnings, there have been four classes of fishes: the jawless, the armored, the cartilaginous, and the bony. The first to appear—and from what ancestors, nobody knows—were the jawless ostracoderms, the "shell-skins." Any typical vertebrate has a good internal skeleton, fins or limbs, and upper and lower jaws to bite with. The ostracoderms had none of these. They were, however, fish-like in general form, with bony scales (and bone is distinctly a vertebrate patent) and, in some of them, a bony head shield. Known evidence of any internal skeleton is restricted to the head region of one group.

So the ostracoderms were not typical vertebrates. However, they certainly were not anything else, and they had at least one unmistakable vertebrate feature: the same kind of three-part brain, and associated cranial nerves leading away from it, as is found in all other vertebrates. They flourished for millions of years in a wide variety of forms; their very variety suggests that the class was already old when the most ancient fossils we know were forming. While they were still flourishing, the armored fishes appeared. Probably these came from ostracoderm ancestors, but they had true skeletons and primitive jaws, and in most cases a body form suggesting that they were faster, better swimmers than their old jawless predecessors. Then followed two higher classes still: the sharks and rays, whose skeletons form only in cartilage and do not change to bone; and the bony fishes we know, with light, strong fins, and good internal skeletons giving them powerful bodies for fast swimming, and fully formed jaws and teeth.

Now in all this evolution the fishes were not becoming more man-like; they were becoming more fish-like. The jawless fishes vanished long ago, except for one or two aberrant relatives like the lamprey. The armored fishes are completely extinct. The sharks, though persistent, have never been dominant. It is the light-scaled or thin-skinned bony fishes which, after several stages of modification, have become the magnificently adjusted, successful and varied tribes we see today. Furthermore, this evolution was not a neat train of successive generations. It was more like a series of experiments. The armored fishes have not been traced right out of the jawless fishes of their time or earlier; there are no clear links, and they appear rather to have arisen separately from a common undiscovered ancestor. And from some similar but as yet unknown stem, doubtless at a higher level, came the two later classes (cartilaginous and bony), to compete with one another and their unfortunate poor relations.

Conquest of the Land

Out of the midst of this sprang the ancestry of the land animals. Pilgrims, so to speak, left the house of the fishes and marched off to found a land house. Like that of the fishes, it was occupied by four classes: the amphibians on the first floor (still pretty damp), the reptiles on the floor above them, and the birds and mammals atop these. Here the architecture of the house must be changed a little: from the reptile floor there is no central staircase, but rather two, leading from different reptile branches separately up to birds and mammals, who are not directly connected. (As a matter of fact, the same design can be applied to the bony fishes and the sharks.)

In the fish house practically nothing is known of those inmates who lived close to the stairs or actually climbed them. In the land house things are much better, and we can now practically see climbers on the stairs themselves all the way up. It used to be argued against the idea of evolution that these links were missing. But modern evolutionary theory, as I have explained, expects the stair climbing to be rapid, and remains of the climbers to be few and rare. And in any case the links are no longer missing. Good examples have been found throughout, even to that famous feathery reptile, that toothy bird, *Archaeopteryx*.

This is how the migration to land came to be made. In their early days, there were already two main branches of bony fishes, both with heavy scales and both with true primitive lungs as well as gills. One branch, the ray-finned fishes, progressively reduced their scales, perfected speed, turned the ancient lung into a swim-bladder, or air ballast tank, and became the multitudes of the modern streams and oceans. The other branch, which may be broadly called the lobe-fins, kept their lungs and had fins which were not membranous with spiny frames, but were fleshy lobes with fringing fins, having a small bony skeleton inside them—a skeleton, in fact, with the first elements of the limbs we have ourselves.

This lobe-finned branch, successful for a while, fell behind the ray-fins and has almost disappeared. One distantly related line led to the three living lungfishes of South America, Australia, and South Africa, who can breathe air during the partial or total drying up of their homes in the dry season. Another stock of lobe-fins, the coelacanths, took to salt water and flourished into the Cretaceous period, after which, over seventy million years ago, signs of their fossils disappear from the rocks. They had always been thought totally extinct, until 1938, when a live one was caught off East London, South Africa. This was no less staggering than meeting a live dinosaur would be. It was sent to the local museum, but the curator was away; some time went by before a photograph reached him and he recognized it for what it was. And a five-foot coelacanth decays with as much enthusiasm as any other five-foot fish. It was taken to the taxidermist and stuffed, with most of its original stuffing, alas, being thrown away. This is all right aesthetically and all wrong scientifically. Luckily the tragedy was made up for. Since 1952 other specimens have been taken from time to time near Madagascar; probably they had been caught at intervals for years without their worth being recognized by fishermen. At any rate, we now know that there has been an extraordinary survival of one or two species in the western Indian Ocean after the general dying off of the group as a whole.

The main stock of lobe-fins, or crossopterygians, lived in fresh water, and from these the amphibians derived. It was made possible by two glorious preadaptations, the lungs and the almost-limbs. I have earlier suggested what happened. A stock of these fish was caught in stagnant and drying inland seas or streams, and they were able to keep alive by breathing while they dragged themselves on their stumpy fins to

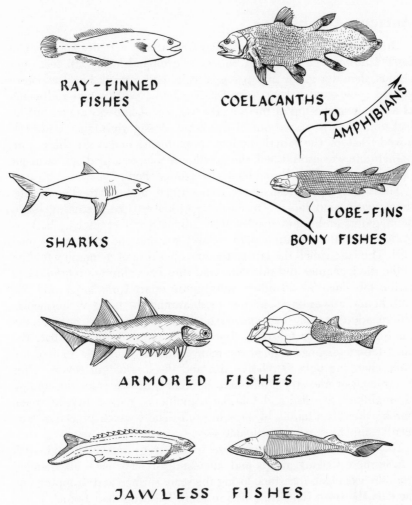

RAY-FINNED FISHES

COELACANTHS

TO AMPHIBIANS

SHARKS

LOBE-FINS

BONY FISHES

ARMORED FISHES

JAWLESS FISHES

Rise of the fishes. Representatives of the four classes, not drawn to scale. The coelacanth shown is the surviving *Latimeria*. After Gregory and Romer.

better water. Without these "limbs," of course, they would have perished entirely, as doubtless other water life around them perished. Perhaps they were persuaded to dally in the mud by such easy prey; perhaps at first they were lured by fresh bodies of water, and later simply by fresh bodies.

Ancient Amphibians

One kind of animal which resulted from this is actually known. The fossil *Ichthyostega* had small but well-developed legs, with feet, and a good shoulder girdle and pelvis. But he had a weak back—a poorly jointed spine—and a long, very fish-like body, with actual rudiments of a fin along the top of the tail. He was a real halfway stage, but he had nevertheless passed out of the fishes. A slightly higher stage followed, that of the labyrinthodont amphibians; and with these, amphibian life was established, the new house was occupied, and a major radiation took place throughout the ground floor.

These early amphibians were well formed, and progressive for the times, with good limbs. The basic type looked like a stumpy lizard or alligator, and some species were about five feet in length. It is evident that they continued to inhabit streams and swamps a good deal. They are called the labyrinthodonts because of a complex folding of the tooth enamel. But this same trait runs back through *Ichthyostega* to the lobe-fins. So do other traits, quite apart from lungs and the limb bones. For example, all had teeth around the edge of the mouth, but in addition they had special teeth in the roof and floor of the mouth, perhaps for grasping slippery fish more firmly. All had the same telltale arrangement of the many bones forming the roof of the skull, changing only in relative size and the loss of gill covers. Thus the tracing of ancestry is no mere inference, drawn from the finding of amphibian-like fish and fish-like amphibians, with a link between. Rather, there is a family likeness in skull details which proclaims true relationship in a most particular way.

You do not see many amphibians today: frogs and toads and, with a little more looking, newts and salamanders. They have all changed from their ancient ancestors, losing the scaly surface and dropping one digit on the front foot, from five to four. The frog-toad branch is exceptionally specialized, with holes in the skull top, a short, stiff, ribless body frame, and powerful hopping legs. So the old amphibians, dominant while they were still the best things on land, have suffered a great decline from which the frogs, in particular, have escaped only by intense specialization. It is obvious that this peculiar path of theirs led to survival, but it is not obvious why. (The advantage of hopping, it has been suggested, lay in a faster escape from land into water when an enemy came by.)

The amphibians, after all, did get us part way out on land, and we should not sneer at Adam for his wardrobe. They added true limbs to the fish torso, with developed limb skeletons in place of the undifferentiated limb rudiments of the crossopterygians. And they gave us the model for an ear, formed from a stretched membrane, and borrowed a small bone from the jaw supports to pass its vibrations inward. But their debits eventually outweighed their credits. Their eggs are still small, like those of fishes, and must be protected from drying up; they must be laid in or near the water, and the tiny tadpole must live in water, using gills, while it grows. And the amphibian lungs are inefficient, as are the heart and the arrangement of arteries. The whole system is a makeshift from something which is really suited to gills and to the water, just as the first venture onto land was a makeshift, not a carefully planned project. The first amphibians were land-going fishes, and they, and the salamanders after them, did not use their limbs alone to walk, but bent the powerful body, fish-fashion, as they put forward a foot, now on one side, then on the other, throwing the spine into S-curves. It is like the first automobiles, which were horseless carriages: a motor took the horse's place, but the carriage was still a carriage, and it was only little by little that the carriage followed the lead of the new kind of locomotion and changed in every way.

The Reptile or the Egg

But if the later story of the Amphibia was stagnation and collapse, the earlier was progress. Even while the labyrinthodonts were making some use of the new world of land, one branch continued to improve its basic structure in what turned out to be the direction of the reptiles. To use the house idea, it was as though this line had barely paused at the ground level before starting up the stairs to the next floor. And again paleontology has caught an animal, known as *Seymouria*, in the act of stair climbing. He had a skeleton much like the basic reptiles in a number of details, but his skull was a good deal the same as that of one branch of the labyrinthodonts, in the number and arrangement of bones. And he had, in the roof of his mouth, some of those special extra groups of teeth which first appeared all the way back in the lobe-finned fishes. Most people call *Seymouria* an amphibian, but some class him as a reptile; nobody knows how to decide the point, without discovering whether he grew from a tadpole or not.

On the landing just above, we find the "stem reptiles," the ancestral group from which, once more, sprang a great and still successful progeny. Now at last there could develop vertebrates who were truly at home on land. In many ways the reptiles improved on the early amphibian skeleton, and stabilized it. They reduced the number of joints in the "fingers" and "toes" of the feet to a smaller, standard number, though not as far as we ourselves have done. At the same time, they had separated from their amphibian progenitors before the latter had lost a digit from the front feet, otherwise we ourselves should now have only eight fingers and thumbs. The spine was stronger and better articulated, and at least two ribs, rather than one, formed the attachment of the pelvic girdle to the spine. In the skull fewer separate bones were retained to form the roof, and the teeth, though still replacing themselves without limit and still accompanied by extra groups in the palate, came to differ somewhat in shape, for different purposes.

But none of this would have made the reptiles more than high-class amphibians, nor would it have allowed the spectacular radiation which followed the stem reptiles. There were other reasons for this. First, there was a greater enclosing of the body, not only through good scales or horny plates but especially through better lungs, better kidneys, and a better constructed heart and circulation. The living amphibians have to get much of their oxygen, and give off some of their waste products, directly through the moist skin, all in damaging admission of fish lineage. This lineage was overcome and cast off by the reptiles in no more positive and important way than in their new kind of egg.

Professor Romer of Harvard, whose explanation I am quoting, considers that in fact the reptile egg came before the reptile. Natural selection would have helped such an egg along as it developed, in the amphibian world then existing. The ordinary amphibian egg is a mere speck of an embryo in jelly, which will quickly dry up out of the water, and from which a tiny tadpole must soon hatch, to swim about and fend for itself, being much more likely than not to be eaten by the first larger creature that comes by. Various modern amphibians have tried[1] to combat this grim destiny by laying their eggs not in water but in damp hollows, or even by carrying them secreted on the body, in little pockets, or bunched around the legs. But some ancient amphibian species (probably like *Seymouria*) managed far better, evolving an egg with a shell, a large egg with plenty of yolk (though the embryo, as you can see in any hen's egg, is as small as ever).

This egg need not be kept wet—the embryo is protected by a fluid mass, within the amnion, which was retained, along with some

---

[1] Of course, they have not "tried" to do anything. For simplicity of statement, I am using here, as at other points, dramatic language and the active voice to convey the nature of adaptations brought about in a species through natural selection.

other membranes, by the birds and the mammals when they in turn arose from reptiles. The embryo in this egg grows and grows, on yolk absorbed by its gut, until it is nearly as large as its egg, and then it steps out into the world fully formed, a small version of its parents. It is a real land animal, not a tadpole. And the possessors of this egg, whether they knew it or not, were free of the water at last.[2] From them came the stem reptiles, parents of all higher vertebrates to follow. The reptiles have even penetrated the deserts, where amphibians cannot exist, and have in fact made them a favored habitat. This alone is a symptom of how, in an egg, the reptiles had found the key to the open spaces of the land.

The stem reptiles were already well established during the heyday of the amphibians, down to two hundred million years ago. Then, with a vigorous expansion in the Mesozoic, the Age of Reptiles, they showed what the reptilian structure could do. In a wonderful example of radiation they invaded the seas and the air, with the ichthyosaurs and the pterosaurs, and on land they produced adaptations of every kind for hunting and defense. They did not, perhaps, give rise to all the types or niche fillers produced by the later mammal radiation, but on the other hand the mammals never produced a form of life to compete with a snake, a turtle, or an alligator.

While these familiar kinds were coming into being, the center of the stage swarmed with monsters, the dinosaurs and the other great ruling reptiles. Surely an observer from space might have thought them the final sovereigns of this planet's animal kingdom, from whose thrall the world was never to escape. Size was the order of the day; many species reached appalling bigness, and most of them were large. The carnivorous dinosaurs were, at the same time, very active by modern reptile standards, some of them becoming adapted to running on their hind legs for greater speed. The giants may have resulted from several forces of natural selection: the protection which size affords, a steadier body temperature in a larger mass, and economy in feeding—greater bulk of food, to be sure, but less constant stuffing. The huge herbivores of the swamps were the largest of all, but their meat-eating cousins, like *Tyrannosaurus*, who could stand nearly twenty feet high, were the most dreadful. Almost every section of the earth shook to their tread, and it would have seemed that,

[2] How much this means is emphasized by Romer as follows: "As far as can be told from the fossil record, the adult structure of the very earliest reptiles showed little if any advance over that of their amphibian relatives and contemporaries. It was solely owing to the amniote mode of development that the evolution of higher vertebrates was made possible." (A. S. Romer, "Origin of the Amniote Egg," *Scientific Monthly*, August 1957.)

in the dinosaurs, Nature had made her last and greatest effort. No wonder that they still compel the imagination of man, who never saw them living.

Certainly they were a success; their adaptability shows it, and they reigned for a hundred million years, no small interval of time. And then they failed. It is by no means clear why. But the suspicion is strong that their size somehow brought them vulnerability, as specialization is so apt to do; that their proudest boast was also their Achilles' heel. They must have been closely adjusted to a warm, moist, lush climate, in which they had developed and which endured a very long time. Giant herbivores, then, needed giant swamps, and giant carnivores certainly needed giant herbivores. There are some signs that mountain building took place late in the Mesozoic, changing climate somewhat and draining swamps, which proved too unsettling for reptiles of such bulk. At any rate, they went, in a short time and from every part of the world.

While the big reptiles held sway, only a watchful eye would have detected other animals in the landscape. They were there, however, apparently constrained from expansion by the saurian success, and probably living in danger, with every sense cocked for the approach of a dinosaur. These were, of course, certain other descendants of the old stem reptiles: the living, non-gigantic reptiles, and the mammals.

3. MAMMALS

CAN YOU now imagine a world without birds or mammals? I mean the modern world, with these animals suddenly removed, not an ancient scene still rumbling with dinosaurs. A landscape with no birds in the trees, on the lakes, on the shore. No bats in the dusk; no deer, no skunks, no woodchucks, mice, or squirrels in the woods; no lions or antelopes or baboons in the plains; no men, women, or children. It would be an empty landscape and a quiet one, with only the seasonal croak of frogs, buzz of insects, or noise of summer thunder, autumn leaves, and winter wind. That is how much the mammals dominate the earth today.

Of course, in the time of the early land animals there was plenty to see and hear. Though noises were perhaps less significant and varied, the amphibians and the reptiles had developed several different ways of picking them up—through an eardrum membrane, or through the jaw or the forefoot—and of passing them to the skull through the stapes, that ear bone transformed in amphibians from the fishes' jaw stiffener (the hyomandibular). Noises arrived at the skull in the region of the old balancing organ of the fish, which was actually a sort of meter to register pressure and movement of liquid, and therefore already equipped (preadapted) to pass along to the brain information about sound waves. So in addition to keeping balance, it became, and still is, the inner ear. But outside, in the middle ear, the stapes got some unexpected help. In typical reptiles the lower jaw was made up of several bones, but in the immediate ancestors of mammals the tooth-bearing bone enlarged, and the others grew smaller until in mammals they left the mandible entirely. But they did not vanish altogether. The hindmost (articular) had been acting as the joint between jaw and skull, in partnership with another small bone of the upper jaw (quadrate).

Now in the transformation I have been describing, the jaw developed a new joint with the skull at a different place, and left these small servants without joint duty. However, they had evidently also been serving to transmit ground or air vibrations, picked up by the

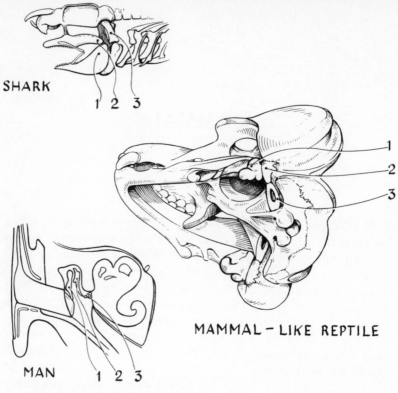

SHARK

MAMMAL – LIKE REPTILE

MAN

Origins of the middle-ear bones in mammals. All arose from gill arch supports of fishes, originally existing as simple upper and lower paired elements. The parts concerned are numbered, as follows:

    1: *articular* which became   *malleus* (hammer)
    2: *quadrate* which became   *incus* (anvil)
    3: *hyomandibular* which became *stapes* (stirrup)

Stage one: cartilaginous skull of a shark. One pair of gill supports has become upper and lower tooth-bearing jaws, loosely hitched to the skull. From the hinder parts of the primitive jaw plates there later developed, in the region of the joint, specific small bones: the articular below, the quadrate above. The upper jaw was also supported behind by part of the next pair of stiffeners, the hyomandibular.

Stage two: skull of a mammal-like reptile, seen from under the left side. The articular and quadrate, though small, still form the surfaces of the jaw joint. The hyomandibular has become the stapes, a separate bone running from the quadrate inward to the side of the brain case. (Note also that this animal has two occipital condyles, on either side of the *foramen magnum,* a mammal trait.) After a model by Watson.

Stage three: cross section of the human ear. The three bones have become very small, making a series carrying vibrations from the ear drum directly to the fluid of the inner ear. After Baer.

mouth and jaw, to the stapes, and they continued in this capacity, though now getting their vibrations from the outer skin, where a true ear developed. Thus in the mammals these two bones (becoming the malleus and the incus) joined the stapes to become the delicate, three-bone mechanism of our middle ear, able to vibrate with great sensitivity to a rich variety of sounds.

This change, though gradual, was striking. In fact, paleontologists, finding a fossil skull of one of these transitional animals, will class it as mammal if the jawbone is single, and as reptile if it still has vestiges of the other bones. This is the one best distinction, in a stage of evolution where lines are hard to draw. But there are certainly better reasons for mammal superiority than mammal ears and jaws. Just as the main key to reptile life was a new egg, so the main key to mammal life was warm blood. In each case, there were many generalized skeletal and bodily improvements, but in each case some leading development gave meaning to the others.

What Warm Blood Means

"Warm blood" is a simple name for a whole complex of things. First of all, of course, it means a high body temperature, and a constant one, maintained throughout the body. The importance of this to the mammals cannot be overvalued, because it is what gives them their activity and organization. Activity comes from a high efficiency in feeding the muscles with substances derived from food, and in being able to release the energy obtained suddenly and in large amounts in response to a nervous command. It also requires a fullness of nervous co-ordination and development. The biochemical processes back of this seem to function best in a constant temperature not far from a hundred degrees Fahrenheit. Mammals all have such a temperature, and the birds, who evolved warm blood entirely independently, have temperatures a degree or so higher. This constant internal warmth makes mammals able to go into any climate, even the arctic seas, while retaining their high organization. But primarily mammals live at a higher pitch, a higher turnover of energy, anywhere and all the time.

Reptiles have no such independence. We call them cold-blooded, which means that their body temperatures are lower and variable. They cannot retain the heat they generate, and so they are greatly subject to the temperature of their surroundings. They are, in effect, stupefied by the cold and rendered inactive, but excessive heat is dangerous for them also. They must have evolved a degree of tolerance for temperature changes as they rose from the fishes, who can stand very little fluctuation, but while the reptiles have some mechanisms for responding to heat or cold, these are inefficient. Their egg gave them the freedom of the land, but this was really only the tropical regions, for they occupy temperate zones at the price of surrender of action for half the year, and to colder areas they cannot go. By way of comparison, you might say that being a reptile is like living in a cave with a fire at the opening, while being a mammal is like living in a modern house, with insulation, a central furnace, and a thermostat.

The thermostat lies in the nervous system and brain. The insulation is provided by hair and fur, a patent of the mammals, and by fat in some places where it is needed. The reverse insulation, for getting rid of heat, lies in a good supply of sweat glands in the skin, to cool us by evaporation. The whole system is backed up by improved circulation. There is a four-chambered heart, which keeps the blood going in a double circuit: to the body and return, and then to the lungs for freshening and return, and back to the body. Thus bright red blood

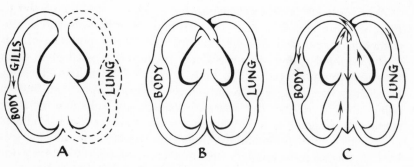

The heart from fish to mammals. A diagram of how the circulatory system was transformed from a single into a double circuit.
A. In the fishes, blood is pumped by the heart through the gills, where it is oxygenated, and then direct to the body tissues and back to the heart. In air-using fishes, some blood passes via the lungs instead of the gills, returning to the heart. This becomes important when air must be depended on.
B. In amphibians the gills are lost, and the lungs begin to be a separate circuit. Freshened blood from the lungs is partly separated in the atrium, the heart's first chamber; however, fresh and stale blood may be somewhat mixed on going to the body tissues. This is not as inadaptive as it seems, since the body (skin and mouth) also acts to freshen the blood to a considerable degree.
C. In the mammals, in whom lungs do all the work, the heart is fully divided into two halves (four chambers), and no mixture of the two streams of blood passing through takes place.

full of oxygen goes from the heart out to the body, unpolluted by stale blood returning to go to the lungs; this complete separation does not exist below the mammals. (The birds, quite independently, evolved the same system, suggesting its importance.) And the supply of oxygen, as a needed fuel, is helped by a bony palate, which separates the nasal channel from the mouth, the channel for food. It is also helped by a diaphragm at the base of the chest, which separates the abdomen from the heart and lungs and is pulled down to suck air in large quantities into the lungs.

Born Alive

Another vital achievement of the mammals is live birth. The mammal embryo grows in a suit of membranes clearly betraying their origin in those of the reptile egg, to which a new one has been added, the placenta. This is a fat disk of blood vessels through which, from the umbilical cord, runs the blood stream of the unborn young. Through the walls of the placenta and of the womb this blood stream comes so nearly in contact with that of the mother, though without mingling, that the two may exchange all the oxygen, nourishment, and waste products which the life of the fetus demands. Basically, it thus lives by precisely the same things as its parent. It is as good as being out of doors, and takes no effort. The fetus is, practically speaking, a pure parasite on its mother.

Consider the virtues of this system. The warmth and protection it furnishes the unborn are useful, of course, but the birds attain the same ends in other ways. Mainly, there is a much higher limit both to the amount of nourishment this piratical proto-infant can requisition and to the time it takes in the process. In an egg it would eat and grow its way outward to the shell, and then it must hatch or starve; and the size of an egg has practical bounds—ask a hen. Among mammals, on the other hand, perhaps only human beings and a few of their relations, with their overloaded heads, are putting the principle of live birth to any strain. The blank check on time and energy permits the unborn a gradual development to a high level, and a decent size, before it must face the harsh world.

And provisions have also been made to extend the protected development for a relatively long time after birth. First are the mammary glands, which produce a concentrated food in the form of milk. They have given the class its name, of course, even if they are not its most important feature. Second are all the natural behavior and strong emotions which lead the mammal mother to care for her nurslings in the most devoted and unselfish manner through their infancy. Except for birds, most other animals never see their children.

Mammal Skeletons

The mammal framework, the skeleton, is built on the fundamental vertebrate one, but is clearly improved over that of reptiles. The improvement is marked by two main trends: reduction of the number of bones used, and differentiation or specialization of those that remain. At the same time, a number of quite new features are present, so that the whole thing is a far more efficient engine than its prototypes, something of no small importance to ourselves. For example, the skeleton is more solid, yet more flexible, because of the high degree of modeling of joints and of muscle attachments on bone surfaces. Furthermore, ossification is very complete, meaning that cartilage is almost entirely replaced by bone. In mammals cartilage serves principally to

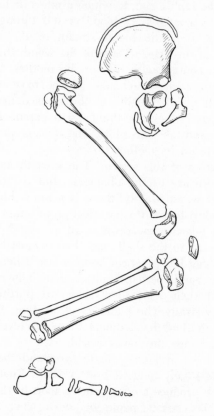

Epiphyses in mammal bones. The immature hip, leg, and foot bones of man, to show the epiphyses and other parts before final union.

line joint surfaces—it provides smooth and tough veneers of gristle so that two bones do not grind directly on one another.

Thus the skeleton supports mammal strength and activity and, by a new mammal invention, does this even during growth. In lower vertebrates the working bones of the limbs and spine take their shape (ossify as bone) within a cartilaginous matrix which blocks out the shape beforehand, so that the center of the shaft or body is bone, growing toward the ends or joints, which remain cartilage, serviceable but less rigid than bone. But the growing mammal has new centers of ossification for the ends as well as for the shaft of the bone, with cartilage between, so that the caps or joint surfaces (epiphyses) are, like the shaft, of bone. This gives the active, growing animal the advantage of a more perfectly formed skeleton during his development, while allowing the bone to grow freely in the cartilage lying between epiphysis and shaft. These parts unite and become a single piece only at maturity, when the animal definitely stops growing.

The mammal spine is reduced, especially in the tail. Ribs are lost except in the thorax, so that the neck is free. The back is arched for support in quadrupeds, or columnar in man and his nearest relatives. There is a flexible lumbar column in the small of the back, very useful for speedy runners. And the sacrum, that part articulating with the pelvis, is a solid block of several vertebrae fused together, so that the pelvic girdle is a strong ring firmly fixed to the spine, instead of being loosely hitched by a couple of sacralized ribs. The shoulder girdle— shoulder blade and collarbone—varies among mammals, but it is flexible and mobile, especially compared to reptiles. This differentiation of the flexible pectoral girdle from the fixed and heavy pelvis is of first importance to man, in whom there is so marked a contrast in the uses of arms and legs.

At any rate, both pairs of limbs are strengthened in mammals, in this and other ways, for powerful action and for ability to take stress. The ancient paw retained the generalized five digits from its ancestry, but considerably reduced the joints in each, to two for the thumb and three for each finger; a piercing glance at your free hand will confirm all this. But many mammals have done away with a digit or so, and the majority walk on either the balls or the tips of the "fingers." This is part of the process of getting the body off the ground, in which the whole limb partakes; such a stance certainly helps preserve body heat, and allows the energy of the limbs to go mainly into actual walking. Reptiles, by contrast, face something of a strain in heaving themselves up in the first place. The chronicle of legs has three stages: in amphibians the side fins of the crossopterygians were bent at a right angle, downward to meet the ground; in the higher mammal-like reptiles they had been twisted, the front ones back and the rear ones forward, so that they do not jut directly out, but instead provide a better leverage for muscles and work in a fore-and-aft line; while in mammals they have been strongly stabilized in this position. Men, of course, have their own peculiar modification of this last stance, which is one of their few real claims to distinctiveness, and the foremost of them. If reptiles appreciated the uses of elbow and knee, the mammals have done the same for "wrist" and "ankle" and foot bones generally. In lower classes of vertebrates these are rather formless and undifferentiated, seeming to be mainly internal stiffeners and hitching spots for muscles. But in mammals they have characteristic and specialized shapes of their own, employed for stability, mobility, length, leverage, or other desired ends, as the case may be in different species.

Mammal Skulls and Teeth

In the skull once more, bones have gone up in complexity and down in number. The lower jaw, you saw, is a single bone (on each side), the other bones having vanished or gone into the ear. The teeth are another mark of aristocracy. The dental array in a generalized reptile consists of a large number of simple pegs or points which may be replaced numerous times during life and which differ, if at all, only in the larger size of some. Mammalian teeth are much more specialized. A mammal has two definite sets, and two only: one, which is smaller in size and number, to grow on, and the other a second, adult set which replaces the first as the jaws become large enough to accommodate it. The teeth of this last set, especially, have hard enamel and are firmly rooted (compared with those of most reptiles) and seem to have been meant to last, with luck, as long as the mammal itself. We, as men, seem to have got out of touch with adaptation here. Perhaps we live too long. Perhaps we are the only mammal which grinds its teeth without putting food between them, a most unadaptive habit.

More striking than the limited replacement of the teeth is their differentiation into four series: chisel-like incisors at the front where the jaws open widest, for nipping and cutting; dagger-like canines at the front corners where they are most available for slashing and piercing; and premolars and molars, the cheek teeth, which are progressively heavier grinders or cutters placed close to the joint of the jaw where, as in a nutcracker, the crushing power is greatest. These last are the most noteworthy. The front teeth are modified merely in shape, but the cheek teeth are distinguished by a proliferation of new

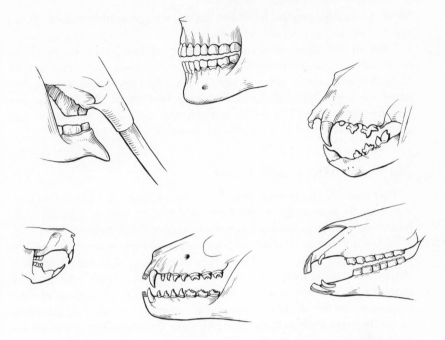

Differentiation in the teeth of mammals. Below, a generalized
mammal set, with 3 incisors, 1 canine, 4 premolars, and 3 molars.
Clockwise from this: a rodent, adapted for gnawing and chewing;
an elephant, with tusks, and with grinding molars which come in
one after another as they wear out; man, without marked specializations; a lion, with teeth for gnashing, slicing, and bone cracking; a horse, fore teeth for cropping, back teeth for grinding grass.
Mostly after Gregory.

cusps, added to the original point, which in different shapes and combinations allow a complex and varied modeling of tooth forms for
different kinds of food. In carnivores, for example, the cusps tend to
be disposed in a fore-and-aft line, changing the primitive reptile point
into a jagged blade for shearing flesh and cracking up bones. Herbivores have, instead, developed broad and symmetrical ridged surfaces,
sometimes with deeply folded enamel layers bonded by cement, for
milling vegetable matter including such tough material as grass. Mammals with broader diets, man among them, are apt to have more
generalized teeth.

A last kind of specialization among the orders of mammals is loss
of some of the original set, believed to have numbered forty-four.
Cows, for example, have dispensed with all their upper front teeth.

More generally, groups have lost an incisor or a bicuspid or so, as have man and his relatives.

Thus in the class of mammals, specialization has been piled on differentiation, and the intricacies of conformation and development in mammalian teeth are very great. Luckily they fossilize well, because of their hardness; paleontologists find them of great interest and use, and so teeth have been much appealed to as a court of last resort in classifying fossil mammal remains.

Mammal Diets and Gaits

This, then, is the ground plan for mice and men, for bison, beavers, and bats. It is actually surprisingly uniform, as anyone can see who takes the trouble to look at a series of mammal skeletons in a museum. It varies not in the number and identity of bones (except where loss has been radical, as in the hind legs of whales), but rather in their shape. The fact is interesting that every single mammal, with three or four exceptions, has seven vertebrae in his neck, regardless of how long or short the neck is. The vastly varied mammals that surround us are the result of a continuous radiation that has been going on for over seventy million years.

It was that long ago, in the Paleocene, just after the disappearance of the great reptiles, that the small and simple ancestors of the modern types of mammals were appearing and becoming distinct from one another. This was the first epoch in the Age of Mammals, the Cenozoic ("recent life") or Tertiary era. Through the Paleocene and the Eocene, mammals were rapidly exploring a wide variety of possible niches, some new, some standing vacant since the doom of the dinosaurs. Gradually they branched out as they grew in size, and the forerunners of the main types of modern animals were plain enough in the Oligocene. In the Miocene and the Pliocene they became what we might term full size and, like a developing photograph, were getting more and more like the species we recognize. An ark full of animals from this last half of the Tertiary could be named off in a general way by any little boy, but their exact appearance, through its unfamiliarity, would make an adult think he was dreaming. Lately there has been only a sort of rehashing of species, without very important changes; and the particular tableau of present mammalian life, in all its details, is a relatively few thousand years old.

The most ancient of the mammals were probably insect-eaters, small animals with a set of teeth which could have led to all the other kinds. At any rate, such creatures today—moles, hedgehogs, and shrews—are recognized as a main division, or order, of mammals, the Insectivora, many of whom are close to those early forms. The great tribes of the herbivores and carnivores have become specialized, but they seem to have diverged from a common parentage, closer than some other orders, in spite of their present unlikeness and animosity. Other lines have gone in for other foods. The Rodentia, from mice through woodchucks up to beavers, will eat many things, but their chisel-like front teeth enable them to gnaw bark and roots and nuts and so to get at foods too difficult for other forms. Others, like anteaters or armadillos, use heavy hooked claws to open anthills, and dig out foods, but have degenerate teeth or none at all, turning their backs on the advantages of mastication. Finally our own order, the Primates, has kept an ability to chew and eat a very broad diet even while it was producing monkeys, apes, and men. There is nothing to prevent us from eating insects except our feelings about eating insects; plenty of people do, though it would be hard to subsist on insects alone. Actually, we are omnivorous, if any animal is.

Locomotion, or the business of getting about, is the field above all others in which mammals have shown their great adaptability, and made clear the fundamental excellence of their skeleton. Some of them still patter around on the original little flat feet, but the others have practically exhausted the more interesting possibilities, short of sprouting wheels. Horses, antelopes, and so on are cursorial—adapted for running—to a high degree. Some of the rodents are saltatorial (i.e., they hop). Whales and porpoises are perfectly aquatic, having become fully streamlined, and losing almost every sign of leg or pelvis. Others, like seals, have followed them, but not so far; seals can still maneuver on the shore. Bats fly and have been partially imitated by flying squirrels, who glide. Moles burrow. A sloth proceeds upside down, hanging from a bough by claws like gaff hooks.

We primates began with the simple four-footed gait, but adapted it to the trees by a growing ability to grasp. Monkeys can both run and jump. Apes, however, instead of jumping, brachiate, or swing hand over hand. Man doubtless was once good at this last, but on starting to become human he specialized intensely, adopting the most singular gait of all. His uprightness is unique, because he has no hindward prop like a kangaroo, and his legs are not really like the landing gear of the birds, whose true vocation is flying. His gait is not the simple handing about of weight by means of limbs, as if he were flying, or hanging by hands, or standing on four feet, because it calls for worrying about equilibrium at the same time. It is related to balancing a cane on the end of your finger. You shift your weight in the proposed direction first, as if you were going to fall down there, and then hurriedly move your legs under your body again to keep this from happening. That is what human walking is, and any trainee, like a two-year-old child, will tell you it is tricky work.

A final feature of the mammal skeleton is of particular interest: the clavicle or collarbone. It is specially developed compared to the reptiles, who have more and different bones in this region. You can trace its course simply enough at the top of your own chest. It is a strut which runs from the head end of the breastbone to a process of the shoulder blade, and it actually creates the "shoulder" by holding the arm socket out away from the chest. A horseman falling on his shoulder breaks his collarbone for that reason. This structure is a great advantage to an arm which is used in movements sideways or in several directions, providing a universal fulcrum for it and for all its muscles. But it is of no particular use to an animal which moves its forelimb only forward and backward along the side of the chest, as in running; and the horses and their relatives lack a clavicle altogether. It varies among carnivores, who are capable of a certain amount of sidewise and crosswise movements and of various uses of the paws. It is well developed in burrowing, clawing, or climbing animals, but it reaches its greatest length in connection with the sweeping wings of bats and the perfectly liberated arm of man.

Marsupials and Monotremes

Now for a small confession. I have been talking, all the way through, about only one kind of mammal, the placental mammals, who form a full-fledged placenta in reproduction and so enjoy, if that is the word, an extended period of gestation or prenatal development. It is true that these are the most important mammals, reigning supreme today as the result of an early victory, and counting us among them. But they are far from being the only recognizable mammals who have existed, and mammal history is not theirs alone, by any means. They are not even the only mammals who survive today.

In the first place, there is the still important tribe of the marsupials, or pouched mammals. Everybody has seen an opossum, the most widespread of them. In the Americas he has few relatives, but in Australia and New Guinea he is accompanied by many, of whom the kangaroos are only the best known, with the koala doubtless next best. The marsupials are, in fact, the true mammal fauna of this region: the only placentals to reach Australia before Captain Cook's time were rats, bats, and men, the last apparently bringing their dogs as passengers. It is interesting, and important, to note how the marsupials had a radiation of their own, much like the placentals, producing similar forms to occupy similar niches. As Gregory has said, these likenesses deceived the English colonists into calling Australian marsupials "mice," "cats," "tigers," "moles," "rabbits," "bears," "badgers," and "squirrels." Probably the leaping kangaroo fills the same niche among marsupials as the hoofed herbivores among the placentals.

Marsupials bear their young alive but, without a well-developed placenta, cannot continue to nourish them internally for a long time, and must bring them forth, tiny and undeveloped. These embryonic objects find their way into the pouch, a sort of incubator, where they live without real consciousness on a milk diet until they have grown into something resembling a newborn placental mammal. They then begin to take short field trips. The marsupial skeleton differs from that of the placental and may have a larger number of teeth; marsupials also have a less complete milk set. But the two branches seem, as we shall see, to go back to a distant common parentage.

More mysterious are the monotremes, also of Australia and New Guinea: the duckbill or platypus, and the echidna or spiny anteater. Their skeletons lack many mammal features and in fact are reminiscent of reptiles. And they lay eggs. But when the young monotreme hatches out, he is nursed by his mother, whom he also finds to be hairy (or spiny) and warm-blooded, though of low degree in this as in other things. The monotremes are mysterious because their ancestry has so far yielded no fossils. Unfortunately there exist only these two odd forms, and more unfortunately still, they have only crudely formed teeth or none at all. So one of the best kinds of evidence for placing a mammal with its proper kith and kin cannot be used.

A History of Mammals

What about mammal history? I have spoken of the Tertiary as the Age of Mammals, but their antiquity is actually much greater, for the Tertiary was only the prime of their life. For origins, and for perspective, we must plunge into the past far deeper than the seventy million years of the Tertiary and look at the time scale of the vertebrates and known life as a whole.

The Paleozoic era, or Primary, not with the earliest life but with the first copious fossils, began half a billion years ago. Its duration was immense. In its second division appeared the ostracoderms, to be followed, midway in its march, by the rise of the bony fishes. Then there arrived the amphibians and the reptiles. Not only were the latter coming into their own during the Permian, last period of the Paleozoic, but the stem reptiles were already giving signs of the advent of the mammals.

That is to say, there appeared a line of reptiles, the Therapsida,

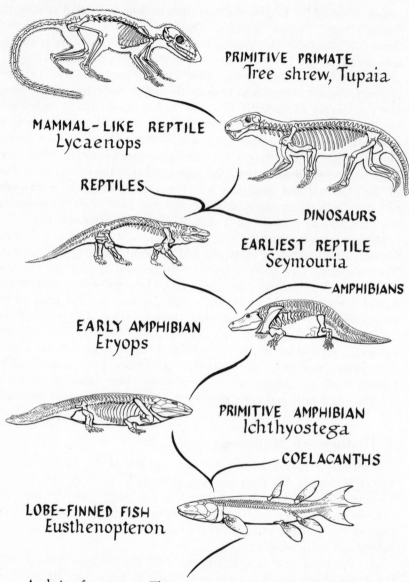

PRIMITIVE PRIMATE
Tree shrew, Tupaia

MAMMAL-LIKE REPTILE
Lycaenops

REPTILES

DINOSAURS

EARLIEST REPTILE
Seymouria

AMPHIBIANS

EARLY AMPHIBIAN
Eryops

PRIMITIVE AMPHIBIAN
Ichthyostega

COELACANTHS

LOBE-FINNED FISH
Eusthenopteron

A chain of ancestors. These are animals lying on, or close to, the line which led to man between fishes and mammals. After Gregory, Jarvik, and Romer.

who were plainly connected with the basic, primitive stem but who also progressed more and more directly toward a mammal form, even before the opening of the Mesozoic, the Age of Reptiles. And in the early part of this new (Secondary) era, when the old amphibians had gone downhill but still before the dinosaurs had made their appearance, the therapsids had come to the very threshold of mammaldom. Then they themselves gave out, surviving only in the primitive mammals who descended from them.

These mammal-like reptiles had got the body permanently off the ground on well-formed limbs, and in many species the joints in the paws were already reduced to the mammal count. They possessed well-differentiated teeth, with multiple cusps in the molars in contrast to the peg-toothed standard reptile, and they grew two sets only. They had, in some cases, a bony palate. And the number of skull bones was reducing and approaching a mammal pattern. Most interestingly, the main bone of the lower jaw steadily grew at the expense of those at the joint region, until in the latest forms these latter were only vestigial strips. In the mammals they vanished, except for the articular, which became part of the middle ear.

These animals, then, were certainly active, and probably warm-blooded (in view of the bony palate—see page 45). The "mammal-like reptiles" were truly intermediate, and nobody can tell if they had warm blood, wore fur, laid eggs, or secreted milk. With only skeletons to go on, drawing a line is difficult, and that is why students have agreed that, if a fossil has a jaw which has finally become a single bone, they will call it a mammal and stop arguing.

So, once more, we have a class of vertebrates rising from the continuously progressing stem of the class below. Once more, the stair climbers seem to have gone on up the stairs without even a pause at the landing where their brothers began to fan out through that floor. In this case, the mammal-like reptiles continued up, approaching the next higher landing at the beginning of the Mesozoic, two hundred million years ago. They reached it early in the Mesozoic, at the end of the Triassic period, so that true mammals have existed the better part of two hundred million years, and not during the Tertiary alone.

Actually, we must stretch the house-and-stair idea a little. For different primitive mammals seem to have risen from the mammal-like reptiles more than once, coming not only up the stairs but up the fire escape, the laundry chute, or any available ascent, with the peculiar monotremes shinnying part way up an unlocated drainpipe somewhere about the house. By the mid-Mesozoic there were five clearly defined mammal groups of different origin, obscure and little known to be sure, while the dinosaurs basked in their own splendor. Three of these groups dropped out of sight well before the Tertiary (unless the monotremes are survivors of one of them), while a fourth, the pantotheres, also vanished after their stock had given rise to

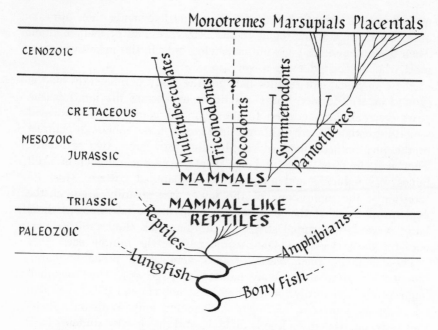

Mammal origins. Mammal-like reptiles flourished in the late Paleozoic and early Mesozoic periods. Several groups of mammals arose from these, but most of them became extinct even before the Cenozoic (the Tertiary, or Age of Mammals). After Patterson.

two daughter lines, the marsupials and the placentals. Then, after this long period of experimentation and development by the mammals—almost in their middle age, so to speak—the dinosaurs vanished at the dawn of the Tertiary, and the world was theirs by default.

It found them small and still rather primitive. Adaptive radiation began, by fits and starts. But the early placentals had already got the upper hand of the early marsupials, leaving as their competitors only the rodent-like multituberculates, the last survivors among the ancient Mesozoic founders of Mammalia. The superiority of the placentals in basic design became more and more insistent. The multituberculates gave up the struggle and succumbed in the Eocene, probably from rodent competition. The marsupials were crowded out of most of the world. But they found their way into the southern blind alleys of the map. The main placental mammals did not catch up with them in South America until a few million years ago and (except for some rats) never reached Australia at all, because of the early isolation of that continent. So the marsupials found a sanctuary there in which to continue their radiation and to survive for our own eyes.

There is probably nothing like a short discourse on the bones and teeth of little proto-mammals to reduce the ordinary person to a state of stupefaction, and probably no subject which contains more excitement and reward for a paleontologist. Again and again, year after year, the pieces come to light which tell the needed parts of the story. Oddly enough, the more perfect and complicated becomes the knowledge, the more difficult it seems to be to make clear the meaning of a new find in the newspapers. Perhaps this is why so little that is fresh can penetrate through the comfortable banalities about dinosaur eggs and "Darwin's theory." And yet the many obscure and unsensational fossils do add up to important conclusions. Certainly, the strong upward surge of several independent original branches of mammals, out of the mammal-like reptiles, tells much about evolution and natural selection, showing with what momentum these forces move when circumstances (environment plus a promising set of bodily mechanisms) open up a broad boulevard of adaptation toward a higher organization.

4. THE PRIMATES

"AND OUT of the ground the Lord God formed every beast of the field, and every fowl of the air; and brought them unto Adam to see what he would call them; and whatsoever Adam called every living creature, that was the name thereof." If Adam reviewed the whole animal kingdom on this occasion, he must have had a tiring day, for the known species number something like a million.

They are numerous enough, at least, so that Linnaeus did a great thing for science by starting, two centuries ago, the formal classification of classes, orders, families, and species that we use today. In this way, he not only provided precise Latin names, to avoid the kind of ambiguity and confusion that Adam's system is liable to, but also put the animals into an orderly arrangement which powerfully suggests their natural kinship, although Linnaeus himself was no believer in evolution. At any rate, since mankind, whether Adam or Linnaeus, has always been in charge of the naming, it is not odd that our own order of mammals was called the Primates: the "chiefs," the "number ones."

This seems only fair. Since a human being is so extraordinary an animal, his relatives should share the credit. Man is a perfectly good mammal, and he did not result from the vertebrates climbing more stairs, or heaving up an entirely new class by some systemic development like warm blood. Rather, man is man because of his brain, and he got this brain, as we shall see later, by being a primate and a descendant of primates. Now the primates range from man and other highly intelligent animals down to little tree shrews, who virtually overlap with the simplest placental mammals known, past or present. And a visitor from another world, happening along seventy million years ago, would probably have laughed at the idea that the Paleocene primates could ever produce a man. But they did.

One of the things which marks a primate, and a thing which was certainly vital in our having emerged on the earth at all, is some ability, great or small, to grasp. Certainly, and said without cynicism, man is a grasping animal. His hands—generalized hands—have kept the ancient five digits of the first tetrapods, and the mammalian three free segments of each finger except the thumb; and they have made the digits flexible and capable of independent movement. Fingers can close over something in a wrapping motion: they are prehensile. The thumb has a base rotated inward from the palm, and it can be set against the other fingers, and wrapped around an object from the other side: it is opposable. And a good grip, even on a most slippery surface, is helped by the skin inside the fingers. This is not smooth, but ridged into fingerprints and kept

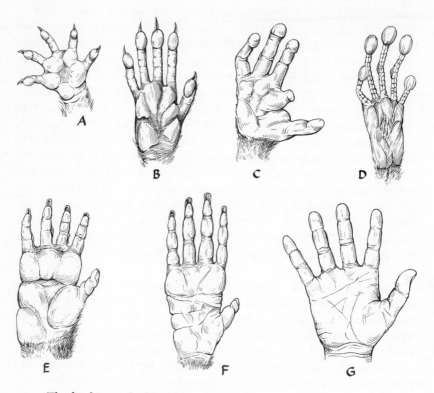

The background of hands.
A. opossum, primitive but mobile.
B. tree shrew, with simple primate proportions.
C. potto, using thumb and 4th digit for greater span (reduced 2nd digit).
D. *Tarsius,* a small hand with specialized enlarged skin pads.
E. baboon, used in running as well as handling, fingers somewhat shortened.
F. orang, lengthened for brachiating, with reduced thumb.
G. man, with short fingers, long thumb, with good opposition.

slightly moist by many tiny glands, while the fine oil which is supplied to the rest of the body's surface does not appear on the palms or soles. Finally, where other mammals have claws or hoofs, we have nails; they may sometimes be a nuisance, but they are no encumbrance to our use of hands in gripping.

So our hands are superb holders, turners, twisters, pullers, catchers, throwers, pinchers, as well as pushers, slappers, or smoothers. Not so our feet, which are only kickers, stampers, or treaders. They have the skin, the digits, and the bones, but our great toe is no longer opposable, a thing which sets us off from other primates. In fact, man is particularly unusual in this—in having hands which are better graspers than his feet. For in other primates it is more apt to be the foot which has a better opposable great toe, and the hand which varies from the plan, being long and hook-like in apes, having a non-opposable thumb in marmosets, and a vestigial thumb or none at all in the spider monkeys of South America and the colobus monkeys of Africa.

But the plan is there in all of them, though realized only vaguely in the lower members of the order. Power of hands and feet to grasp a bough, or manipulate an object, is enhanced by other features of the limbs, features which are also refinements of an ancient heritage. For example, the two bones in the forelimb were present, and independent of one another, in the earliest land vertebrates. But among mammals it is virtually the primates alone who have kept and fostered the ability to twist the radius (on the thumb side) on the ulna, until the human hand can be flipped over, or rotated, through a full semicircle, without moving the elbow or upper arm at all. Hold your right elbow with your left hand and twist your right hand, to see what this means to your use of fingers. In evolution it has meant: without primates, no human beings.

Otherwise, primates are unspecialized. They lack peculiarities like the teeth of rodents, the wings of bats, or the hoofs of horses. An expert may recognize a primate skull by its teeth, and even a tyro might know it by the bridge of bone from the edge of the brow to the cheekbone, making a full ring around the eye socket, though this ring is not exclusive to primates.

In general, then, it is actually more enlightening to follow Le Gros Clark and note that the primate order is distinguished rather by certain tendencies in its development. While there is a wide range, and some members are very primitive, the whole group has shown an increasing propensity toward large brains (as indeed have most mammal orders), toward refinement of the use of the hands and feet, and toward reduction of the number of young born at a time.

More characteristically yet, primates have tended to sit up; to poise the head more vertically on the spine; to reduce the sense of smell and its instrument, the snout; to increase the sense of vision and bring the eyes near each other in the front of the face; and to pull the jaws down.

These trends are the real coat of arms of the order of Primates. They are prominently displayed in monkeys, apes, and, above all, men. They are much less visible in our simplest relatives.

Prosimians: Below the Salt

There are two main divisions of primates. The lower consists largely of the "lemurs," which I put in quotes to signify a general kind of animal, scattered through the Old World tropics from Africa through Madagascar to Southeast Asia, living in trees, mostly nocturnal in activity, eating fruit and insects, furry in coat, and about the size of a cat or smaller. They are appealing in appearance, and interesting animals, but they are hard to see in the wild and not much more satisfactory in zoos because they are apt to sleep all day. They are more properly called prosimians, since this suborder of the primates is named Prosimii. They vary more than the above simple description may suggest.

The true lemurs all live on the island of Madagascar, which abounds in species running from the size of a cat to that of a mouse. Typical ones look rather foxy, though they have hands in place of paws, and spring about actively at night. If you can get one to open his mouth, you will see a peculiarity of his lower teeth: the six at the front are long and narrow and lie projecting forward close together to form a "comb," which he actually uses to clean his fur. There are other kinds of lemurs on this island, including the deliberate, stump-tailed indri and the extremely aberrant aye-aye, who has a long and skinny middle finger for spearing grubs in holes in the bark of trees and a rather rodent-like set of teeth, to help him get at the grubs. On the whole, lemurs are friendly and gregarious. They will eat many foods and are partial to insects. And they are good little fighters for their size, and have tough constitutions, surviving unexpectedly long when badly wounded or very ill.

But a search for signs foreshadowing humanity will be frustrated. Lemurs have hands, but they are better at grasping boughs than in handling objects; prehension is poor and clumsy and the thumb is hardly used in opposition at all. If you offer a bush baby a raisin, he will pull your hand toward him and take the raisin with his teeth instead of picking it up.

As to brains, furthermore, lemurs are a disappointment. This is clear to the specialist from the restricted size of the cerebral cortex, or outer shell, of the brain and from the fact that this is smooth, lacking the convolutions or folding which add vastly to its total surface area in a monkey or a man. And the actions of lemurs betray only commensurate mentality, with no hint that they are related to the four most intelligent animals in the world. The lemurs are, in fact, very ordinary small mammals, simple and rather primitive, who are, we might say, not making much of an effort to be primates. We can appreciate them more in hindsight; like other primitive or basic types we have already seen, they have only simple forms of the potentialities which their higher relatives developed and expanded.

In addition to the true lemurs of Madagascar, there is a mainland family, composed of the lorises of Asia and the galagos, or bush babies, of Africa. The former are wide-eyed, short-faced, long-limbed creatures who climb and clamber carefully and are rather monkey-like in a few ways. Their cousins, the bush babies, resemble the lemurs, active jumpers with strong hind legs. Taken together, the lorises have puzzled zoologists somewhat, by some minor but striking anatomical and dental differences from the lemurs, which argue that they have had a long separate history. That may be so, but otherwise they are the same general kind of animal, and of primate. They have at any rate developed the same peculiar lower front teeth. Perhaps the differences are not so great. What is really interesting is the evidence of evolution fanning out in the primates, in this simple stage.

If all these "lemurs" are primitive, tending to carry the primate line back toward the first placental mammals, the tree shrews virtually bridge the gap. They are a family (Tupaiidae) of species living in southern Asia and the Indies. They are small with long tails and pointed faces, all but one species flourishing by day, and they live on fruit and insects. They certainly are not much removed from the tiny mammals of the Mesozoic. They look, act, and eat like the other little insectivores of the past and present, and were for a long time classed with that order, the Insectivora. But later close inspection disclosed two things. One: the members of the Insectivora are not as much alike as they seem; and they share primitiveness, small size, and an insect menu more than they share anatomical features. Two: the particular features of tree shrews, when at last perceived, turned out to be the first suggestions, in a basic mammal, of primate features. Small though they are, their brains and eyes are slightly enlarged. In the cortex of the brain the part serving sight is a little increased

Prosimians. Above, tree shrew and bush baby, or galago. Below, *Tarsius* and a lemur. After Le Gros Clark and Wood Jones.

and that serving smell is reduced. And the skull has the beginning of a downward bend in the middle, like primates generally.

Other body details also whisper "primate," particularly features of the reproductive system. And the paws, though clawed, can be spread out and used in the beginning of a grasp. Disagreement continues, it is true, as to their classification as primates, but there is little about these shrews which debars them from our own order, even if they have not developed all of the few "typical" traits of primates generally. And that is how we ourselves can be joined directly, in our "ancestral" line, to the oldest of mammals. In any book about unmissing links, this is one of the most unmissing of any.

On the other side of the main lemur group we find the oddity known as *Tarsius*, the spectral tarsier, who dwells in Indonesia. He evidently has no immediate relatives today within the prosimians. He looks something like a chunky rat, for size and color. But he perches upright, by clinging, in bamboo groves. And his round head has a short face surmounted by enormous eyes, facing fully to the front; he has large ears which can be stuck up or furled (as have galagos and some lemurs); and he can twist his head around so as to look right out over his spine. So it is evident that he has well-developed senses, and his large brain bears this out. In other ways he also seems more "advanced," or at least more monkey-like, than lemurs: his eye sockets have a complete back wall and not only a ring, and he has a real upper lip. That is, it is a single lip, free of the gum below it, like ours, and not split in the middle, like a dog's, with a region of naked, moist skin around the nostril (a rhinarium), which is what the lemurs have. With this lip we can make faces, and so can *Tarsius*. Lemurs cannot.

In still other less noticeable ways *Tarsius* seems to approach higher primates. But in his limb architecture he is much specialized, for grasp and for hopping. Instead of having the inner side of his tiny elongated fingers and toes continuously lined with friction pads like ours, his pads are separated enlarged disks, very efficient for the animal's size. In leg and foot he is still more modified. He gets his very name from the fact that the hinder part of his foot (the tarsus) is greatly lengthened. Various other mammals have long "feet" (horses and rabbits), but they are lengthened in the forward or metatarsal part, corresponding to the instep, or to the palm of your hand. But *Tarsius*, in extending the back segment instead, is true to primate tradition, because the whole forward, working part of the foot remains a grasping, hand-like organ on the end of a long lever. So he is rather like a miniature kangaroo with a whole little hand where its toes should be. And this peculiar combination, in so small an animal, gives it a powerful leg leverage without sacrificing the ability to grasp. *Tarsius* can make a jump that is almost a snap, flitting from bough to bough with surprising suddenness. He is designed principally for upright perches, not for flat surfaces, on which he is clumsy.

Tarsius has been upgraded and downgraded in humiliating fashion as knowledge of him, of other primates, and of fossils has increased. In fact, he is a good example of how our understanding of nature is apt to advance, not directly but by an erratic course, as students apply the best interpretation possible at any time. At first acquaintance the tarsiers were put down as unusual lemurs. Later, on appreciation of his relatively large brain and eyes, his lip, and some internal features also pointing toward monkeys, *Tarsius* was taken up front to a place of honor and given a suborder of primates all to himself, sandwiched between the lower and the higher divisions. He was considered by some (such as Dr. W. K. Gregory) to be the ideal source for the higher primates generally and even, in a foray by Professor Wood Jones, made the ancestor from which the human line had sprung direct. All this was put forth with the understanding that the specializations of the living tarsiers are to be discounted, and only their progressive and general features used in the ancestor.

Lately, however, while he is still considered to be suggestive as to our ancestry, he falls more easily into place in the broad spectrum of fossil prosimians. He is more freakish than most of them. But his principal interest is in showing that the whole lemur-like stock ran from something as primitive as tree shrews to something in which higher, monkey traits were foreshadowed. Furthermore, the lorises have expressed vague tendencies in the same direction, while the galagos have also independently imitated the lengthened ankle bones of *Tarsius*. Accordingly he has been sent back, with apologies, to the prosimians.

The Higher Primates

The higher primates are put in a second suborder named the Anthropoidea. Here at last we are turning in at the gate, for it contains ourselves as well as apes and monkeys. This whole aristocracy represents a distinctly higher grade than the Prosimii. Its progressiveness is marked, while on the whole its nature is rather generalized, at least compared to many of the living lower primates.

There is not much that is distinctive about them, once you have said that they are higher primates. They are diurnal, or day-living in habit. As in *Tarsius*, the back wall of the eye socket is well closed in, separating the socket from the depression in the temple region just behind. Much more importantly (and once again this is a progressive trait which *Tarsius* shares), the eyes themselves have a "yellow spot" (macula lutea), of particularly acute sight, in the retina opposite the pupils; and they have stereoscopic vision.

The latter is what gives us a sense of three dimensions. Both eyes, entirely at the front of the head, cover the same field of vision— finality of a primate trend—and they also produce in the brain a single unconfused image of what they jointly look at. This last is managed by a splitting of the nerve fibers from each eye so that about half go to each half of the brain, where the impulses from the two eyes merge in consciousness. (Such splitting, less complete, is found in other animals; it is apparently limited in *Tarsius*.) And yet, at the same time, the slightly different direction from which each eye views an object is also registered, as in a stereopticon or a range finder, which allows a very precise judgment of distance. As if this were not a magnificent enough present from evolution, the Anthropoidea also see a fuller range of different colors than do other mammals.

From its inferiors this suborder differs otherwise mainly in degree. The brain is larger, with ever increasing emphasis on the cerebral cortex, the seat of all higher functions, which extends backward more and more to cover the rest of the brain. Actually, some of the small South American monkeys have the largest brains of all, relative to their body size, as small animals tend to do. But making allowance for this, the effective brain supply increases toward man. Evidently the important thing is a brain which is large both relatively *and* absolutely, for this is where we outdo both little monkeys and whales, whose brains are larger than our own.

The skull becomes rounder, and more like ours, and spine and mouth have come alarmingly close to each other underneath. The face of man, obviously, has moved ninety degrees down from its position in a quadruped, being on a plane with his chest, so that a dog with a human face would be looking straight at the ground. Thus in an ordinary mammal the snout is directly at the front of the skull and the joint with the spine is directly at the back, while in the primates both snout and *foramen magnum* ("large opening," for the spinal cord) have tended to move downward and toward one another below the skull. These shifts, only hinted at in lemurs and affirmed in *Tarsius*, become manifest in monkeys and extreme in us.

Apart from brain and eye, the higher nervous organization of the Anthropoidea is reflected in the growing independence of the hands, not only from the chores of support and walking, but also from each other. This means we can readily use them to do different things at the same time, supplementing one another, as when you hold a nail with one hand and hammer it (the nail) with the other. It was a major step toward man when primate hands became as interested in grasping movable objects like apples as in grasping fixed objects like boughs.

The higher primates are typically much larger in size than the lower, with four giant animals (orang, chimpanzee, gorilla, and man) at the head of the whole order. Taken all in all, however, their very obvious higher status is not accompanied by clear-cut and striking skeletal differences from the prosimians, and a student of form is almost driven to the teeth in order to distinguish them unmistakably. In prosimians, as in primitive mammals generally, the small lower molar crowns have spiky cusps and deep recessions (are "tuberculosectorial," in case you would like to flatten the next person who asks what you have been reading lately). In higher primates the crowns are broader, more level, with shallower, blunter cusps.

Families of Our Relatives

The Anthropoidea are divided, or classified, in several different ways because of several different kinds of relationship among them. This is most useful for experts and most upsetting for college students. To begin with, there are five families: three of monkeys, one of apes, and one of men. These are split, in the monkeys, into those proper to the Eastern and the Western hemispheres respectively. The former, of the Old World (men, apes, and one monkey family) are called catarrhines (downward-nosed) from the fact that their nostrils point down and are close together. They also suggest relationship by sharing the same dental formula, or count, of the several kinds of teeth: 2-1-2-3 (two incisors, one canine, two premolars, and three molars, on either side of both jaws). The remaining monkeys, who live in tropical America, are called platyrrhines (flat-nosed), their nostrils facing front and being well separated, with little in the way of an actual nose showing. They have one more premolar tooth in each series. This is a sign of relative primitiveness; there are others, and the platyrrhines and catarrhines differ in small details of the skull, important but not visible on a trip to the zoo.

The five families are also arranged another, slightly different way, into superfamilies. Here the two families of New World monkeys, the platyrrhines, are grouped as the Ceboidea, the Old World monkeys are set off as the Cercopithecoidea, and the apes and man put together as the Hominoidea. This is actually the most important arrangement from our point of view.

Groups of the Prosimii or Lower Primates

TREE SHREWS

LEMURS

LORISES

TARSIUS

Families of the Anthropoidea, or Higher Primates

superfamily
Ceboidea
{
NEW WORLD MONKEYS,
the CEBIDAE

MARMOSETS,
the CALLITHRICIDAE
}
the Platyrrhines

superfamily
Cercopithecoidea
{
OLD WORLD MONKEYS,
the CERCOPITHECIDAE
}
the Catarrhines

superfamily
Hominoidea
{
APES, the PONGIDAE

MEN, the HOMINIDAE
}

A chart of the Primates, to show the main groups, and how they are arranged or classified.

If you see a monkey hanging by its tail, it is from the New World. Not all of them can do this, but the trait, a sort of fifth hand, is found only in the platyrrhine monkeys. It serves them as an excellent safety device against loss of footing, or handing, by the four regular prehensile "hands" in the dangerous tropical forests. The alert, intelligent cebus monkey, the organ-grinder's friend, is probably the best known, but the larger howling monkey, the long-limbed and agile spider monkey, and the woolly monkey are some of the varied members, followed by others of smaller size and lesser familiarity; altogether there is a good deal of variety and evolutionary divergence among them.

All these are members of the family Cebidae. The other family, the Callithricidae, is that of the marmosets, small squirrel-like creatures hardly recognizable as monkeys to look at, with banded fur of black and yellow or red, and in several species tufts of hair at the sides of the head or all around it, making a mane like a toy lion. The marmosets are strange in that they have claws instead of nails (except on the great toe) and have lost the opposability of their thumbs. They have two molar teeth only, not three like other primates. And they have twins at every birth. After a certain amount of perplexity over them, and suggestions that they are perhaps the primitive parents of the other higher primates, it is now generally agreed that they are simply backsliders, being actually built on the same basic plan as the Cebidae, with their claws having resulted from the compression of nails in very small feet. Furthermore, the rare callimico just about bridges the two families; he has, practically, the body of a marmoset and the skull of a cebid monkey. Even the unopposable thumb is not much of a difference, since in the platyrrhines generally opposability is good in the hind limb but poor in the hand. The howling monkeys, for example, are apt to separate the first two digits, not the thumb alone, from the rest; the spider monkey has no external thumb at all.

Across the oceans are bigger monkeys, throughout Africa and southern Asia. All of them belong in the family Cercopithecidae, which is also treated as a superfamily for the sake of neatness, the Cercopithecoidea. Most familiar to us are the populous tribes of macaques and baboons. Any large cageful of monkeys in a zoo is apt to turn out to be rhesus macaques, and the medical laboratories also swarm with these hardy animals. They and other macaques live around the world all the way from the Strait of Gibraltar to Japan. Baboons, largest and fiercest of the monkeys, are found in various forms almost everywhere in Africa; indeed, the baboon would make as good an emblem of that continent as would a lion or an antelope. His name, pleasant and euphonious, and sounding a little silly, does not do justice to a magnificent and formidable primate. He is a cunning animal, but his reputation has outrun him, crediting him with nearly human social activities and with military maneuvers in groups, such as ambushes, hollow squares, councils of war, posting of sentinels, and so on. A grain of salt is indicated. Excellent studies made

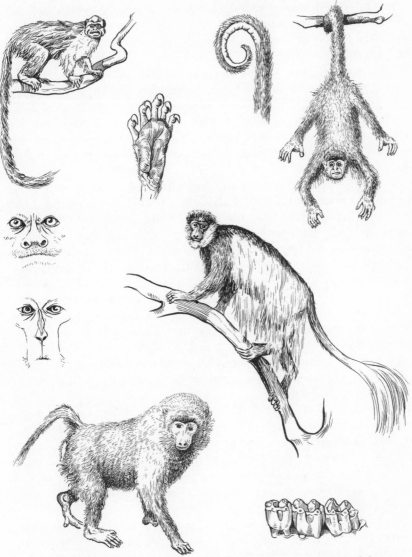

Monkeys. Above, left, a tamarin (marmoset), and detail of fore-paw, showing claws, and non-opposable thumb. Above right, a ce-bus monkey with prehensile tail. Below, right, a colobus monkey. Below left, a baboon. Details show facial difference between plat-yrrhine and catarrhine monkeys, and bilophodont teeth of latter.

recently in the wild, however, show rather complex individual re-lationships of the members of a troop, obviously the basis for these older stories.

The Old World monkeys are quadrupedal and quite generalized in body form. Some species have hands of very human proportions, not long in the fingers or short in the thumb, and with good opposability. They are not as strictly tree-living as the New World monkeys. The baboons, indeed, have left the boughs entirely, inhabiting such un-forested regions as North and South Africa, and the Abyssinian high-lands, in particular. Obviously to face the dangers of ground life, they have become savage fighters, with long snouts and heavy canine teeth in males. But you will see that the snout has grown out in front of two thoroughly primate eyes, near together at the root of the nose.

The cercopithecoid monkeys are decorative and varied in externals like fur and skin color, many of them being strikingly beautiful, like the Diana monkeys or the black and white colobus. Others are bizarre as well as beautiful, like the proboscis monkey with his pendulous nose, red fur and gray shirt front, in Borneo, or the crested "black ape" of Celebes. The family also has certain definite specializa-tions, four in particular. The most obvious is ischial callosities, paired patches of tough, fibrous substance, in effect almost as though the ischial part of the pelvis were protruding through the skin, at the place where the back of the leg begins. These callous areas are evidently specializations for sitting and, S. L. Washburn thinks, for sleeping in trees. Some species, and above all the baboons, have rose-ate skin and even colored fur in the same region, giving them strik-ingly effulgent behinds.

A second specialization is the possession of bilophodont (two-crested) molar teeth. The molars all have four cusps (except the last, with five) and are square in plan, with the two forward cusps joined by a crossing ridge (loph), as are the two back ones, so that the whole molar set makes a series of transverse ridges and troughs. This is a specialization away from the arrangement found in the rest of the Anthropoidea.

The two remaining special traits belong to two different main groups. The tree-living leaf-eaters, mainly Asiatic, have sacculated stomachs, divided into a series of sacs by circular bands of muscle. The other branch, more general feeders, has cheek pouches, which expand to hold food that cannot at once be chewed up and swal-lowed, very useful in getting more than your share and putting it where nobody else can reach it. Thus equipped, such monkeys can give rein to their natural avarice, bad manners, and disgusting selfish-ness. They can make a banana disappear in seconds, only to reappear as a collar of bulges around the throat. Their actions are everything you would want to stamp out in your own child. But the rhesus monkeys flourish like a green bay tree.

Apes and Men

Now to the Hominoidea. Here is our own clan, the superfamily containing the family of men, Hominidae, and the family of apes, Pongidae. It is an important group (obviously), with an important name. Unfortunately the name sounds, especially when you say "hominoid" to speak of a member of the group, as though you meant "man-like." So we might note that it has no such particular meaning and is only a name following from the rules of classification. According to these, the name of a family or superfamily must be based on some animal (genus) within it. The genus *Homo* is a name of respectable age, going back to Linnaeus himself; at any rate, its family is Hominidae, and the superfamily takes its name from it also, rather than from the Pongidae and *Pongo*, the orang. This does not necessarily mean that man is the most typical, the oldest, or anything else; it is only a way of choosing a name. Consequently "hominoid" does not really mean "man-like" appearances to the contrary; it simply means "pertaining to the Hominoidea," or any member of the group.

All hominoids are catarrhines. But our own relations with the Old World monkeys are simple and general; with the apes they are more specific. The reader is implored to assimilate the distinction at once and never again to point to a chimpanzee and say, "See the big monkey." It would be a far less hideous blunder, zoologically speaking, to confuse an ape with a man. There is nothing new in this idea; Huxley stated it, but the point has been popularly ignored, nevertheless: apes are more like men than like monkeys.

Of course, the distinctions are not so plain at a glance. The average person, asked for the difference between an ape and a monkey, will cast about in his mind and end by responding that apes have no tails. Quite true; they have only the same internal vestige (the coccyx) as man, recurved beneath the pelvis and even smaller and more degenerate. Also, apes lack the cross-crested molars of the Cercopithecidae, having instead, together with man, their own plan of a more basic primate pattern. And they lack other monkey specializations, although gibbons and many chimpanzees have ischial callosities, and female chimpanzees, like baboons, have an additional conspicuous periodic swelling, a sexual phenomenon.

But the important distinctions are broader. The hominoids (apes and men) differ from the monkeys in the torso and in the shoulders and arms. Men differ from apes, as we shall see, in the pelvis, leg, and foot. The monkeys, whether of the New World or the Old, are true quadrupeds. Men walk upright, as true bipeds. The anthropoid apes fall in between, to a degree, but actually they are neither quadrupedal nor bipedal. They brachiate: when it comes to locomotion in the trees, they are bimanual, swinging hand over hand from limb to limb.

This is a primary distinction, but not an absolute one. Many monkeys are part-time brachiators, in varying degrees, especially the spider monkey of South America. Among the apes, chimpanzees and gorillas

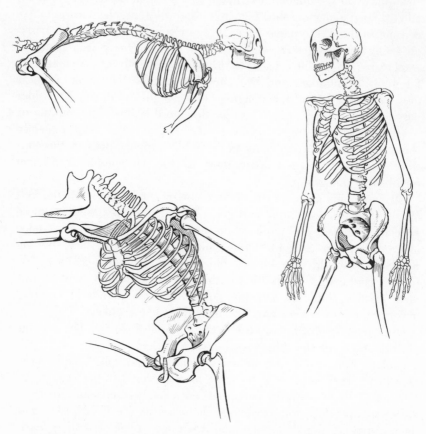

The trunk in monkeys, apes and man. Above, a monkey, showing small and narrow rib cage, and long lumbar section of the spine, with processes of vertebrae inclined toward a central point in the lower back, related to springing motions. Below, orang, showing powerful and broad shoulder girdle, especially at the collar bones; also large rib cage, short lumbar spine, and splayed-out pelvis. Right, man, with broad, flat chest and shoulders, strong lumbar column, and rounded, basin-like pelvis.

are essentially ground animals. They stand erect easily, and walk bipedally with some facility, though never for long distances. The gorilla, with his great bulk, goes in trees very little and must brachiate seldom if at all; such "brachiation" as he does is probably horizontal, bulling and pulling himself through jungle growth in very uneven countryside. Like chimpanzees, gorillas go mainly on their feet and knuckles. But this is obviously a kind of secondary quadrupedalism, in animals who are large-bodied ground livers, and whose ancestors were clearly not quadrupedal, like monkeys, in the trees.

In spite of the living gorilla and chimpanzee, the basic habit of the apes, the home adaptation, is an upright, suspended body. A primate trend has been carried almost the full distance: monkeys sit rather erect whenever they are not on the move, but the apes are typically erect even when on the go. It is true that, on the ground, they assume a stooped-over posture, leaning on their knuckles. Nevertheless, their internal organs, and ours too, are arranged differently from monkeys, being slung from the upper chest and spine in accommodation to a vertical trunk. And the whole skeleton has responded to their way of life, for brachiating serves to throw emphasis on the arms and remove it from the legs.

In their evolution the arms have been encouraged to lengthen, and the fingers too, since within limits the longer the arm, the longer and more effortless the swing, or "stride," it can take. Shoulder and collarbone are also strengthened, facing outward and slightly up, as a pivot for arms which work in almost any direction. Monkeys have a high freedom of the arms, of course, but since they use them to so great a degree as legs, their shoulders remain narrow and face downward rather than outward, and their chests are deep and pointed. But ape (and human) shoulders are broad, with the effect of having been pulled out to the side of the body. The chest has become flattened in front, instead of being pointed, so much that the breastbone of hominoids is broad and flat and rather short, while in the monkeys and other mammals it is long and rod-like, with no breadth to speak of.

The spine in a monkey, or any four-footed animal which runs and leaps, is long and springy in its free (non-rib-bearing) or lumbar part; it acts something like a bow with different sets of muscles as bowstrings. But this part has quite a· different function in man and apes, in whom it serves to support the upper part of the body on the lower or, when brachiating, to attach the lower part to the upper, with the muscles acting as guy wires. Here a limber lumbar spine would be a weakness; and in the hominoids, both ape and human, it has been compacted and solidified somewhat, partly by getting rid of some of the actual vertebrae (and thus the joints between them) and partly by widening the remainder. This evidently beneficial effect has come about by having one or two of the last lumbar vertebrae captured by the sacrum (the block of fused vertebrae which forms the keystone of the pelvis), which has become relatively longer and heavier to suit these larger animals. The shortening has gone furthest in the orang, the most given to brachiation among the great apes. But it is also marked in man, so that what helps in brachiating helps in walking too.

The anthropoid pelvis, compared to that of monkeys, is broadened out in such a way as to reinforce the spine in its work of holding things together and giving underpinning to the swelling torso in its upright position. Monkeys, narrow in the hips, have a hipbone whose forward blade, the ilium, is extended toward the head, parallel to the spine, which helps in giving a leverage to the muscles which pull the leg forward. With the broadening anthropoid trunk, these blades are also extended outward toward the sides. Thus advantageous points of attachment are provided for trunk muscles to support the heavy torso and knit it to the pelvis.

So in shoulder, chest, spine, and pelvis the apes exhibit a complex of features related to their brachiation. Some of them are copied, on a small scale, by the spider monkey of South America, who brachiates a good deal also. Most of them are very evident in man as well. Does this mean that he was once a brachiator? Please read further.

5. MAN AND THE ANTHROPOIDS

$\mathbf{N}$OW WE COME to man, the hero of the tale. In spite of the fact that you already know and admire him, we shall have to review some elementary facts about him and his nature. Furthermore, we shall consider him along with the apes, for they all form a natural group. Apes are the animals most like him anatomically, and so they give us a perspective on him which we can get in no other way. Two of them, the gorilla and the chimpanzee, live in equatorial Africa, and the other two, the orang and gibbon, live in Southeast Asia and the Indies. There is a considerable separation, other than the geographical, between the Asiatics, who are strictly tree-living and highly adapted to brachiation, and the African pair, who spend the major portion of their time on the ground.

Gibbons inhabit southeastern Asia and much of southern Indonesia, living in solid forest. They move about from tree to tree well above the ground, and neither in the lowest nor the highest branches. Here they are property owners, in a sense. A mated pair of gibbons stays together permanently, with such children as are not mature, and this family keeps within a span of tree territory which it defends against other family groups. (They are thought to have an infant about once in two years.) Good humor prevails within the family, but they seem to be ferocious little fighters, inflicting serious gashes (they have done this to human beings, on suddenly getting angry) with their long and spiky canine teeth. They eat fruits, buds, insects, and birds' eggs and nestlings.

Gibbons are quite distinct from other apes, both in size and in some other traits, being both primitive and specialized. They have small ischial callosities (those built-in seat pads), like the Old World monkeys, and a thick coat of fur, while the other apes, like man, have only coarse hairs on the skin. Their fur may be gray, black, or cinnamon; the skin itself is a dense black. The gibbons proper weigh between twenty and thirty pounds and are less than three feet high. A larger form, the siamang, has partly webbed toes and an air sac in the throat, but he is essentially the same animal. To the slender,

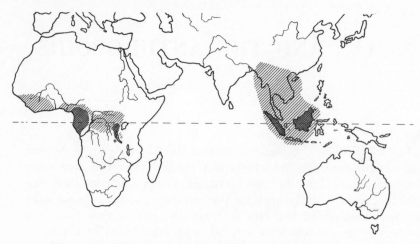

Habitats of the anthropoid apes. Africa, chimpanzee and gorilla, with latter heavily shaded. Southeast Asia, gibbon and orang utan, with latter heavily shaded.

wasp-waisted body are attached limbs which are long and spidery, especially the arms. The gibbon is the greyhound of the apes, while all the rest of us—the "great apes" and ourselves—are heavy, thick in the midriff, and relatively sluggish. And when you see this small ape actually brachiating, you understand the meaning of specialization in terms of action very well. He is the world's finest aerialist and a breathtaking thing to see, describing flowing festoons in the air as he swings from limb to limb, occasionally making long jumps across open spaces. So easily does he swing on his lithe but strong arms that even when going along beneath a single bough he may be free in the air between handholds, not clinging with one hand until he has a grasp with the other, but actually making a series of open swing-jumps.

Thus his elongated arms express his adaptation to a very special sort of locomotion. So do his hands, which are likewise long and narrow. He uses them hook-fashion over a bough instead of grasping, as we would, which must be more efficient in his quick flight; and his thumb is relatively short and not good for opposing against the other fingers, human-style. His legs, though not like his arms, are not short; they are usually carried drawn close up when he is brachiating, and if he is a she, there may be an infant cradled in her "lap," living dangerously. The foot has a good first toe which is separated further back than in the other hominoids, being well made for grasping a bough as the gibbon walks along it, which he does from time to time. Gibbons walk upright readily enough, with their long arms outstretched and their hands dangling, in a burlesque ballet style which helps them balance. They can do this well on the ground, especially if they have begun when young, but on the flattest of surfaces they still look as though they were walking carefully along a bough. As a copy of human erectness, it is a fake, since the gibbon has no bend in the spine, like ours, to straighten him up, but simply throws his trunk back on his legs and bends his knees.

The Careful Orang Utan

The lonely orang utan (Man of the Woods) keeps to the forests of Borneo and Sumatra. Nobody knows much about his family life; he has been seen only in very small groups, and most animals are probably solitary. A big male orang is as heavy as a big man, though with much shorter legs and a much larger trunk. His head is curiously domed, giving him something of a brow which lacks the beetling ridges over the eyes of the other apes and of primitive men. His eyes are beady, and his nose and mouth project sharply. If he is a full-grown male, he will have two half-moons of flesh flanking either side of his face, greatly broadening it, as well as a big pouch of skin below his jaw, looking rather like a goiter. His hair is long, especially on his back and arms, and it is ginger-red; his beard is orange and his skin a chocolate-brown. His gaze can be direct and withdrawn at the same time, and you will have a hard time deciding whether he is a misanthrope or an engaging clown at heart. In a zoo you will find that he likes to play with things and will mull them over with long slow thoughts.

Whether or not he is slow-thinking, he is certainly slow-moving. He is very much a brachiator. But there should perhaps be two different words to signify the brachiating of a gibbon and the brachiating of an orang, for they are as different as a series of *grands jetés* in ballet on the one hand, and crossing a shaky gangplank on the other. Not that the orang is unskillful or inefficient, but he is as heavy as six or eight gibbons, and he moves deliberately and cautiously, holding firm and not jumping. Furthermore, he even comes close to brachiating with his feet, if we are not dealing in absurdities; that is to say, he shows no aversion to being upside down, and he has a good "handgrasp" with his foot, which he often uses to hang by. This is exceptional in the apes and is perhaps an extra safety adaptation, like the grasping tails of some of the platyrrhine monkeys. Along with this he has another peculiarity: he lacks a certain ligament, the *ligamentum teres*, which binds the thighbone into its place in the hip socket in the other apes and in man. Although this lack may weaken the total stability of his leg, it allows him to stick the leg out in directions impossible to us, and makes it that much more arm-like.

Once more, anatomy expresses locomotion. Orangs are spidery in their own way, being potbellied, with exceedingly long and strong arms and equally small and weak legs. The hands are long, and hooked somewhat in the actual bones of the fingers, and the thumbs are short and degenerate (orangs vary in these things). The feet are strongly hand-like, as you would suspect from the account of their use in trees; at any rate, they are miserably suited to use on ground, and an orang stands upright by using the curled outside edges of his feet rather than the soles. If you can imagine trying to walk on a foot which is a hand, with long fingers which will not flatten out, and with a heel so short it is almost like your wrist, you will see what an orang on the ground is up against. He is a tree animal, pure and simple, but he is so large that he has problems aloft as well. All this applies to the adults, in whom size and curving of the fingers is most pronounced. The young are much more agile.

The Apes of Africa

The African apes, by contrast with the Asiatics just described, are more suited to life on the ground. Although they are animals of the equatorial forest, their forests are less dense, and the chimpanzee occupies country in West Africa where the woods are quite broken. Technically speaking, both chimp and gorilla are brachiators, and they are very much at home in trees. Their brachiating is what we might imagine doing ourselves, but better, and with the advantage of a foot having an opposable great toe. Both apes sleep in nests, but while those of chimps are all built in trees, in suitable crotches, some of them fairly high up, a gorilla band makes its nests on the ground, except for an occasional few in bushes or low branches, probably made by juveniles. Both apes actually spend most of their waking time on the ground, the gorillas virtually all of it. Both apes are free moving; they may stay within a general range of territory, but in West Africa at least they have been seen to cover long distances, and their traveling is done on the ground and at a good pace. Their gait is one using the flats of their feet and the knuckles of their hands; it is not quite the same in the chimp and gorilla, but there is no essential difference.

Therefore, these apes are compromisers, and perhaps they are not actually as arboreal as they appear to a purely terrestrial animal like a man. Are they brachiators who have been impelled to remodify themselves for an important amount of ground life? Or are they apes which,

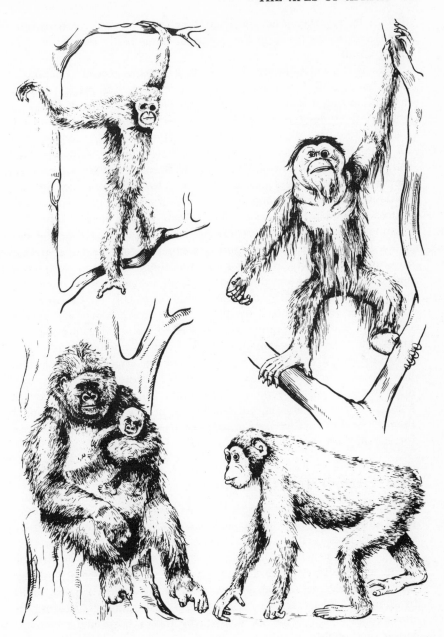

The four anthropoid apes. Above: gibbon and orang utan. Below, gorilla and chimpanzee. (Gorilla based on a photograph by Maria Hoyt.)

though having the basic ability to brachiate, have never committed themselves to the trees to the point of being badly embarrassed on the ground?

This is a good question, but we lack a good answer. Looking at their hands and feet does not tell us by precisely what paths of adaptation they got to be what they are. Chimpanzee and gorilla are both relatively long-armed and short-legged, though by no means like the orang or the gibbon in these proportions; in fact, compared to torso length, some chimpanzees are not longer-armed than man himself. Their hands are not hooked like an orang's, and the thumbs are longer and more useful in our sense, i.e., for picking things up and working with them. Chimp hands are fairly long, but gorilla hands approach human proportions when seen in the flesh, with good thumbs and broad palms. Feet are used flat on the ground in walking, and a look at their skeletons shows a much bigger heel region than an orang's, especially in the gorilla. And the great toe is lengthened and the side toes somewhat shortened, again more so in a gorilla. Such feet are quite distinct from hands, especially in the development of the heel region. This distinction between hands and feet is much less obvious in orangs. But these African ape feet are still not human feet, by any means—they have simply copied a little.

At any rate, it would be a mistake to suppose that natural selection has played these species false, and that they are essentially tree animals forced to the ground by their bulk. Chimps are obviously at home in a tree or below it, and gorillas seem well adapted to hauling themselves—brachiating horizontally, so to speak—through the dense forests they occupy.

The Extroverted Chimpanzee

Chimpanzees live all through West Africa and much of the Congo forest and beyond, and up to now have been numerous. They may wander in twos or threes, occasionally forming larger groups, or they may go about in well-knit bands of various sizes, feeding on quantities of wild fruits, seeds, and pods of a large variety of kinds, foraging for these in the trees. Such groups make a good deal of noise, both by shouting and by crashing through the bushes and by beating on stumps and logs. It does not seem to be talk, i.e., specific communication of thoughts, like ours. It probably acts as a kind of simpler social communication. And it surely is also a personal emotional outlet, for the pleasure it gives them to make a noise and to express a vague sense of well-being or, as the case may be, annoyance. If it serves any general, day-to-day purpose, it is to keep them from getting separated in the dense grass and growth, because an absent-minded soul, picnicking by himself, could note that the communal din was receding in a given direction and could hasten after it. Actually, they dislike any outside interference intensely, such as being spied on by human beings, and they are very alert to detect it. When they do, all noise stops at once and they take themselves silently off. They probably give more cues to each other—communicate in simple fashion —from expression and gesture than by voice.

Young chimps in cages or other civilized surroundings show that this ape is mercurial, ebullient, demonstrative, affectionate, and on the whole sanguine. They have impressed old hands with the fact that they vary markedly among themselves in temperament, intelligence, and behavior, as we ourselves do. It is true that adult chimps are not so uninhibited as youthful ones, becoming more serious, perhaps dour, so that a full-grown animal conscious of his powers and dignity is not something to be trifled with. (A full-grown chimp, by the way, though smaller than a man, is still an animal of a hundred pounds and very strong, quite different from the familiar television performers.) But it appears likely that chimpanzees are like men and a little less inhibited.

The Self-Contained Gorilla

Gorillas, on the other hand, are apparently more inhibited, though this can hardly come from an inferiority complex. Small chimps shriek with laughter or delight and seize human friends, new or old, with crushing affection. Small gorillas chuckle and are coy and shy. In their own forests gorillas are no more approachable than chimpanzees, but while chimps will flee from man, a gorilla group is apt to retire while one male remains to intimidate the intruders. George Schaller and others have proved that the old stories are wrong: in spite of bluff charges a gorilla will not actually attack unaggressive human beings (particularly if they are not accompanied by hunting dogs, which seems a sure way of infuriating the apes), though he will give a fearsome exhibition by a series of rushes, by thrashing with broken branches of a tree, standing erect, beating his chest with his hands, barking and roaring, swinging his fists, and even chucking himself under the chin to rattle his teeth.

Since he is the largest living primate, this menacing behavior is impressive. His size has often been exaggerated, though it is hard to see why this was necessary. Grown males are probably about the same total height as men of today, with occasional specimens six feet or over. In man, of course, this height is half legs. In gorillas it is largely torso, and male gorillas weigh from 350 to 450 pounds or beyond (even more in zoos, where they get fat; Mbongo at San Diego weighed 640). Compare this to the weight of large human athletes and you can estimate gorilla strength; in fact, comparative tests on all the great apes indicate that it would be folly to pick on an anthropoid your own size, or anything like it. The outstretched arms of the gorilla may span as much as nine feet; in a man this reach is just about equal to his height, i.e., six feet or less.

Gorillas support their bulk on vegetable food, and so they are necessarily prodigious eaters. This is especially so in the eastern part of their range, where their main diet is soft lush plants growing on the mountain slopes. A gorilla will set himself down in a likely spot and, without stopping, eat every piece of vegetable matter which he can reach with his arms, so that he winds up in the middle of a small clearing. They eat energetically and steadily, stripping leaves and soft material from tougher stalks with their teeth, making less noise and waste than chimpanzees. In view of the unnutritious nature of this diet, eating is serious business, and Gregory and Raven, collecting for the American Museum of Natural History, report emptying "pail after pail" of such stuff from the stomach and intestines of one specimen. But it is interesting that these vegetarians can be kept on more concentrated and richer foods, meat included, in captivity; that is, on a human diet.

Gorillas are rare animals. In spite of protection for some time by the governments concerned—colonial and now African—they are subject to poaching and, worse, contraction of their territories through expansion of native agriculture and pasturage. Today they live in two unconnected habitats. The western one runs from the Cameroons, at the angle of the Gulf of Guinea, southward to the mouth of the Congo River. The other area is the highlands and volcanic mountains of Kivu Province, in the eastern Congo. It is surprising that gorillas, who have been delicate in captivity, should flourish in this cold, damp forest at altitudes upward of six thousand feet. The western gorillas, called Coastal or Lowland, have shorter hair than the eastern or Mountain gorillas, who appear to be larger as well and to exhibit other slight differences. This distinction has sometimes been stressed to the point of calling the two types different species, but this is quite unjustified, and the types are probably best looked on as races.

There has been similar discussion about chimpanzees, who manifest a good deal of variety in color of skin, from pink and mottled to black (all gorillas are black-skinned), and to a smaller degree in color of hair. But these differences appear more individual than anything else, and it may not even be possible to divide them into local races satisfactorily. Chimpanzees simply vary. However, there does appear to be a clearly defined pygmy chimpanzee living south of the bend in the Congo River, about whom all too little is known as yet. He has been labeled a separate species, *Pan paniscus*, but even this is probably unjustified, since we have pygmies within our own species, and the same is true of some species of monkeys.

In fact, there are those who would bring gorillas and chimps closer together, as two related species of the genus *Pan*, instead of leaving them in a separate genus for each (*Pan* and *Gorilla*). Of course, to the practiced eye they appear quite different: the chimp with his jug-handle ears (not crimped as they are in man, gorilla, and orang), his smaller size and longer hands, and his thinner hair, especially on the head; and the gorilla with his black hair and skin and his peculiar nose, which has fleshy wings as does our own, but with these wings, so to speak, turned upside down and placed below the nostril.

On the skull the crossbar of bone across the brow, over the eye sockets, is very prominent in the chimp. It is prominent in the gorilla as well, and of entirely the same nature, but in his case the crown of the head appears high in the living animal and the brow ridge does not appear. This is because of his temporal muscles, for the jaw, which pass up under the cheekbones and attach themselves to the roof of the skull. In our own head they make a thin layer on and above the temple, where you can feel them as you chew. In the gorilla they are so massive that they reach to the very top and above, since a bony crest rises along the middle of the skull, meeting another crest across the back, for further areas of attachment for the muscle.

This crest formation reflects the size of the animal and his jaw: it is feeble or missing in female and young, merging with what is found in some large male chimpanzees. So it appears that this, and many of the differences in the skulls of chimp and gorilla, are the effect of different body size up and down the scale, influencing a fundamentally similar structure throughout. Now, if an extremely large chimpanzee thus begins to have a skull like a gorilla, a lot of apparent differences boil down to a main difference of size, which tends to bring the two animals closer together in actual relationship. In any case, there is no question as to their generally close kinship and their apartness from the orang, let alone from the gibbon.

Where We Differ

Now as to man. This animal has long ago forgotten where he originated, but he is a catarrhine, of the Old World; his anatomy shows it all over. And he is a hominoid; his anatomy brings him close to the apes. But he is no tree-living brachiator, and his anatomy reflects that too. He is, to let the cat out of the bag, a walker on the surface of the ground.

There are various things about us that must make us seem, to the eyes of other primates, freakish if not comic. There is our hair, cascading out of the tops of our heads and almost absent elsewhere from our naked skins. However, on giving our skin close scrutiny (and they love this kind of work), an ape or monkey would find the hair was there, and in the same pattern as on themselves, but in a rudimentary downy form on most of us. They would see our inflated heads, pushed-in faces, pointed breathing apparatus, and so on. Chimpanzee yokels might giggle and gape at all this, but a really educated anthropoid would direct his gaze at our feet, for these are what make us human. And now merriment would change to chagrin, as it dawned on him that we had curiously become adapted to a niche far more promising than his own way of life: that we had taken advantage of primate and hominoid potentialities and pushed them to a new conclusion. Being at home on the ground, we have added human feet to

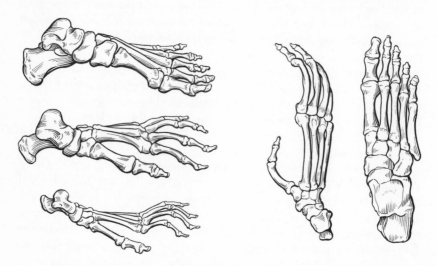

Foot skeletons, to show form and function. Left, from the top, feet in profile of man, gorilla, monkey; man shows long arch and long great toe; gorilla lacks an arch and a long great toe, but has a good heel; monkey has a more hand-like foot still, but with a long great toe. After Gregory. Right, feet of orang and man from above. The orang has a strongly hand-like foot, with long side toes, small great toe, and small heel and ankle region (tarsus). Man has a large tarsus and weight-bearing surface, and a large great toe with shortened side toes. From specimens.

hominoid uprightness and primate hands, and made a perfect division of labor: walking on our legs, we use our arms entirely for other things. There you have the essential, the *hominid* trait. And at last our ape may be gnashing his teeth (and fine teeth he has for gnashing) at seeing what a mistake he has made in using his otherwise skillful arms and hands for brachiating and allowing them to lengthen and change shape for that purpose.

Let us look over his shoulder. He will be observing that apes and men are alike, differing from other primates in the torso and arms and showing clear adaptations for brachiation; and that it is from the lower spine on downward that apes and men differ, more and more— above all, in the foot. The human foot has actually become a new segment of the leg, giving extra distance and special strength to the steps we take. The large great toe is the only one in the primates which has lost its opposability, now lying next to the others, with its joints working vertically. The other toes do not, as they do in apes, grow longer and beyond the first toe, like the fingers of a hand extending beyond the thumb. Instead, they actually become relatively shorter as we develop, and the result of this is to bring all the joints at the base of the toes in line, making a ball to the foot. This ball is the secret of our walking, and it is also made possible by the formation of two solid arches behind it. One arch is crosswise, making the middle of the foot a small vault; the other is lengthwise, from the ball to the end of the heel, raising the instep off the ground and carrying the ankle joint—the whole body!—on top of it.

The compact fitting together of the bones of the foot makes it act essentially as one piece. The muscles of the calf of the leg run down to the projecting heel, pulling it up and so forcing the ball of the foot down against the ground and lifting the body. This is what makes our long and effortless strides. An ape, with his hand-like, uncompacted foot, can do nothing of the sort; he simply cannot rise on the ball of his foot because he hasn't got one. The middle part of his foot is movable, and so his step takes place mostly at his ankle. The gorilla imitates us to a degree, having a longer heel and shorter side toes than other apes: and he can also give the best imitation of walking erect like us. But all this, both anatomy and performance, is imitation and not the real thing.

Our legs follow out the theme of the foot. They are, for primates, of exaggerated size. It is true that legs may be relatively as long in some chimpanzees or gibbons, but that is neither here nor there, for our legs are straight, columnar, and heavily muscled, and quite extreme in these ways. The bones rise vertically from the ankles, and

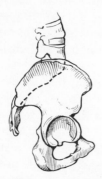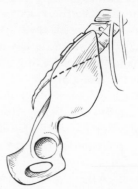

Pelvis and lumbar spine of man and chimpanzee, showing the nature of the lumbar curve in man in relation to posture. Viewed from the right side. Compared to the chimpanzee, the human spine angles back sharply above the pelvis. The contrast in the two, in the relation of the sacrum and the upper part of the ilium (hipbone) to the hip joint, is evident.

above the legs in turn it has been necessary to swing the upper half of the body back into position directly over the same points.

This has had a whole train of effects. Because of the insertion of the thigh bone in the hip joint it was not possible simply to tilt the pelvis back as needed. Actually, the pelvis faces forward at some forty-five degrees, about as it does in apes. Instead, two main things took place. The lumbar spine, of five vertebrae, leaves the pelvis in a forward direction, as in apes, but then turns sharply back to point upward, describing what is known as the "lumbar curve" and so carrying the torso back into position above the hip joints and the legs. And in the pelvis itself the hinder portion of the hipbones, where they are joined by the sacrum, has been bent downward and pulled back, so to speak, until these bones have a shape very distinct from the anthropoid apes.

This last important move has two effects. One is to help bring the sacrum, and thus the weight of the spine and the upper part of the body, into position over the legs. The other is to give a protruding point of attachment—a better leverage, as the heel does in the foot— to the muscles of the buttock and the back of the thigh, so that a powerful force can be applied to the engine provided by the legs and foot, pulling them back to push us forward. And so the whole human skeleton, with its muscles, has been perfected from the waist on down, both in design and in motor power, to allow us to proceed, serenely erect, with our peculiar gait, upon our peculiar feet.

The hipbones also curve well around the sides toward the front, and form a better supporting basin than in apes, as well as giving more efficient attachment for muscles of the upper trunk, to hold it upright in its turn. But above the waist we come to that zone of likeness among the hominoids. Here, in fact, it is man who is the more generalized, with his simple hand, and the apes who clearly have a story of specialization to tell. It is not until you come to the head that we suddenly look remarkable once more.

Head and Profile

Now it is quite possible to put up an argument to the effect that these head differences are all an accident and of no importance. Nothing could be more absurd, of course, since without the contents of this head I would not be writing a book nor would you be reading it. Nevertheless, a lot of its nobler features are somewhat secondary in the evolutionary sense. For example, our nose does nothing an ape's nose does not do except get broken. As you will see further on, men are men and apes are apes because of the different adaptations of their hands and feet, and not because our brains got bigger than theirs. That happened later.

Of course, the human skull is very different from what sits atop a gorilla's spine. Yet both of them are catarrhine skulls, differing, like the limbs, in emphasis rather than basic parts. Aside from housing

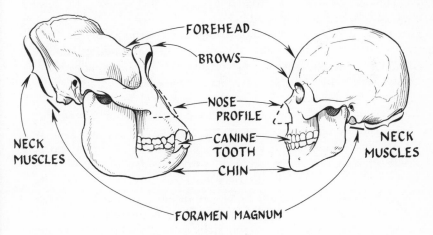

Skulls of gorilla and man compared for various features. Notice that the actual profile of the nasal chamber is similar in both.

organs of sense in likely places, the main business of the skull is to make a platform of bone, supporting above it an envelope for the brain and below it a squeezing apparatus lined with teeth for mashing food as it passes the portal of the digestive system. The several sizes and forces of brain and jaw explain the special shapes arrived at in man and ape. Both kinds of animal carry to extremes the primate trends to large brains and to bent-down faces, but man, extreme in erectness, is also extreme in poising the head perfectly on the spine, helped by a lightening of the jaw at the front. And man, toward the end of his career, has greatly expanded his brain from the size possessed by the already large-brained chimp or gorilla to something three times as large.

So much for the high dome above the seat of mind. The human face, from its ancestral form, has undergone an equally startling pulling-in under the forehead, probably beginning with a shrinking of the size of the teeth. Not only has the dental arch become smaller; it has been further reduced in its length by spreading apart at the back. This broadening may be connected with chewing; we chew with a swinging motion of the lower jaw, from side to side. We are able to do this because the crowns of our teeth are all on one level, and our canines do not project, while in apes the long canines interlock, inhibiting the side-to-side motion to a considerable degree. Along with the shortening of both upper and lower tooth rows, and the lessening of squeezing force between them, the whole facial skeleton deflated sharply; even the eyes have tended to recede under the swelling forehead. But in this shrinking there were two spots which could not very well deflate, and that is why we have a nose with a bridge, and a chin.

The nasal cavity, for the moistening and warming of air, is a narrow chamber in the middle of the face, like a standing triangle running fore and aft. This fits nicely into the sloping profile of an ape's face. But, while the face in general diminished, the nasal cavity itself could not be reduced in size, in an animal as large as man, without losing its efficiency as a clearing chamber for air coming in. And there is no other place in the architecture of the face to put it. So, when the whole cheek region shrank back, the nasal cavity was left sticking out in its original position under a sort of shed of its own, looking like an annex to the face.

The chin evidently emerged in similar fashion. In the open space beneath the long anthropoid lower jaw there is plenty of room for the muscles which work the tongue, help in swallowing, etc. We are animals of giant hominoid size, and we need this muscle space at least as much as apes do. In our case, then, the lower rim of the

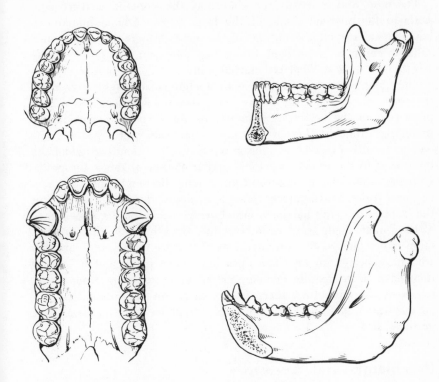

Comparison of upper and lower jaws in man (above) and gorilla. This contrasts: form of dental arch; size of canines; presence of diastema (gap) in front of gorilla canines; general size of lower jaw; nature of chin region; simian shelf in gorilla. After Gregory, and specimens.

mandible seems to have remained roughly as it was, while the teeth and the tooth-bearing part of the bone drew back over it. But the middle of the jaw is exposed to special stresses, especially to a sort of pinching action by the muscles which pull the jaw back and shut it, as though you pinched the two ends of a wishbone together. As the bone of the jaw lightened, it appears that extra bone in the form of a chin arose on the front, as a response to these stresses. There is a reinforcement in the jaws of most apes also, a flooring of the foremost part of the open space below the tongue, called the "simian shelf." This is on the inside, not the outside, but in such a long jaw this evidently is no disadvantage to the space available.

The nose, and in a way the chin, may therefore be seen as sign-posts to the onetime shape of the face. If you take a human sil-houette and extend the outline of the nose, bringing it round in a suitable curve to come back under the chin, you will get a profile which will suggest what we started with.

This does not mean starting with a chimpanzee. When we view the teeth of men and apes, we see certain differences other than plain size, or the heavy ape canines. In apes, we see a particularly projecting front portion of the jaws, and one which has become widened, with extra large incisor teeth. Such a dentition seems to be geared to the coarse vegetable and fruit diet of the anthropoids, with the canines being important in opening the tough rinds of many of these fruits. Furthermore, there is evidence that the widening of the front of the jaws has been largely responsible for the appearance of the simian shelf, as an extra truss for strength. Now, all this leads to an interesting point, easily overlooked: we are not the only animals who have been evolving. The apes have been evolving too. And if they have been steadily evolving broad and projecting front teeth, as seems the case, then there is no reason for supposing that our ancient snout goes back to what we see in today's chimpanzee or gorilla.

Brachiators and Ancestors

This is taking the outer wrappings off the large problem, for what applies to the teeth applies to the rest of anatomy. What *was* our ancestor like? More of that later. But how do we seem to be related to the apes, just on the basis of anatomy? Is it all mere parallel adaptation that we share similar torsos and have lost our tails, because we all became upright creatures, though of different gaits? That is, did we arise separately from a simple monkey-like primate or even something lower? Or are we really close relatives, which implies that man got his uprightness and his longish arms as an adaptation to brachiation? Granting that our ancestor was no "gorilla," no "chim-panzee," no "orang," no "gibbon," are we nevertheless all "hominoids" by descent as well as by classification?

It is a problem with several aspects. Did the intensely human foot actually come from something like a gorilla's, or are both merely moving in the same direction? Our arch must have come from a grasping foot, probably with a good first toe and probably rather ape-like; but much of the musculature is like a monkey's, not an ape's. Is the torso with its wide shoulders and flat breastbone an adaptation encouraged by brachiation? Or contrariwise does the brachiation of apes follow from the flattened, widened torso: did such a form, in animals already upright, suggest brachiation as the suitable adaptation to tree life? That is to say, did our common ancestor possess such a torso before any hominoids became actually specialized for brachiation?

The human hand is very generalized. No signs of brachiation there. But the shoulder, before birth, points high up, like an ape's (who seems so short-necked because of this). This position is a brachiating adaptation. Gradually it grows down to its human position.[1] Actually, the freedom with which we move and raise our relatively long arms, and the strong resemblance in so many parts of our torso to the apes, powerfully suggests that our early ancestor was indeed an arboreal brachiator and considerably adapted to the habit. Once again, we must assume that the great apes and ourselves have both been evolving: the orang utan at least, and probably the chimpanzee, toward a greater insistence on brachiation while we have receded from what may very well have been a more marked adaptation of our torso to that habit.

Now the above discussion revolves around the question of adaptation and brachiation rather than of actual relationship. There is more to it: apart from the wealth of anatomical correspondence, there are common hominoid features having nothing to do with brachiation. One is the basic cusp pattern of the teeth, lacking the cross-crests of the Old World monkeys. Another is chemistry of the blood proteins. These have always allied us consistently with the apes, but recent studies have shown such an astonishing correspondence in the serum proteins of man, gorilla and chimpanzee—making them all definitely closer than any is to the orang—that one worker has invited these apes to leave the Pongidae and join us in the Hominidae, which is taking a rather one-sided view of classification. This is very important evidence showing us our nearest kin, and the closeness of the kinship. But it does not after all tell us about our own immediate ancestor, who may not have been very much like the living apes of Africa.

This is as good a point as any to recall what Darwin said about human origins, in 1871, in the *Descent of Man.* He said it carefully and judiciously. You would never guess from the hot rebuttals of

[1] This may be a false interpretation. Dr. Gottfried Kurth points out that the early hunched-up shoulders are probably a simple adaptation to the cramped pre-natal space and to easier passage of the large infant through the birth canal. A similar doubt holds for the meaning of our early ape-like limb proportions: longer arms, shorter legs. Dr. Georges Olivier of Paris, an embryological anatomist, believes that this results, not from a deep-seated brachiating adaptation, but merely from a fetal growth gradient in which the head end of the body takes the lead, with the hind end catching up later.

the next few generations how reasonably he had set it forth, nor how acceptable his view is today, a century later.

Reviewing the nature of man, he noted that we must be classed with the catarrhines, rather than with the platyrrhines. (He believed, it is true, that all these higher primates, New World and Old World, had come from the same extremely ancient progenitor, while most students today, I am sure, consider that platyrrhines and catarrhines arose independently from prosimians, and not necessarily from the same prosimian source.) "If the anthropomorphous apes be admitted to form a natural sub-group," he continued, then man possesses such peculiar characters in common with them that "we may infer that some ancient member of the anthropomorphous subgroup gave birth to man." And, he pointed out, a naturalist would feel obliged to classify such an ancient form, which possessed many characters in common with the higher primates generally, as an ape or a monkey. Therefore, "as man from a genealogical point of view belongs to the Catarrhine or Old World stock, we must conclude, however much the conclusion may revolt our pride, that our early progenitors would have been properly thus designated. But we must not fall into the error of supposing that the early progenitor of the whole Simian stock, including man, was identical with, or even closely resembled, any existing ape or monkey."

That is the substance of his conclusion. Darwin was right.

6. PRIMATES IN THE PAST

As THE ROYALTY of primates, we have in the last two chapters been looking around upon our vassals. (Here you have the editorial, the royal, and the human "we," all rolled into one.) Nearest the throne we see the apes, the royal dukes; beyond them are the barons, the monkeys of the Old World and the New World, and beyond them in turn a clownish peasantry of prosimians. This little hierarchy seems to make a nice "family tree" for us, and much writing has been based on such a view. But the view is too simple, because it pays more attention to primates in the flesh and less to primates of the past, to whom I am now turning. Because of this distinction, certain common useful phrases can be dangerous and misleading, such as "family tree," "ancestor," "forerunner," or "missing link." Like guns, they will do the right thing in the right hands, but they are loaded, and ordinary citizens without Ph.D.'s are not the only ones who have accidents with them. Many a specialist has shot himself in the foot when he thought he was only cleaning a paragraph.

Take "forerunners," for example. I have been presenting the other primates, and the lower animals generally, as shedding light on stages of development through which the ancestry of man passed. Such stages may be termed forerunners as long as they are not necessarily supposed to be direct ancestors. Indeed, forerunners is not the best name for runners who are behind the leader in a race, and so they might better be called hindrunners.

Similarly, take "ancestors." Obviously no living animal can be our ancestor, and this point should never be forgotten. Nevertheless we must have had a series of true ancestors in the past, who were akin to various living animals. Therefore the proper notion is one of continuous specialization and evolution away from a parent form, a true ancestor, which ancestor we share with some animal we are regarding as "ancestral." We must have had a common ancestor with a lungfish and a coelacanth. But that ancestor can only be an ancient fossil form, and the lungfishes and coelacanths have been descending from it as long as we have, though they have changed less. If it is known, or evident, that our ancestor at some point must have been rather close to some living animal, it is appropriate to speak of that animal as a "surviving structural ancestor." If you were one of those who believed us to be "descended" from *Tarsius,* you could call him a structural ancestor in the sense that he represents a stage in our evolution in his brain and parts of his anatomy, after you have discounted his own very specialized legs.

Or take "missing link." This is not a fortunate term, but it is graphic and compelling. You are herewith licensed for its use if you use it only for forms which lie in a true ancestral chain. These must therefore be fossil, not living. That is, it signifies animals not yet discovered as fossils, but animals which must in fact have existed. You may find missing links between man and mammal-like reptiles. But you could not find a missing link between a chimpanzee and a man, because *Pan troglodytes,* the twentieth-century chimp, is not, and cannot be, an ancestor of man. He cannot be an ancestor of anything but future chimps, even if they should stand erect, wear clothes, and begin to talk real nonsense in place of the imitation nonsense they now emit. The only sense of a missing link would be a true parent of both man and chimp, so far back along the line as to be different from either of them. This animal would not be something halfway between the kinds we know; instead, it would in general lack the special characteristics of both men and chimpanzees, even though it might superficially seem more like one than like the other. In this example, it would surely seem more like a chimp at first glance, since he is the more primitive of the pair, with respect to brain size, hairiness, and certain other traits.

Forgive these dry precepts. They are important, as is the main fact that most of the primates are extinct, not living. It is hard to realize how greatly the vanished forms outnumber the survivors, and yet it stands to reason. The true picture is one of a whole bush with radiating families for branches. Most branches are dead throughout, but there are a few green leaves at the ends of some, representing the species of today. We could hardly get a sound idea of the bush as a whole if we looked only at those leaves, so let us see what we can of the dead branches. You understand, of course, that to see the entire bush we should need fossils of every primate of the past. Actually we have pitifully few, even though they already outnumber the living types. They are spread throughout Tertiary time, which has the following divisions (with the number of years ago each began):

Paleocene	70 million
Eocene	55 million
Oligocene	35 million
Miocene	25 million
Pliocene	12 million

Golden Age of the Prosimians

Primates have one of the longest histories of any order of mammals. Unquestionably they rode on the mammalian *Mayflower*. Their general simplicity ties them to those early placentals who, with other primitive kinds of mammal, were beginning to make their way in the middle of the Mesozoic, the Age of Reptiles, at least a hundred million years ago. And the tree shrews, as I have indicated, not only hark back to this stage, representing those ancient forerunners, but also provide a fine "structural ancestor" for all the later ones.

So the primates came into the Paleocene, the opening of the Tertiary, with a full head of evolutionary steam, already splitting up into various prosimian lines. Some were lemur-like, some were tarsier-like, and there was a fairly broad range of other kinds, now extinct, who could have been parental to nothing later. Some were rather specialized, others were more generalized. The ancient lemurs, for example, lacked the procumbent tooth comb of the modern ones. And those which may have foreshadowed *Tarsius* indicate that the last living survivor of this group is especially peculiar. Thus the paleontologists are already acquainted with a surprising spectrum of prosimians, some primitive, some progressive, and some decidedly specialized or aberrant. One effect of this acquaintance, as I said earlier, is to fill up the seeming gap between *Tarsius* and other prosimians, and to put him in the same family portrait.

This was the happy childhood of the primates. In those times all mammals were small and primitive, many of them in fact being the still flourishing survivors of the multituberculates, one of those very ancient offshoots from the mammal-like reptiles who were not even members of the marsupial-placental stock. In the Paleocene, as far as the mammals were concerned, the world was young and the going was easy. For the little primates the competition was not stringent, and they flourished over most of the world, especially in North America. They lived mainly in trees, as they do now, but there are signs that they lived on the ground as well and had a wide variety of diets, rather like squirrels and other small rodents of today.

This idyll carried on through most of the Eocene, and then calamity struck. The multituberculates vanished completely, and so did some early orders of placentals. Extinction also swept away the main body of the prosimians: they disappeared from Europe and North America, and in Africa and Asia they were reduced to a small number of lorises and galagos and the isolated *Tarsius* of the Indies (and of course the tree shrews). Prosimians are almost unknown as fossils through the rest of the Tertiary.

What had happened? The answer is that a new tide of mammal development had risen. More modern types like carnivores, and above all the rodents with their powerful teeth, were coming into being, and reaping the rewards of specialization. Generalized forms may be resistant, and also relatively adaptable on a broad evolutionary scale, but they are apt to be exposed to the onslaught of specialized cousins competing for some of the same niches. The infantry is the irreplaceable Queen of Battle, but the best infantry in the world will have a rough time when assaulted by heavier armor.

Anthropoidea Inherit

Rats and cats are doubtless not the whole answer; these enemies and competitors would probably not have been so destructive to the more arboreal primates. Here the prosimians contained the seeds of their own decline, in giving rise to the higher primates: the monkeys and hominoids. These new animals, also on the whole generalized but progressive, would have been living in the same forest and eating the same foods as their prosimian contemporaries, and so would have provided the really corrosive competition which would explain the losses. This is, of course, based on presumption, for the known fossils are too few to tell the whole story. But the higher primates must have begun developing just then, during the Eocene, and they begin to be known from the early Oligocene, when the prosimians had collapsed.

In the very manner of their going the prosimians showed the breadth of their possibilities for progress in a monkey-like direction. On the continents of the Old World they declined or vanished, but they gave rise to monkeys and apes. Only the lemurs, in a curious way, kept the old days alive. Becoming entirely extinct on the mainland, they managed to get to the island of Madagascar, probably on floating masses of vegetation, where they survived and flourished with their old vigor to the present. In fact, in very late times they even evolved a new series of monkey-like and other forms, in a special radiation, though these are now largely extinct. One of them, the extraordinary *Megaladapis*, got to be as large as a donkey and, if native tales can be believed, may have lived right down into our own centuries, becoming extinct about the same time as its Mauritian neighbor, the dodo.

In the New World also, prosimians gave rise to monkeys in South America, which was then cut off from North America. In the latter, prosimians were long thought to have died out in the Eocene, but one

line (known from poor finds in South Dakota) continued into the
Miocene, millions of years later. And in 1964 Professor John Wilson of
the University of Texas found a beautifully preserved prosimian skull
in Oligocene deposits in that state. *Rooneyia* (as he named it) evidently had *two* upper premolars, not three (a tooth count of 2-1-2-3),
and a clearly progressive brain (but no back wall to the eye socket).
An Old World monkey in the New World? No; an imitation Old World
monkey, in the form of a decidedly advanced prosimian. But this
promising animal did not survive; it cannot be a relative of the monkeys of South America.

So we are in a zone of advanced prosimians and primitive higher
primates, but the lines of ascent across the zone are not clear—the
links are missing. The Anthropoidea might have come from ancient
cousins of *Tarsius;* they might have come from the lemur-like family
Adapidae; or they might have come from the Omomyidae, to which
Rooneyia probably belonged, and which was a broad and progressive
group. All of these had members in both hemispheres in the Eocene,
and any might make an acceptable structural ancestor. At present, the
fossils do not decide.

How Many Kinds?

From all this it does seem clear that higher primates came on
the scene at least twice. This is hardly surprising, if you remember
that "mammals" arose from the mammal-like reptiles several times
over. But it is interesting in showing that early primate potentialities
could give rise, not only to monkey-like lorises and tarsioids, but also
more than once to true monkeys. That is to say, while platyrrhine and
catarrhine monkeys are both classed together as Anthropoidea, they
are not actually such close kin, being related only through their lower
primate parentage. For the indications are that no primates crossed
from the Old World into the New, or vice versa, after the first part of
the Eocene, which would seem to isolate the hemispheres before
higher primates had ever appeared.

Therefore, "monkey" can be taken to mean not only a kind of existing animal but also an abstract grade of primate organization, a way
of primate life. As it had for proto-mammals, an open possibility
existed, provided there was a suitable environment and a basic primate pattern as furnished by the prosimians. And the possibility was
realized independently, in the Old and the New Worlds. This may
seem like a persnickety point, and a digression in the story of man,
but it is the kind of thing that makes evolution fascinating as a study
and as philosophy.

At this crucial time, the early Tertiary, the two Americas became separated from one another, and the present Isthmus of Panama did not exist. A prosimian or prosimians unknown crossed from North into South America, perhaps by floating on natural accidental rafts of vegetation, like the lemurs to Madagascar. From these, in South America, monkeys developed, and in a rapid radiation the several main lines of the platyrrhines were established. When, toward the end of the Tertiary, the Isthmus of Panama made a bridge to the north, some of them crossed over into Central America, getting as far up as Mexico. Actually, fossils of these monkeys are almost lacking, but those recovered do indicate that the stock had a typical early expansion and evolution, and a stable later history. Certainly this was true of other mammal lines in South America, which arrived there in the Paleocene and had their own special histories of radiation, without interference from the rest of the world until they were overrun late in time by competitors from the north.

As to the Old World monkeys, even less is known of their past. But they too must go back to unknown Eocene ancestors, and they may have acquired such specializations as they have, including the bilophodont molars, early in the game. Nothing, at any rate, now points to the contrary. There are a few good fossils, all of which are late. It is a guess, in the face of ignorance, that the history of the catarrhine monkeys, after their first appearance, was rather uneventful.

You would not say this about the hominoids, however. In the first place, we are now considering a group which did not go on as decent, God-fearing quadrupeds but began as, or became, semierect animals. This in itself suggests greater evolutionary experimentation, and such experimentation certainly seems to have taken place. Luckily the fossil record is very much better in this, our own ancestry, than in either monkey line.

The hominoids are evidently, for reasons already given, more closely related to the Old World monkeys than either lot is related to the monkeys of the Americas. But we cannot say whether this is because they arose from the same kind of prosimian, independently, or whether there once actually existed a primitive "higher primate" or catarrhine (which could be classified with the Anthropoidea), from which monkeys and hominoids both descended. If the latter, there was an almost immediate split, and all the hominoids avoided such things as bilophodont teeth. Nothing more is going to be known on this point until the right fossils come along. But, a little later, fossils have plenty to say.

The Earliest Apes

The hominoid line—the founding of the ape-human dynasty—goes back, we can be quite sure, to the late Eocene. For from the Oligocene, and possibly from the Eocene itself, has come a striking group of fossils from Egypt and Burma. Numerous, but consisting only of teeth and jaws (with the sole exception of a frontal bone) they are fragmentary, poorly preserved, and in some ways puzzling. But taken together they hint strongly at a series of evolutionary experiments toward forming the higher primates, especially the apes. And they fall in just that time, around thirty-five million years ago, when the prosimians were dying off, and after which we can see well-defined lines of anthropoids leading to those of today.

Perhaps the best way to begin is to report on two lower jaws described in 1911 by Schlosser, found in the Fayum depression in Egypt and belonging, supposedly, to the early Oligocene. He named them *Parapithecus* and *Propliopithecus,* and because of their interest as the earliest higher primates known they have been starred with almost perfect regularity in every book and treatise touching on human evolution since that time, and with justice.

Propliopithecus, like most of the others, has the catarrhine tooth count and is instantly recognizable as a hominoid. (He got his name as a supposed forerunner of the later *Pliopithecus,* who in turn was clearly a kind of fossil gibbon.) His teeth are marked by simplicity of pattern, by a fairly short and light canine, and by particularly unspecialized bicuspids or premolars, not skewed in the direction either of later apes or of strongly "bicuspid" man. Those writers who did not consider him specifically a very early gibbon thought he might in fact be an ancestor of all apes and men together, a basic, simplified, but quite positive hominoid.

Parapithecus was still simpler in nature, thus jostling *Propliopithecus* for the position of generalized ancestor. In fact, his incisors, canines and premolars all shaded into one another so gradually that it has never been decided which was which. For a long time the dental formula was accepted as being 2-1-2-3, making *Parapithecus* the perfect emerging hominoid. But Schlosser himself thought, as do some very recent students, that the formula was *one* incisor and *three* premolars, so that at best he would be a dubious hominoid and perhaps not even a primate at all (some ancient and primitive herbivores had similar teeth).

Eventually, as fortunately is often the case, the light provided by new fossils grew stronger. First, *Amphipithecus,* a little fragment of jaw from the Eocene of Burma, was described as a very likely tiny ape still keeping a small third premolar tooth in the front. If this is what *Amphipithecus* was, he indicates that the late Eocene was indeed the time when some progressive prosimian evolution was producing an early model of "ape." Even without him, however, the very important mass of fossils lately collected by Dr. Elwyn Simons of Yale has shown the same thing: the laying down of tracks leading to major later forms of hominoids occurred before the Oligocene was well under way.

Simons proceeded on the modest assumption that Schlosser's collector had not picked up all the fossil jaws in Egypt, and that there might be more of these exceptionally important specimens there for the finding. (Unfortunately exposures of Oligocene deposits are not common, and no other is known in all of Africa.) I am sure that he was far more successful than he expected to be. Not only did some of his pieces represent new individuals—and apparently new species —of *Parapithecus* and *Propliopithecus*, the latter later in the Oligocene than thought previously. In addition, he discovered three totally new kinds of hominoid distinct from the above and from each other. Important as they are, I can only give their names and say briefly what Simons makes out from them.

Aeolopithecus, smaller than *Propliopithecus*, was nevertheless more gibbon-like, with its spikey canine teeth and rather small third molars. In other details as well it suggests closer gibbon relationships, via *Pliopithecus*, than does its neighbor *Propliopithecus*.

Aegyptopithecus. This was somewhat larger, already being approximately the size of a modern gibbon, and already giving signs of a more definite resemblance to the present-day large apes than any of the others I have mentioned. Its third molar was large, not small, and in other details of this kind it forecast the fossil apes of the Miocene and Pliocene, to be described on the next page or so.

Oligopithecus lacks the kind of suggestive resemblance to later animals which the two above have, and instead has some faint resemblances to the little-known *Amphipithecus* of the Eocene. This, as Simons notes, tends to strengthen the credentials of *Amphipithecus* as a real hominoid, but reveals little else at the moment.

Apidium, which I have not mentioned, is still another of these early Egyptian forms. He was first named from a single fragment in 1908 but, while recognized as a catarrhine, remained mysterious because of his peculiar characteristics. Simons found more pieces of this creature, as well as specimens of a smaller, earlier species of the same genus. *Apidium*, like *Amphipithecus*, and perhaps *Parapithecus*, still had three premolars, suggesting that this trace of prosimian parentage had not completely dropped out of the catarrhine stock. As will appear, it is likely that *Apidium* also had a later hominoid descendant, *Oreopithecus*.

If we add to the above collection *Parapithecus* and *Propliopithecus*, we see that Simons and his predecessors have produced a really extraordinary sampling of the hominoids, or at least the catarrhines, not long after their radiation into several lines. The various forms were still of small size, and while varied they tended to have a community of primitive traits showing them to be still near the beginning of the radiation. If Simons is right in classifying them as he does, this implies that more different genera of hominoids were present than are known to have existed at any time since. Lines were already leading to three branches of ape-like animals (if we include *Oreopithecus*), and there may have been others now extinct. As to *Propliopithecus*, he seems to have lost his place as everyone's ancestor, especially if he belongs well along in the Oligocene, and Simons has another interesting suggestion as to his meaning, which I shall divulge further on.

An Ape with a Tail

I have mentioned *Pliopithecus* as a kind of extinct gibbon, existing in the Miocene and Pliocene of Europe. Another form, *Limnopithecus*, lived in East Africa in the Miocene, and is known from two species and a number of skeletal parts. The skulls of all these apes ally them to the gibbons of today, and if only jaws and skulls were known— the usual case!—they would be put down simply as gibbon ancestors. But their skeletons reveal something interesting. *Limnopithecus* had limbs more generalized and less elongated than gibbons, and a little monkey-like; clearly he was not a brachiator of the extreme type we might expect, but a more general climber, though surely able to brachiate efficiently. This alone suggests *Hylobates* (today's gibbon) may have become long-armed and specialized in quite recent times.

Pliopithecus however provides bigger surprises. This is no new fossil; his first remains were found in 1837, in the Miocene of France, and other discoveries, of at least one other species, and from the Pliocene as well as the Miocene, have taken place since then, particularly recently in Austria. Long ago it was remarked that this ape—a "gibbon" in skull and teeth, all agree—had astonishingly monkey-like hand bones in association with these teeth. Then very good, more recent finds produced nearly complete skeletons with "monkey" stamped all over them: in limb proportions; in a humerus, or upper arm bone, of exceptional primitiveness and recalling that of certain lemurs; in an ulna (of the lower arm) with a long funny bone, not found in apes; in a long lumbar part of the spine (behind the ribs) consisting of 7 vertebrae, not 5 as in living gibbons and in man; and in a primitive pelvis generally. But all this did not prepare students for the final blow. Recently Dr. Friderun Ankel of Zürich has been carefully analyzing the sacrum (the spinal keystone of the pelvis—see pp. 47, 75) in apes and in short-tailed and long-tailed monkeys. She finds that, in this bone, the canal for the spinal cord virtually pinches out at its lower end in man and the apes, with their vestigial tail bones, but in tailed primates the same canal has a cross section at the tail end which is at least half that at the head end, the size depending a good deal on the size of the tail itself. Now, no tail bones have been found for *Pliopithecus*, but his sacrum shows he must have had a tail! And not a short one like a baboon either, but a well-developed affair of 10 to 15 vertebrae, and comparable to that in the tree-living African monkeys.

So *Pliopithecus* had the head of an ape and the body of a monkey, in marked contrast to *Hylobates*, to whom he is nevertheless related. (One authority, however, has removed him outright from the gibbons and made him a separate new family of hominoids.) While he could probably brachiate as well as any known monkey, he was doubtless essentially a quadruped, something of a black sheep among apes. It is most unlikely that he was in or near the direct ancestry of modern gibbons. Was he a primitive holdover from the early days of hominoids? Does he emphasize an early separation of gibbons from other hominoids? He hardly suggests the opposite.

The Jaws of Dryopithecus

So we have some satisfactory if surprising early relatives of the gibbons. What about the later forerunners of the large apes? From the beginning of the Miocene, the remains are really copious, even though they consist very largely of jaws and teeth. A great array of these has been found from Spain to China, representing the kind of animal from which chimpanzees and gorillas must have come, as well, some think, as man himself. Only the ancestors of *Pongo* cannot be found among them.

In a century of discovery, these many finds have been put in twenty-eight different genera and twice as many species, and this has long suggested a vigorous burgeoning of the apes here in the late Tertiary. However, Drs. Simons of Yale and David Pilbeam of Cambridge University have gone over them carefully and decided that the differences among the "genera" are quite small. They have therefore placed them all in not more than seven species of a single genus,

Dryopithecus, this being the name given in 1856 to the first known find. The largest distinctions they can find allow only the status of a subgenus, and they recognize three of these: (*Dryopithecus*), essentially European, (*Sivapithecus*), essentially Asian, (*Proconsul*), essentially African.

This varied genus shows the large anthropoids at an interesting stage.

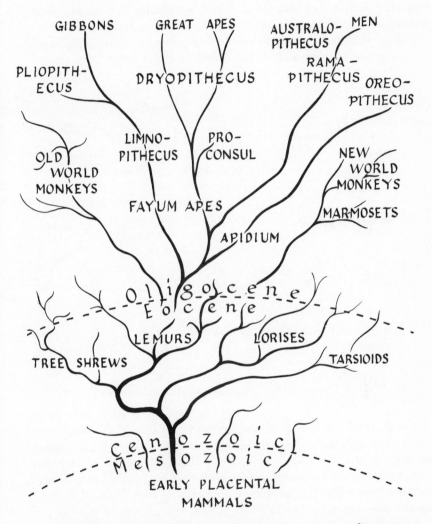

Evolution and relationships in primates. The connecting lines are emphasized, for the sake of showing the general pattern clearly. In reality, few of the connections are known so positively, and there should be many more branching lines.

They had attained, perhaps recently, large size, the largest already being that of a gorilla. What they were actually doing by way of brachiating, or not brachiating, we can hardly tell from broken jaws. But we can see more clearly the growing trend toward a specialized enlargement of the front of the mouth, for the eating of coarse fruit, which eventually in the gorilla reached an exaggeration which Gregory aptly called "swine-like." The incisors were widening and the canines becoming deep-rooted tusks, and with this widening the "simian shelf" was appearing as a reinforcement at the base of the chin.

Just behind the lower canine is the first premolar. (This is bicuspid, or two-cusped, in our own mouths, with a larger outer cusp, as you

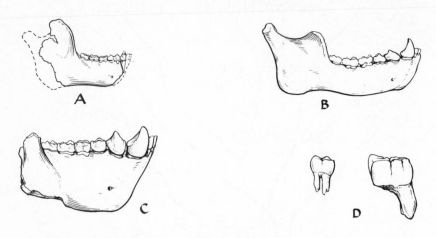

Ape jaws and teeth, all ½ natural size.
A. *Propliopithecus*
B. gibbon
C. *Dryopithecus*
D. *Gigantopithecus:* molar tooth compared to modern man. After Gregory and casts.

may feel with your fingers if you are the proprietor of the tooth concerned.) In apes the upper canine bears on this tooth, projecting down between it and the lower canine. And this first premolar tooth has joined up with the canine group by becoming long from front to back and also pointed and canine-like, with a cutting edge forward to work against the upper canine tooth.

Now all these traits are not unique to the great apes. They occur in gibbons and monkeys, perhaps by independent development, perhaps from common ancestry. But it is possible to see that they have become more marked in the living apes as a result of gradual specialization, and in this light we may consider that our teeth are more generalized than theirs. That is the real point.

As to the molar teeth of these fossils, Dr. Gregory has invested them with particular importance by his studies. Analyzing the arrangement of their cusps, ridges, and fissures, he discerned what he named the "Dryopithecus pattern," and he showed how it exists today in modified form in man, gorilla, chimpanzee, and orang. In fact, if the molar teeth were considered alone, this pattern would seem like a generalized one from which all the others, man's included, could have been derived. A "structural ancestor," in other words. This is the kind of thing which puts teeth into the meaning of "Hominoidea," grouping man and apes together. With his other special features, however, *Dryopithecus* seems to be pointing more definitely in the direction of chimpanzees and gorillas.

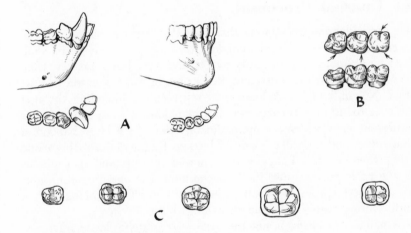

Teeth in apes and man.

A. Canine-premolar teeth, in side and crown views. In a pongid the canine is large, and the first premolar imitates its shape, differing from the second premolar. In hominids the canine is small, and both premolars are bicuspid.

B. Remnants of a basal cingulum in upper molar teeth of a chimpanzee.

C. The Dryopithecus pattern emerging. These are lower right molars showing cusp pattern. Left to right: a prosimian, with fore cusps well separated from after cusps; an Old World monkey with cross-crested pattern; *Dryopithecus* with 5 cusps and a Y fissure in the middle; gorilla, a larger version; man, who often has the pattern but also often has reduced to the four-cusped "plus" pattern shown here. From Gregory and specimens.

One other feature is the common prominence of the cingulum in the molars or premolars. This is a sort of low collar of enamel all around the base of the tooth, out of which the cusps arise. It is a main trait of more primitive teeth and is thus a sign of primitiveness when it occurs in the hominoid line, which has developed higher crowns largely devoted to the cusps themselves. Vestiges of a cingulum appear rarely in man and rather more commonly in chimpanzees and other apes.

So there we have a toothy genealogy of the large, or "pongine," apes to put alongside that of the gibbons. We catch sight of them as they were budding and flowering in the later Tertiary. It is striking to see how widely they flourished compared to the present day: chimp-like apes in Europe and Asia as well as in Africa, and near-gibbons in Africa and Europe as well as Asia.

The Unusual Proconsul

Of particular interest among these are the forms previously put in the genus *Proconsul*. These remains have been recovered in soul-satisfying abundance, principally by Dr. and Mrs. Louis Leakey, from lower Miocene stream beds along the shores of Lake Victoria in East Africa. Not only is his skeleton well represented, including the first skull ever found of a Tertiary ape, but he is known from three species of different sizes, which are approximately those of a large baboon, a chimpanzee, and a gorilla. Many of his jaw fragments probably came to rest when crocodiles caught him, chewed him up, and spat out his less digestible portions into the Miocene mud. But one proconsul, per-haps the best specimen of all, preserved himself by falling into a rapidly silting water hole and drowning, bless his heart.

His name, *Proconsul*, is not the gesture of stately classic reference it sounds like. Dr. Hopwood, of the British Museum, his original describer, thought the first fragments had the traits of a chimpanzee forerunner, and named him forthwith in honor of a living chimpanzee, a popular favorite in the London zoo, named Consul. But while *Proconsul* may represent the ancestor of the chimps, and the gorillas as well, he was both primitive and general. His teeth have the basic Dryopithecus pattern, but they are primitive, with a pronounced cingu-lum. He had heavy canine tusks, but without the broad muzzle; his chin was narrow, with no simian shelf. The skull, belonging to a mem-ber of the smallest species, lacks ape-like brows, and has a somewhat monkey-like face.

More important than this, he was a little monkey-like in his skeleton as well. His hand was especially so, although his arm contained slightly

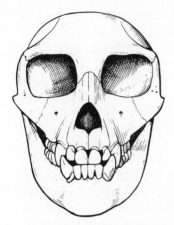
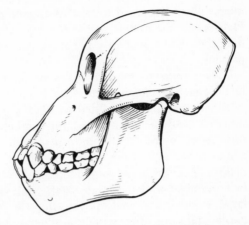

The skull of *Proconsul*, ½ natural size. After Le Gros Clark, Leakey, and Robinson.

human features, and seems altogether to have been generalized and primitive and not the forelimb of a practiced brachiator. His leg bones agree in nature and altogether suggest a capacity both for scampering on all fours and for standing erect with some efficiency.

What have we here? An ancestor ("structural") for both man and apes? It is reasonable to think that the present apes did go through a stage like this—did have such a forerunner, or even direct ancestor— and perhaps even more likely that the human line went through the same stage, at least for the skeleton, preserving generalized hands. It is probably only a minor question whether *Proconsul* himself is the actual ancestor, since he may have lived at a time when more fully developed and advanced ancestors had already arrived.

Gigantopithecus

Perhaps the strangest ape of all was *Gigantopithecus*. Professor von Koenigswald (of whom much more later) found him, or rather bought him. Among quantities of fossil teeth, of all kinds, which he purchased in Hong Kong drugstores (where such "dragon's teeth" are sold to be ground up for medicine), he discovered at least four teeth, from 1935 on, belonging to some kind of a hominoid and bigger than any higher primate teeth ever seen anywhere. Their vanished owner was, by some, even considered to have been an early man: the molars have the high crowns and the blunt cusps of actual hominids (members of the family Hominidae). At any rate, the late Dr. Weidenreich seized upon them as evidence for his theory that man had passed through an early giant stage, just before settling down to something about our size. The main difficulty seemed to be that *Gigantopithecus* lived in the Middle Pleistocene, the middle of the Ice Age, after all the fossil apes I have described had apparently perished, and man himself was very much present.

Gigantopithecus puzzled everyone for twenty years. In some parts he became a legend, a monster twelve feet high. Then in 1955, Chinese scientists themselves decided to have a go at the warehouses where dragon's teeth are assembled for market. They found no less than forty-seven more *Gigantopithecus* teeth and later recovered three actual lower jaws from caves. As far as described, these new finds make *Gigantopithecus* a good pongid, with a somewhat canine-like first premolar and a simian shelf. And yet he had only moderately large canines and incisors, lacking the "swine-like" muzzle of the gorilla and some other pongid exaggerations. So he seems to have been a conservative pongid, doubtless a ground-dweller, who grew larger than a gorilla and lived on into the Pleistocene, the Age of Man, defying the fate of most of the rest of his family.

Oreopithecus

This peculiar primate is probably not related to the main story, but that hardly diminishes his interest. His remains come from marshes turned into coal (lignite) in central Italy, and date from the Lower Pliocene, with an age of about ten million years. The strange thing is that his first fragments (all lower and upper jaws) were found in the late eighteen sixties. They were duly examined in the light of the knowledge of the day. It was decided, because there is a tendency for the cusps on his molars to line up in crosswise pairs (to be bilophodont), that he was a sort of half-baked monkey, and he was assigned by the majority to the Cercopithecidae, the Old World monkeys, and put away on the shelf.

There he sat for a couple of generations, until he was rescued by Dr. Johannes Hürzeler of the Natural History Museum of Basel. Hürzeler was studying a more primitive primate fossil, whose emphasis of a particular molar cusp put him in mind of the reports of *Oreopithecus*. He got hold of the original specimens and discovered how badly they had fared in paleontological annals. Not only were the available plaster casts, previously used by him and others, very poor. He concluded that, out of some eighty papers and monographs written about this supposedly well-known fossil, only eleven, all ancient, gave evidence of having been done by people who had actually seen the specimens themselves. The rest were all the work of writers looking over one another's shoulders. This is some kind of a moral lesson.

Enthralled by his redisovery, Hürzeler put himself to the task of collecting more specimens. He located coal mines containing them, near the Tuscan shore of central Italy. He soon found that *Oreopithecus* was in fact a common animal in the fauna of his time and place. It cannot yet be said what kind of a place it was, except for being marshy. At any rate, *Oreopithecus* was the only primate in the countryside.

In the face of difficulties and frustrations (most of the fossils were apt to wind up on the coal heaps) Hürzeler found a number of new fragments, and eventually, in the summer of 1958, a miner exposed the flattened but almost entire skeleton of an *Oreopithecus*. Hürzeler had already concluded that the creature was no monkey and that it was not only a homin*oid* but a homin*id*. Everyone agrees that he is right as to the monkey question: fragments from the upper end of the ulna (funny bone) of *Oreopithecus,* and of his lower spine, are quite unlike a monkey and are instead suggestive of the mobile arm and the supporting vertebral column of men and apes. Skull and jaw, as far

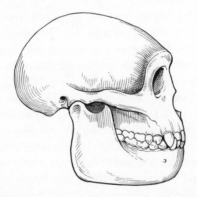

Skull of *Oreopithecus*. Not to scale. The skull is based on a restoration by Hürzeler and on unpublished photographs, through the kindness of Dr. Hürzeler.

as they are known, agree and ally *Oreopithecus* with man in a very vague and general way. They exhibit a relatively vertical face, as shown by teeth, chin, angle of jaw, and the lower border of the nose; no gap (diastema) in the upper tooth row to receive the lower canine, so important in later pongids; low if sharp canines, not bent like those in apes; and premolars which are all bicuspid, though decidedly sharp, with no modification of the lower first premolar toward the form of the canine tooth. *Oreopithecus* apparently had strong brows and jaws, but no ape-like muzzle. In body form he appears to have been something like a smallish chimpanzee, rather stout in the torso and with long arms and, as would be expected, no tail.

Thus we have an unusual animal, pongid in the body, vaguely homonid in the head, and certainly not a monkey. However, his teeth give trouble. Most of them have a marked cingulum around the base, a very conservative trait. More important, the molars lack the Dryopithecus pattern and have a special cusp toward the center of the lower molars, the cusp in fact which drew Hürzeler's attention to him, which is not found in any of the hominoids. This is strong medicine in paleontology, and has caused later opinion to remove him from close connection with either pongids or hominids. He is now generally given a family all his own (Oreopithecidae).

Strange as he is, he seems to have one relative. Simons has pointed out how closely his molar teeth resemble those of the equally peculiar *Apidium*, who is known from two species belonging to two different periods in the Oligocene, among that flourishing group of early higher primates in Egypt. So Simons believes that *Apidium* was the direct ancestor, over millions of years, of the later *Oreopithecus*, making a line which was separate from monkeys, from gibbons, from dryopithecines, and from hominids.

Looking over all these bygone apes we see a kind of diversity unsuspected only a few years ago. In *Pliopithecus* we find a gibbon imitating monkeys. Does this mean that the early Oligocene fossils (not only *Aeolopithecus*, the gibbon-like one, but his contemporaries also) were tail-waving quadrupeds, closely related to monkeys? Or even that *Dryopithecus*, known so largely from jaws alone, may be under such suspicion? I think not, though it is well to remember: you can look in a horse's mouth to read his age but you cannot look in an ape's mouth to read his kind of locomotion. *Pliopithecus* aside, the trend to uprightness in the hominoids was very strong; it was followed over a long period independently by the living gibbons, by the great apes, by *Oreopithecus*, and probably by hominids, at least in later stages. How *Gigantopithecus* looked, ate and walked about, it would be a pleasure to know.

At any rate the tendency to an upright position—not actual brachiation, or specialization for it, but a bias toward verticality of the trunk—was probably established early, perhaps in prosimian forebears. This made the range of hominoid locomotion very broad, but tended to accent brachiation of one kind or another. Nevertheless, given *Pliopithecus* (and with less significance *Proconsul* and *Limnopithecus*) it seems within the possibilities that the Old World monkeys, instead of being a completely separate line, are actually still another early offshoot from the hominoids which reverted frankly to quadrupedalism, developed specialized teeth, and then underwent a limited radiation.

7. DART, BROOM, LEAKEY, AND AUSTRALOPITHECUS

SOUTH AFRICA has been blessed with two remarkable and determined men who brought to light the most important fossils, for man's ancestry, of this century. They are Raymond Dart and Robert Broom, and they found *Australopithecus*.

Professor Dart studied anatomy first in Australia, and later in England under the greats of the early nineteen hundreds, Sir Arthur Keith and Sir Grafton Elliot Smith. Those last two will walk our stage again, for they devoted much of their own lives to fossil men. As for Dart, he went in 1923, at thirty, to the Medical School of the University of the Witwatersrand in Johannesburg, where he turned out to be the supremely right man in the right place at the right time.

The curtain was not long in going up. The play starts with a fossil baboon skull—and before 1920 no such skulls had ever been found in South Africa, or anywhere in Africa outside of Egypt. A student of Dart's, Miss Salmons, found the baboon skull sitting on her host's mantelpiece when she was at dinner one evening in 1924. Her host, a Mr. Izod, was a director of the Northern Lime Company, and the trail led to the limeworks at Taung, northwest of Kimberley, where great bluffs of limestone were being blasted down for the kilns. Dart, in some excitement, asked his geological colleague, Professor R. B. Young, who was scheduled to go to Taung the next week, to find out if any other such fossils were to be had. There were, and the mine manager sent a box full of pieces of limestone, enclosing bones, up to Johannesburg. At once Dart saw a fragment representing the brain cavity of something like a chimpanzee, a natural cast of the inside of a skull, formed by lime-cemented sand. By good fortune this morsel fitted another block which, when the limestone was cleared away six weeks later, yielded the whole face, jaws, and teeth of a juvenile "ape."

Dart was startled and a little disconcerted: he was in those days not well acquainted with fossils. (He began as a nerve-and-brain man, having presented his first scientific paper in 1919, on fish and reptile brains.) But he saw his duty and he did it. He realized this was no ordinary ape. He estimated that the brain was too large for a chimpanzee child, or even an adult. The face was less squared-off and protruding than a young chimp's, and, above all, it lacked even the beginnings of a brow ridge. He believed that the teeth, though large, were not ape-like; and that the roundness of the skull even suggested an erect posture. Dart named the find *Australopithecus* (Ape of the South) *africanus,* wrote up a description in which he drew attention to the human, non-ape characters of the fossil, and even suggested it be put in a new family midway between Pongidae and Hominidae. He sent his note off to the English scientific journal, *Nature.*

This now famous paper was published February 7, 1925. But the reaction in the great world was not favorable, even from Dart's old teachers, and some writers were inexcusably caustic. Dr. Broom, who agreed with Dart from the start, never forgave these last, and long afterward wrote, "I was never able to discover what were Prof. Dart's offences. Presumably the most serious was that when he found a very important skull he did not immediately send it off to the British Museum, where it would have been examined by an 'expert,' and probably described ten years later, but boldly described it himself, and published an account within a few weeks of the discovery."

Keith and Elliot Smith, both of whom later changed their minds, gave their opinions that *Australopithecus* was simply a new anthropoid ape, of the chimpanzee-gorilla line, though admitting the presence of some slightly human traits. Now of course it is difficult to form sound opinions far away from the specimen itself. More important, it is difficult to judge much about adult form from a child of five or six. And we should bear in mind that *Dryopithecus* and *Pliopithecus* were, at the time, the only well-known fossil apes of the later Tertiary. Perhaps Gregory's brilliant studies of them had obsessed the anthropologists of the day into assuming that any fossil type showing the Dryopithecus pattern would best be put with the apes. Nevertheless, the anatomists should have been warned by the first permanent molars of *Australopithecus,* already erupted in the little skull, for, though large, the generally human form of these four teeth is unmistakable. And other careful studies have since shown that the milk canine and milk molar of the Taung specimen can hardly be confused with those of apes, though this would have been too much to recognize in 1925.

Broom and Paranthropus

The limestone at Taung ran out, and no further trace of the fossil child or his parents ever came to light. Years went by. Enter Dr. Broom.

This medical general practitioner, with an almost impenetrable Scottish burr, was already famous as a part-time paleontologist because of his studies of the mammal-like reptiles abounding in the Great Karroo. In 1934, General Smuts (egged on by Dart) asked him to give up private practice, to become curator in Pretoria's Transvaal Museum, and specifically to devote all his time to the search for further evidence of *Australopithecus*. Now if Dart was a lucky man, in snatching what may have been an isolated fossil from loss, Broom had something like the Midas touch. Not that what he handled turned to fossils, but that fossils came to his hand in the most extraordinary way.

Where should he begin? There were plenty of limestone caves containing breccias, or consolidated masses of earth and fossil bones. Students of Dart's drew Broom's attention to the limeworks at Sterkfontein, not far from Pretoria and Johannesburg, and drove him out to have a look, on a Sunday in 1936. At the limeworks these students had found baboon skulls not differing greatly from those at Taung. Arriving at the place, Broom learned that the manager, Mr. Barlow, had once worked at Taung, and that he was saving out fossils at Sterkfontein to sell to tourists. This put the acquisition of fossils on a financial basis, luckily a field in which Broom was not unskillful.

At any rate, he needed to make only two more visits when, on August 17, 1936, Barlow handed him a fine brain cast and asked, "Is this what you're after?" Said Broom, "Yes, that's what I'm after." During that day and the next Broom himself found the impression of the

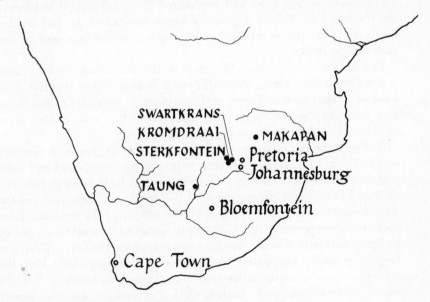

Map of South Africa showing sites of *Australopithecus*.

top of the same skull, as well as its actual base, with parts of the forehead and side walls. Can you detect a note of satisfaction in these remarks of his? "To have started to look for an adult skull of Australopithecus, and to have found an adult of at least an allied form in about three months was a record of which we felt there was no reason to be ashamed. And to have gone to Sterkfontein and found what we wanted within nine days was even better."

As blasting of the limestone continued, Broom kept an eye on things, finding in the next two years a few further pieces, including the knee end of a thighbone. But nothing turned up to match his first skull. Then in 1938, Barlow handed Broom an upper jaw, having one tooth in place and showing fresh breaks. To Broom it was evidently a new kind of man-ape. Barlow was mum about just where it had come from, so Broom returned on Barlow's day off to speak to the workmen and discovered that none of them had even seen it. So he came back again and gave Barlow a talking-to.

Barlow admitted that the fossil was not from Sterkfontein and that it had been given him by a schoolboy, Gert Terblanche. Broom set out for the boy's home and learned he was at school; he went to the school and found Gert at once, "with four of what are perhaps the most valuable teeth in the world in his trouser pocket." School was not yet out, so Broom lectured the entire student body on fossils until closing time. The Ancient Mariner having had his will, he collared Gert again, who took him to a hill at Kromdraai, less than a mile from Sterkfontein, where Gert had hammered his fossil out of a breccia. He produced for Broom a piece of lower jaw which he had hidden there, and the spot eventually yielded much of the face and of one side of the skull.

Broom perceived enough difference in the Kromdraai skull to name it a distinctly new genus, *Paranthropus robustus*. But it was the same kind of animal as the Taung and Sterkfontein specimens, and these new finds emphasized the human qualities of the teeth and of some marks of the skull, such as the jaw joint.

And so at last the barriers of objection began to give way. Gregory and Hellman came from New York to inspect the fossils and lent their authority to the view that the creatures were at least midway between apes and men; and Gregory supplied the apt term "man-apes" for the Australopithecinae, as the group is known officially. The evidence from these battered pieces (Gert had simply whacked *Paranthropus* out of its limey nest with a rock) was far from complete. However, Dart was beginning to be vindicated, and Broom was saying flatly that the man-apes were upright-walking, ground-living near-humans. But the supply of fossils stopped: Barlow died, Sterkfontein was shut down, and the war had come. At the war's end, however, Smuts asked Broom especially to renew the search, and things began booming in the Transvaal once again.

Man-apes Aplenty

I mean precisely "booming." Broom had long experience with lime-stone caves and breccia deposits, and for excavating he adopted Barlow's method as the only practical one: dynamite. But he fell afoul of the Historical Monuments Commission, which now had authority over important fossil sites and which took the stand that Broom's explosive approach might ruin significant evidence of stratification and thus of age. So Broom, who had been awarded a medal in geology at Glasgow, was ordered to work with a geologist or stop working. Smuts was out of the country. Broom was furious and was restrained with difficulty by his own Museum authorities from flouting the Commission. Smuts came back and at once told Broom to go ahead, while he, Smuts, patched things up. So Broom went to Kromdraai, early in 1947. In due course there came a permit to work at Kromdraai, whereat Broom, not a forgive-and-forgetter, stopped work and moved along the valley to Sterkfontein, for which he had no permit.

At once, valuable new fossils began describing small arcs in the air to the tune of his blasts, and before the month was out he had discovered a nearly perfect skull of *Australopithecus*, complete except for the teeth and lower jaw, and unwarped. When the Monuments Commission read the newspapers, they invoked the law and stopped Broom from working at Sterkfontein. He tried a new place, with no success. Then the Commission finally concluded that there was no stratification at Sterkfontein and issued him a permit. This left Broom with no site at which he could defy the authorities, and so back he went to Sterkfontein, continuing his finds there.

During the next year, 1948, an expedition from the University of California opened a third site in that vicinity, on the farm Swartkrans. Having no luck, they asked Broom to help. The Broom magic uncovered a lower jaw almost at once, and the Swartkrans deposit eventually produced a number of skulls and other parts of a new kind of *Paranthropus*. At the same time, Dart had re-entered the action, at a cave far to the north.

A hundred and fifty miles from Sterkfontein, near the town of Potgietersrust, lies the valley Makapansgat. Here in 1833, Potgieter and a Boer force besieged Makapan and two thousand of his Bantu warriors in a huge cave, in a month-long struggle which cost the lives of Potgieter as well as of Makapan and most of the Africans. Known today as the Historic Cave, the place still shows signs of attempts by the Bantu to defend and fortify themselves within its mouth.

But this was not the only cave in Makapan's valley. During the last million years or so, many others have been formed by water seeping down through the dolomite cliffs which form the valley's sides. One cave of moderately ancient vintage, the Cave of Hearths, was old enough to contain the fires and rubbish of Stone Age men. Another, still older, the Limeworks Cave, had a fine stalagmitic layer of limestone and a filling of breccia containing animal bones. Here a lime company had for a long time been blasting out the good lime, and throwing the useless bony material on a waste heap, until part of the roof of the cave fell in and operations became unsafe. Dart had learned of the Limeworks Cave fossils in 1925, as an aftermath of his announcement of *Australopithecus*. But only in 1945—again through the discovery of a fossil baboon of early type—did he and his associates realize that the age of the cave was promising for finds of the man-apes. Two years later, in 1947, among the lumps of discarded bone-bearing material from the long-abandoned workings, they turned up the back part of such a skull. Dart thereafter kept a staff painstakingly picking over the Limeworks dump continuously, and every now and then another piece—face, jaw, teeth, skull bone—has come to light. Dart recognized this as another variety of the original *Australopithecus*, though there may actually be no difference from the original baby at all.

So it is that after 1947 the fossil famine became a feast. The wonderful Dr. Broom died in 1951 at the age of eighty-four. So eager and so active to the end of his days was he that his young assistant and successor, Dr. John Robinson (now of the University of Wisconsin), was some years in freeing specimens, detected and brought in to the Museum in Pretoria while Broom was still alive, from their limey matrix. Swartkrans yielded parts of at least thirty-five different specimens of man-apes, including more than two hundred teeth. Sterkfontein has been equally rich, and all three sites, once thought to be rather limited, are now believed to have large remaining deposits, doubtless with plenty of man-ape bones still entombed and there for the taking. (Unfortunately this costs money.) So Dart and Robinson had plenty to do without looking for new deposits. And the flood of fossils has changed the general view of the australopithecines completely, or rather, brought it close to the original view of Dart and Broom. It has confirmed what the Taung child, in his general form, hinted—indeed, what he actually said, in a small voice, with the shape of his six-year molar teeth.

Dear Boy and the Leakeys

East Africa has also been blessed with two remarkable people, Louis and Mary Leakey, who have even raised sons to be successful finders of fossil hominids in addition. Dr. Leakey himself was born in Kenya, though educated at Cambridge, and since his youth has devoted himself to all phases of natural history in East Africa, but principally to the prehistory of man from quite recent times back to the Miocene and *Proconsul*. And it was Mrs. Leakey who discovered the one good skull of that ape. This creates the impression of a Midas touch, like Broom's, but is really the result of the location of sites, of the training of African assistants, and of the arduous and persistent search and the experienced eye. Like many things that sound romantic, it is just hard work.

In recent years the Leakeys have been devoting their efforts particularly to Olduvai Gorge in northernmost Tanzania. This is a miniature Grand Canyon gouged through the deposits of a basin which was filling up, partly with lake sediments, partly with volcanic ash and other material, over the last few million years. In places three hundred feet high, the walls of the gorge have been divided into five beds, the lower two being the most interesting at the moment. The bottom of Bed I was laid down approximately two million years ago, and this general period continues into the lower part of Bed II, where there is a break, with a change in animal forms marking the beginning of the Middle Pleistocene. In 1959 Mrs. Leakey found the well-preserved fossil skull of a new kind of *Paranthropus* in the upper part of Bed I, and the Leakeys were so glad to see him that they nicknamed him the Dear Boy at once, and provisionally made his scientific name *Zinjanthropus boisei*. In 1964 one of their African assistants, Kamoya Kimeu, working with Richard Leakey fifty miles away at Peninj on the shore of Lake Natron, discovered a fine lower jaw which is such a good match for the skull that it must belong to the same form. The striking thing here is the evidence of apparent difference in date, the jaw being at least a million years younger than the skull, which if correct is an important matter.

What is probably the oldest fragment of any of these creatures yet found was picked up in 1965 by my Harvard colleague Bryan Patterson. Working in an early Pleistocene deposit at Kanapoi, near the southern end of Lake Rudolf in northern Kenya, he discovered the lower end of the humerus or upper arm bone (the elbow joint) of a hominoid of some kind. Now this piece of skeleton is almost identical in man and chimpanzee, and very difficult to assign all by itself. But the fragment is from an animal of this size, and it does seem to be more like man's than *Pan's;* furthermore the antelope remains recovered at the same site make it unlikely that this was a forest, and hence that the arm was a chimpanzee's. It must be assumed to be *Australopithecus* or *Paranthropus,* or a close relative of both. The fauna gives signs of being older than the oldest at Olduvai, and the date is 2.6 million years or more; so the find carries the man-apes back to a time near the beginning of the Pleistocene.

The Nature of Australopithecus

Australopithecus, then, is no mystery. We can describe him clearly and confidently, even though there is still much to learn about some parts of his skeleton. First, take a quick look at the skull. We see a small brain case, hardly, if at all, larger than an ape's. We see a large deep jaw. Now such a combination is bound to look like the cranium of an ape, and we can see why students in the twenties and thirties, knowing only the skull of a child, or broken specimens without front teeth, should have been hesitant about ranking such a being anywhere near man himself. But today only a very quick look indeed would allow us to rank him with the chimpanzees and the gorillas. For the face is shorter, the brain case generally higher and rounded at the back, and the *foramen magnum,* with the joint for the spine, is well forward under the skull. In some details the socket for the jaw joint and the opening for the ear are markedly human. But the teeth give the man-apes away entirely.

The molar teeth are massive. Like those of all apes and men, they show the Dryopithecus pattern, in an exuberant development of the enamel. But these molars are relatively short and broad. In various other ways also they have a human character: the cusps are blunt and rounded, rather than pointed, which is the ape tendency; and the crowns are high, not low. Moving forward along the jaw, we find the canines are not tusk-like and do not even protrude above the other teeth, and the premolars are all bicuspid like ours, though they are larger and better developed and tend to have an extra root. And the incisor teeth, at the front of the jaw, are small and narrow. Strangely, in the larger man-apes, from Swartkrans, the lower incisors are as narrow as our own.

So that complex of ape traits—wide incisors, big canines, lower first premolars imitating the canine teeth, all involved with a spreading front to the jaws—is totally missing, along with any sign of a simian shelf. And the teeth were worn down on even, flat surfaces, as they wear in men who eat coarse food. This is in contrast to apes, whose interlocking canines prevent the kind of rotary and side-to-side chewing which causes such flat wear. It would be hard to imagine a less "ape-like" dentition in a higher primate. The man-apes, in these general proportions, not only veer in a "human" direction. They go beyond us: they are more "human" than we are.

This is striking evidence of their relations with us. But we must ask how they got around, since we do not walk with our teeth. The skeletal remains are far from complete, but they include hipbones of

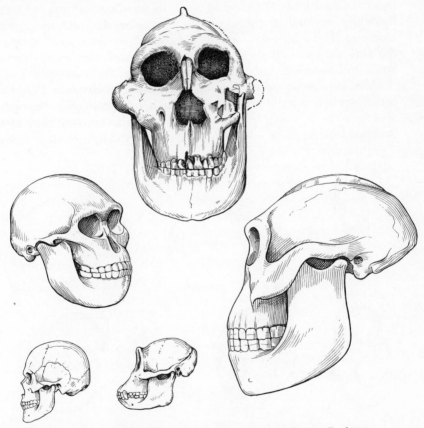

Skulls of the Australopithecinae. Top, "Zinjanthropus" from Olduvai, a *Paranthropus*, from a photograph, with jaw supplied by modification of the Peninj specimen. Left, *Australopithecus* from Makapan, after the restoration by Dart. Right, *Paranthropus* from Swartkrans, based on various photographs and casts. Notable features of *Paranthropus* are the great jaw height and the short crest along the mid-line of the skull. All approximately ¼ natural size. Human and chimpanzee skulls are sketched in for reference.

five man-apes, from three of the sites, and in one case a whole pelvis with much of the spine above it. Now if you remember the special qualities of these bones in ourselves, you will recall that they form a round ring, and the hinder portion of the hipbones is not high and straight as in apes but is bent downward and backward, carrying the sacrum and the spine with it. This is a principal adjustment to upright walking, on the human kind of leg. And that is the nature of the australopithecine bones. They are not exactly like ours in every detail, but they are not at all like an ape's: they are *not halfway between*. Evidently our kind of gait, as an adaptive niche, does not accept half measures. These hipbones are sufficiently like our own so that, when the first were found, some authorities suggested that small human bones had somehow got into the same cave as the man-apes.

There can be no uncertainty or argument. The shape of the head had suggested uprightness before, though less positively. The man-apes were true, erect, ground-walking animals, nothing else. How shall we look on these animals? They were certainly not apes, unless

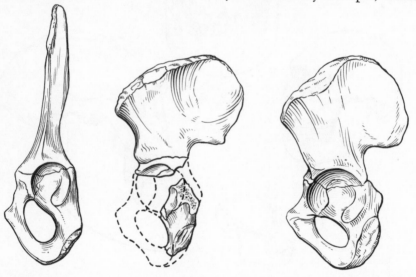

Hipbones, left, in side view, of chimpanzee, *Australopithecus* (Makapan), and man (Bushman). After Dart.

you were to take a simple-minded and erroneous view that any such crude, large-jawed, small-brained thing is to be called an ape. That would be wrong, because the apes are a specific kind of tree-hanging, forest-living hominoid, with particular teeth, pelvis, hands, and feet. We now see that "man-apes," Gregory's simple term which I have been using, is not really appropriate—though no one has thought of a better —since the man-apes were not really part ape.

Australopithecus was no "pongid"—he had none of the special traits of living apes. Nor was he something more generalized, like *Proconsul*. He was our kind of animal. His locomotion was walking, and his teeth were like ours in detail. Though small his brain and large his jaw, he had nothing which cuts him sharply off from us. He can be placed nowhere but in the family Hominidae. You will shrink from calling him a "human being," and you should. But we can be scientific and give him his proper term, which is "hominid," meaning that he shares our line of descent and has to be put with the other Hominidae, ourselves. And so there is no escaping it, he was an early, primitive "man."

Australopithecus vs. Paranthropus

Now I have been using "he" in a rather broad sense, for the remains from the several different sites actually represent somewhat different types. Many people now put them all into one genus, *Australopithecus*, with species *africanus* from Taung, Sterkfontein, and Makapansgat; *robustus* from Kromdraai and Swartkrans; and *boisei* from Olduvai. The last two forms have considerably more in common, however, and Robinson has unremittingly argued that something like *Australopithecus africanus* is the source of later mankind, while the other two represent an extinct side branch; also that these branches differed significantly from one another in anatomy and way of life; and therefore that the two original genera, *Australopithecus* and *Paranthropus* should be preserved. With some others, I think he is right, for the reasons given below and further on. (However it is often convenient to refer to them all collectively as *Australopithecus*, or australopithecines for their joint subfamily.)

Australopithecus proper is indeed most like us and seems to be a perfectly good structural ancestor. That is to say, he betrays no features which do not either point in our direction or might have become modified in that direction. He was rather small in size, apparently with a marked difference between males and females, as in baboons. Certainly the best partial skeleton, a female, must have been that of a tiny "woman," less than four feet in height, and about fifty pounds in weight, a willowy little creature with a slender trunk. There are several other particular features of the teeth and skull which reinforce the likeness to *Homo*.

Paranthropus, on the other hand, both from Swartkrans and Olduvai, looks like a more specialized offshoot of the stem. In the first place, he was considerably bigger, though how large it is difficult to say. The face was long, and the jaw very deep and powerful; and the brain case was low, so that the eyes are close to the top of the skull. Robinson talks of *Paranthropus* as a "hominid gorilla" in a slightly different sense, referring to the massive jaw development. Some of the Swartkrans skulls have a small ridge or crest along the top of the skull like a gorilla, in response to the jaw muscles, and this is more pronounced still in the Olduvai skull. But the form and placing of this ridge emphasize contrast to the gorilla, not likeness, since they relate to large molar teeth, not to large canines. A particular note of specialization appears in the teeth themselves, where those of the front are reduced relatively more than our own and where the first milk molar has departed further from *Dryopithecus* in form than has ours. So, if "human" were to be taken as the opposite of "ape-like," which would be quite proper in this case, *Paranthropus* had carried a human trend to a point which we have never reached ourselves.

As the English anatomist John Napier points out, the rest of the skeleton also shows some striking differences. The thumb of *Paranthropus* was apparently somewhat ape-like, being short but strong in gripping. The upper end of the thighbone is unusual in shape, and the head of this bone, with the corresponding hip socket, was surprisingly small. The pelvis of *Paranthropus*, in spite of its hominid form, is special and in some ways suggestive of a gorilla's. Apparently it would not allow its owner the full striding gait of modern man; Napier thinks his walk was a rolling "waddle," and suggests that in his evolution he remained a forest animal longer than did *Australopithecus*, emerging a less perfectly evolved biped. From the existing evidence of skull and skeleton, then, *Australopithecus* and *Paranthropus* must have differed at least as much as chimpanzee and gorilla, a degree of difference which makes their later histories easier to understand.

Life and Times of Australopithecus

So far we have been dealing with actors on a bare stage. Let us look at scenery and props. The scene is the open country of East and South Africa. The time is the early part of the Pleistocene. This epoch is called the Ice Age, because of the glaciations in other regions, especially the Northern Hemisphere, although here in Africa there was nothing like this, and only moderate fluctuations of climate; in addition, *Australopithecus* pertains mainly to the early Pleistocene, before the colder phases appeared at all. Things were, indeed, much like today, and the generally similar kinds of animals throughout the Pleistocene show that this is so. Species and genus were not the same, but there were antelopes, hyenas, hyraxes, and lions, a familiar collection. Baboons still haunt the sides and the cliffs of Makapan's valley, and baboon bones are found in all the man-ape sites.

In fact, it appears that *Australopithecus* was a meat eater, or at least a general feeder like us, not a fruit eater like the apes. He had the teeth for it. And Dart, refusing to believe that carnivores, especially hyenas, could be responsible for all the animal bones in the caves, has found evidence that the baboon skulls had been crushed by blows, to kill them or to get out the brains, in a way that only a hominid could have managed, that is to say, with a club. Robinson holds that *Paranthropus,* on the other hand, was a vegetarian, at least to an important degree, from a peculiar bit of evidence. Various of his teeth show the scars of tiny flakes chipped from the top of the crown down the side of the enamel. This does not result, he believes, from crunching hard but resilient animal material, like bone. It would, however, take place in animals biting with great force on vegetable matter, if this contained pieces of very hard grit which acted as pressure points just at the right spots near the edge of the tooth.

As to props, it is possible that the man-apes used tools, in some sense or other. Dart has for some time been investigating the likelihood that *Australopithecus,* especially at Makapansgat, did not let the teeth and bones of dead animals, perhaps his own kill, go to waste, but used antelope jaws lined with teeth for scraping, and the heavy bones of the leg for clubs, and so on. He holds that these natural objects are what such a beast, with a small brain but with hands, would make use of in place of the shaped stone tools of later man. A fair enough proposition, though by its nature it is not an easy one to prove. The opposition to Dart's idea has been almost complete, since there might be other ways by which the majority of these possible "tools" might have got into the caves, and since signs of actual use on such natural objects are hard to find. However, Dart has lately produced some indications of polishing from use, as well as several examples of smaller dagger-like bones being thrust through rings formed from larger bones, for what purpose it is hard to imagine. But this cannot all be accident.

The other part of the problem is the actual fashioning of tools out of raw stone, as was practiced by later men. Perfectly good tools (of the so-called Oldowan industry) have been found in association with bones of australopithecines, particularly at Sterkfontein and at Olduvai. Now of course we cannot tell simply by looking at their skulls whether the man-apes were capable of such fashioning of tools. The evidence, as Professors Robinson and Tobias have been pointing out, seems to run thus. In sites where an australopithecine is the only hominid, no stone tools occur. When they do occur, there are indications, however slight, of the presence of a more advanced kind of man. Fragments of such men, or other hominids, are now acknowledged to have been found both in East and South Africa. Thus the position is: the australopithecines may have used natural bone or stone for tools, but did not shape them; and *Australopithecus* (certainly at least *Paranthropus*) and other kinds of early humanity were living at the same time.

Be that as it may, we have been looking back at a stage in evolution when the basic upright ground-walking human form had been fashioned but before brains had become significantly larger than those of other hominoids. Before we see what happens next, let us simply note that we have reached, not a No Man's Land, but a Some Man's Land, the recognizable beginnings of humanity proper.

8. EVOLUTION IN THE PRIMATES

We CAN TAKE the fossils of the hominoids and make up the beginnings of a family tree. They show us dimly the nature of our most important predecessors. But there is more to history than dates and kings; there is also how and why. We can plainly see that a tree shrew is a hairy, four-footed, air-breathing, warm-blooded, live-bearing, tree-going fish. But how do you get from a tree shrew to a man?

Granted that he shows some very faint suggestions of promising primate trends, a tree shrew remains a pretty unpromising object for a grandfather. Luckily it is all over now, and we can use hindsight. This suggests strongly that the answer lies in certain opportunities for natural selection.

That is to say, tree life acted on a little mammal which was extremely generalized and plastic, encouraging it to develop along lines not usual in mammals. The paws did not develop strong claws, which are efficient both in trees and on the ground, but which foreclose the appearance of good grasping fingers. And curiosity came to be served by sight, not by smell. With these conditions, Professors Wood Jones and Elliot Smith long ago developed the "arboreal theory" of primate evolution.

Consider a tree. To us it is something lovelier than a poem, a provider of shade, perchance of apples. To a chimpanzee it is a gymnasium, a place to sleep, and, above all, his larder. But to a little prosimian it is the whole world, not the flat one which we and other mammals tread, but one in three dimensions, a network of separate pathways, some vertical, some horizontal. Imagine a primitive tree shrew, a basic primate, exposed to new kinds of adaptation by such a world. According to the arboreal theory, his evolution now proceeds as follows.

First of all, the thumb and big toe herald later developments by beginning very slightly to rotate, and thus to oppose the other fingers and toes. Even in an opossum, let alone a tree shrew, these first digits can be widely separated from their fellows. Now a terrestrial animal goes its way with no concern over falling out of a tree, and without attempting to grasp the ground with its feet, or even to choose its footing with especial care. The natural working axis of its foot is along the middle, so that the digits to either side are of less importance and may even be lost in evolution, as has happened in the horses.

But this is not so in a small tree animal which, to assure its footing, is trying to cover as much of the curve of a bough as possible. It has come about, probably by accident, that in the primates the working axis has tended to fall between the innermost digit and the rest, the inner one being set off from the others. (This has been more true of hind feet than forefeet, in spite of the state of affairs in man.) When an animal puts weight on such a foot in such a position, on a rounded bough, the innermost digit and the outer four tend to fall a little in opposite directions and thus to oppose each other, no matter how flat the foot was to begin with. Since this helps the grasp, feet eventually became adapted in this direction, further and further.

Freeing the Forelimb

This makes a creature which proceeds through the trees on four clutching hand-like paws, whose digits wrap themselves around whatever they can grasp. Its forelimbs are the explorers, while the hind limbs are in territory which the forelimbs have already covered. So the forefoot is, theoretically, the more tentative, but in any case it is closer to consciousness, and more careful attention is paid to it. The support of the body, therefore, particularly when resting, comes to be mainly the responsibility of the hind limbs, which become heavier and lose some of their freedom of movement (which was never as great as in forelimbs). The forelimbs, however, evolve in a contrary direction, becoming more mobile and less used for support. This is all a tendency which would be natural if not inevitable in arboreal animals with grasping feet, but far less emphasized in ground animals. The process is what Wood Jones considered something of great importance, terming it the "differentiation of the limbs" and pointing out that, to an animal with aspirations, to be four-handed is almost as bad as to be four-footed.

Hot on the heels of this is a consequent tendency, the "emancipation of the forelimbs." The more the hind limbs accept the chore of supporting the body, the more the forelimbs have other opportunities. They are still used, of course, for locomotion, but they are freed for a certain amount of purely academic investigation as well: touching, feeling, and testing. This is another aspect of the differentiation of the limbs, and the more pronounced it becomes, the more the creature tends to sit upright when not on the move, perching on its hind legs and using its forelimbs freely, as true arms and hands. With them it can feed itself, hold and feel objects, and scratch and groom, which is no mean occupational pastime. Supposedly, then, arboreal life opened new vistas for a developing hand. Only grasping paws and sensitive fingers could have started such a train, and only through this train could the men of our planet have developed.

Shrinking the Snout

Sitting up, evidently, must have been an early tendency induced by climbing or resting on vertical tree trunks or limbs. So the tendency to sit and the tendency to use the forelimbs must have been reinforcing one another all the time. Wood Jones traced certain developments in the spine and the rest of the trunk. But it is the skull which is the great area of the further adaptive effects of arboreal life, after the hand has tasted freedom and the animal has sat up.

It will be recalled that progress in the primates has been marked by an ever larger brain and by a diminishing snout (remembering that the anthropoid muzzle, like that of baboons, has apparently become secondarily enlarged). Now a snout exists in an ordinary four-footed mammal to serve a variety of purposes. It does almost everything connected with eating: the mammal arrives at its food, whether animal or vegetable, on its legs, but the latter are of little further use. The game is broken up and chewed, all by means of the jaws and teeth. In leisure moments also the muzzle is the most useful part of the body, because an animal, investigating something, does so by smelling, by nosing, by licking, or by nibbling. Thus it is that the snout is long for various reasons: partly to give the jaws power for fighting, killing, and crushing, and partly to put distance between its tip and the eyes, so that while the owner is exercising the senses of smell, touch, and taste, it may also use that of vision and see what it is doing with its own snout. This would not be possible were the mouth directly under the eyes.

It is actually difficult for us to imagine how the powers of perception in ground mammals are concentrated in the snout. But consider how matters change in a tree, and for an animal with a grasping hand. In the first place, the olfactory sense loses a great part of its value. The air that blankets the unbroken ground surface is a world of smell, but in the trees there is less for scent to cling to, and the paths of travel are narrow. Therefore the power of smell has hardly more than an aesthetic excuse for being. Second, see how the snout is discouraged from being used for feeling. A creature walking gingerly along a bough cannot sniff and nuzzle everything that excites its curiosity without losing its balance and falling out of the tree. However, it may touch and pluck far more of such things if it can use its hands to this end. And it can hold these things, be they buds, fruits, insects, or eggs, and turn them over or pull them apart, at various convenient distances from its eyes instead of only at the fixed focus, so to speak, of the eye-snout combination.

Therefore a fuller co-ordination is possible between sight and touch, particularly when stereoscopic vision is thrown in. Certainly our own education is of this kind. As infants we touch things and look at them simultaneously, until we have gradually learned to tell how anything would feel just by looking at it, and on seeing something unfamiliar we almost automatically reach out and feel it. (The "Please do not touch anything" signs are provided for the more infantile of us.) But we seldom smell such things, and we really know very little about how things smell. In all of this we are simply acting like primates.

The trees, therefore, diverted their primate guests from smelling with snouts toward feeling with forepaws. As the snout became less important to the senses, it also became less important in eating, because the developing hands could be used to convey the food to the mouth, in place of the older fashion of conveying the mouth to the food. This being so, the jaws did not have to procure the food but only to chew it. The eyes, therefore, did not have to watch the snout but watched the hands instead. The higher primates eat precisely as we do, if less fastidiously. We, or they, ensnare a piece of food in the hand, or some extension thereof, like a fork. We then look at it, instead of smelling it, and having approved it for consumption, stow it in the mouth and chew it up. The snout, once responsible for all of these operations, now performs only the last.

A long muzzle, instead of being necessary, thus becomes excess baggage, which is its evolutionary passport to reduction. This is one theoretical explanation for the shorter faces of the higher primates. There is that apparent embarrassment in the massive jaws of the great apes, who seem to fall out of the trend. But there are explanations. First, it is a well-known rule that in a group of related animals the large forms have disproportionately heavy facial skeletons. Otherwise their bulk, their cubic measure, would outstrip their chewing and swallowing areas. Second, the large apes have, from *Dryopithecus* on, grown exaggerated canines and foreparts to their jaws, perhaps mainly in adaptation to a diet of coarse fruit and vegetables. They do not have snouts in the primitive sense, since their faces, like ours and monkeys', are somewhat bent down, with the nose region strongly diminished and the eyes brought together at the top.

Those, then, are the tendencies which would have been directing the evolution of the various prosimian lines in their early days. Now it is plain that such animals, still generalized, offered natural selection the chance to produce a more advanced grade of animal on the same lines, i.e., development of hand, eye, and brain, as well as uprightness. The force of the trend shows itself in the fact that the prosimians made several thrusts in a monkey-like direction, among the lorises, among the tarsioids, and in very late (Pleistocene) times among the lemurs on Madagascar. But the results of such experiments were still prosimians; the breakthrough came with the true monkeys and the hominoids.

Higher Primate Habits

The Old World monkeys would seem to be the more faithful disciples of the main trend, with their generalized and capable hands (though some have lost their thumbs) and their uncomplicated arboreal and quadrupedal nature. The New World monkeys on the other hand went in for more reckless experimentation, producing animals with prehensile tails, or with imitation claws, or with brachiating habits. They also dropped the insistence on opposability of the first digit, so that in some cases opposability has been shifted elsewhere (as in howling monkeys) or even lost entirely.

The hominoids similarly went off on a tangent. This is not easy to understand. But their trend of evolution was dominated by uprightness, which is after all a legitimate primate trend. For some reason it included the loss of tails. Mainly, however, it broke the hold of quadrupedality, of the tendency to go on all fours when running or climbing. And so it may have produced an undecided but still rather monkey-like hominoid, who could manage both kinds of posture, quadrupedal and bipedal. Perhaps this was encouraged by environments with high grass and only thin woods, like much of present Africa, the high grass persuading the little "apes" to stand and walk erect.

All this must be guesswork. And we cannot easily presume that the tree-using pongid apes of today actually started on the ground, that is, passed through a ground-living stage. In fact, we have always in the past gone on the opposite presumption, that the descent to the ground was made by man alone, springing down from a brachiating tree stock. However, the indications are turning against the idea that brachiation, the basic adaptation of the modern apes, was basic to begin with. If the hominoid or "ape" stock from the early Oligocene to *Proconsul*, or even later, was actually not very agile in trees, no more so, perhaps, than the slow loris—neither monkey-like nor ape-like—then some upright venturing on the ground would seem more likely to have taken place at that point than later, after gibbons and chimps had begun to fly through the trees with such very great ease.

But all this is full of pious "would seems." Nobody yet knows. One thing we can be sure of, as a result of the australopithecine discoveries: man did not, as once thought, emerge as a sort of black sheep *Dryopithecus*. For, by any sensible interpretation, *Dryopithecus* already reveals the trend of adaptation to the pongid apes, with their particular teeth, whatever his limbs may have been like. As for the australopiths, they not only show us hominoids who were walking erect, they actually show us creatures who had achieved this stage quite fully, and long enough ago to have given rise to two fairly distinct forms (*Australopithecus* and *Paranthropus*). Especially important are their teeth, which were already completely hominid, and apparently well established in form, not something new. And while you might argue that these teeth are in some respects primitive compared to ours, they are in no sense ape-like.

So we find ourselves with the realization that there have been two distinct lines of development, hominid and pongid; and we are faced with the problem of tracing them back to the point where they diverged. The australopiths, though recent themselves, suggest by their evolved teeth and upright skeleton that this point was not recent. And the dryopithecines, who were already quite definitely like today's great apes, suggest indeed that it might have been at the beginning of the Miocene, or even before. Such a time, verging on thirty million years, is a high estimate compared to those which have generally been made. Nevertheless the fact that the gibbon group had become an independent stem considerably earlier than this makes it seem not unreasonable. At the same time, the biochemical likenesses of man to chimpanzee and gorilla is an argument for more recent separation from them.

But the main point is this: a split existed when the pongids had become strongly committed to tree brachiation and to a definite modification of all their front teeth, while the hominids were becoming walkers (or at least holding back from the brachiating trend) and retaining different and more generalized tooth patterns, probably reducing the canine teeth as well. Man, the man-apes, and all their ancestors back to that fork in the road should be termed hominids, just as the large apes and their ancestors should be termed pongids, or, better, "pongines" (members of the subfamily Ponginae). At that point, and before, there were neither pongines nor hominids, only parental gibbons and generalized parental hominoids.

This makes a fine theoretical ancestry for us, but as far as fossils go it is nearly a void. The pongine lineage runs back through the dryopithecines to the early Miocene and beyond. On our own branch we find the australopithecines, far along in development and falling within the last few million years, although as structural ancestors they may easily be considered to represent a human stage going back at least into the Pliocene. (How times have changed since 1925, when Dart was getting his knuckles rapped for saying *Australopithecus* was different from the apes!) But we are only just beginning to see signs of anything ancestral to them.

Ramapithecus, an Earlier Hominid

This most important development is not the find of a new fossil; rather, it results from Dr. Simons' continuing demonstrations that it pays to beat up the dust in the parts of museums not open to visitors. The story is almost comic in its complications.

In 1934, among fossils freshly recovered from the Siwalik beds of India, Dr. G. E. Lewis of Yale described part of the upper jaw of an "ape" naming it *Ramapithecus brevirostris* (i.e., short-faced). He drew attention to the evidence of a short and upright face, a small canine tooth, and a parabolic or rounded dental arch. Both he and Gregory agreed that its characteristics were strongly hominid. However, this was as close to man as it got, for several reasons. In the first place, a different *lower* jaw was also assigned to *Ramapithecus* and this jaw contained a premolar tooth having the canine resemblance I spoke of earlier, a pongid trait. This seemed to exclude the fossil from the family Hominidae. Secondly, the date was taken to be late Pliocene, or even Pleistocene, which would be very recent for any primitive human ancestor. Thirdly, Dr. Hrdlička of the National Museum wrote in a sharply worded article that the hominid likenesses were an illusion and a mistake. Nevertheless, the human characteristics of the upper jaw continued to be alluded to, and to stick in people's minds, for almost thirty years.

Then Simons re-examined the fossil and satisfied himself that its hominid features were quite positive; in fact, he showed, it could not be restored into a whole arch to form anything except a short and rounded one, unacceptable as pongid. At almost the same time Leakey found other jaw pieces, almost identical in form, at a site called Fort Ternan in Kenya, which he named *Kenyapithecus*. These dated from the Lower Pliocene, not the Upper. But Lewis had also reviewed the date of the original specimen and found an error. This, like the African specimen, is doubtless early Pliocene.

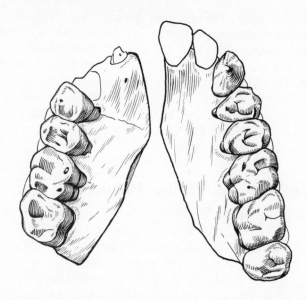

Ramapithecus: palate and teeth, after Simons, as represented by the original fragment from India (left) and *Kenyapithecus* from Africa, combined. Approximately natural size.

That was the point at which Simons began to raise the dust. Long before any of this, in the days when fossil apes were being named right and left, Pilgrim had described *Dryopithecus punjabicus,* also from the Siwaliks. This consisted of upper and lower jaw parts, not of the same individual, but having tooth traits which Pilgrim argued were strong evidence for associating them (that is, lower with upper). However, Lewis later described another fossil "ape" form, *Bramapithecus,* appropriating Pilgrim's *punjabicus* lower jaw for it along with several other mandibles which had turned up at Yale. In the last act, Simons examined the *punjabicus* upper jaw, and decided it was another specimen of *Ramapithecus.* That was the end of *Dryopithecus punjabicus.* Then, agreeing with Pilgrim's earlier logic, he once more associated the *Bramapithecus* mandibles with the upper jaws, as the lower jaws of *Ramapithecus.* Since *Bramapithecus* had consisted of lower jaws only in the first place, that was the end of *Bramapithecus.* Finally, picking Leakey's pocket, Simons added the African specimens to *Ramapithecus,* and that was the end of *Kenyapithecus.* (The species is now *Ramapithecus punjabicus,* since *punjabicus* was the first species name applied to any of the material included.) This is all a beautiful and logical simplification of valuable material which had been masquerading as assorted pongids. Simons has shown more or less conclusively that it all hangs together, that *Ramapithecus* must be excluded from the Pongidae, and that it should be accepted as an early Pliocene member of the hominid lineage, which thus had clearly become distinct from the dryopithecines before the Pliocene. Of course, there is no concrete evidence as to how *Ramapithecus* may have stood or walked, but the short face and front teeth imply that the hands had more work to do in feeding than they have in chimpanzees or gorillas.

Simons, under whose cool brown eye superfluous genera of apes dissolve, is none the less capable of venturesome suggestions. Noting that *Propliopithecus* of the Egyptian Oligocene seems to have lost its place as a very early pongid ancestor, because more definite pongids were already on the scene, he ventures this:

If *Propliopithecus*, with his generalized teeth, is not the ancestor of the big apes, of the gibbons, or of *Oreopithecus*, is he perhaps the Oligocene hominid?

The Brain Expands

To go back to the arboreal theory, there is one more aspect of it which is really the Hamlet of the piece. This is the brain. For, when all the niceties of hominid teeth and feet had been achieved, they had led to nothing more than *Australopithecus*. And, since he fell short of us in brain, the world is getting along without him very well. Our brain is not known to be different from his, but it is much bigger.

The secret lies in the huge cerebrum, the furrowed cerebral hemispheres, surfaced with gray matter; and also in the rise of the neopallium and the association areas. Now on our brains (or on a monkey's) it is fairly well known which parts of the shell or cortex relate to a given sense or muscular region—sight, hearing, arm, tongue—while there are large areas between these parts of which the exact function is very little known. However, they certainly have something to do with higher mental processes.

In the lowest vertebrates the cerebrum is only a small smooth pair of lobes at the forepart of the brain. From them project bulbs which receive sensations of smell, and the cerebrum itself also gets these and other sensations. The cerebrum was evidently first founded on the sense of smell, and most other functions and responses are left to lower parts of the brain. Reptiles have a more advanced cerebrum, and a small new patch on its surface, the neopallium. Not only does this begin to assume more sensory and motor functions, but it exists specifically as an area where associations connected with these can be built up. Here especially, emphasis can be transferred from reflex ac-

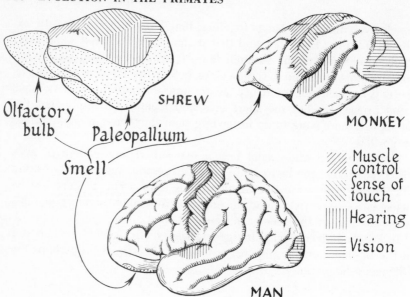

Olfactory
bulb
Smell
Paleopallium

SHREW

MONKEY

Muscle
control
Sense of
touch
Hearing
Vision

MAN

Brain increase, and expansion of the neopallium. Cerebral cortex, seen from the left side. In a primitive mammal (insectivorous shrew; not to be confused with the primate tree shrew) most of the cortex is related to smell (dotted area); the paleopallium is large and there is a prominent olfactory bulb in front to which the olfactory nerve leads from the nose. The neopallium, above, is still relatively small. In a monkey (macaque) the neopallium is greatly expanded, being all that is visible externally, and the olfactory areas are recessed under the forebrain. There are considerable association areas between those devoted to special senses. In man the brain is much larger still, and highly convoluted; association areas form a larger proportion of the cortex. The brains are not drawn to scale.

tion and simple conditioning toward "thinking," or at least the forming of patterns of action from stored associations. The mammals have expanded the neopallium greatly, and the whole cerebral cortex as well, so that it extends back over the other parts of the brain and increases its own surface area by being folded in upon itself, in convolutions.

The higher primates, and men above all, have carried these things to extremes. Evidently the association areas have greatly increased with the enlarging brain, since there has not been a corresponding growth of the primary centers. There is a vast capacity in which associations (memories, impressions, patterns of action) can be stored, so that successful past actions are consciously repeated (that is, they are not simply the result of conditioning), and even brand-new combinations can be formed mentally. To quote Wood Jones roughly, the original centers are those by which an animal sees things and does things, in the surrounding association areas it remembers what it has seen and done, and in other areas still it imagines what might be seen and done.

This is where the arboreal theory makes its contribution. The primate secret of success is arboreal life. This fostered, in the first place, an acute sense of vision and a free grasping hand. And this in turn opened a new field for natural selection in mentality. An ordinary mammal, without hands, however intelligent and successful it may be in its sphere, simply lacks this possible outlet. A snout, no matter how sensitive it is for feeling, smelling, and the like, is not much of an instrument, nor does it carry out many actions from which the eyes can profit. A true hand has a much greater range of movement, and it can open and shut, turn and twist, push and pull, all with far greater facility than teeth and jaws. And, with the addition of a pair of stereoscopic eyes watching and making notes on what the hand is doing, perhaps you can see how older limits to the usefulness of association areas become obsolete.

Finally, if the brain responds by expanding and improving, and so once more endows hand and eye with greater sensitivity and ability, then skill fosters wisdom and wisdom fosters skill. A sort of benign upward spiral comes into play. Here seems to be an adequate evolutionary explanation of the higher primates. And I should not neglect to mention my conviction that the social actions of monkeys and apes are also involved in this mental progress. For exhaustive observations of these animals in the wild have been revealing a complexity and subtlety of the coordination and interaction of individuals which seems like a truer expression of their obviously high intelligence than any rudimentary manipulation of "tools" or the solving of such external problems as they may face.

All this relates only to the development of the brain in the higher primates, the platform from which man took off. Explaining the great leap forward, the rapid expansion of man's own brain in less than two million years, is something else again. The internal capacity of the skull—the most serviceable measure of the size of the brain—in the large apes is about five hundred cubic centimeters. It is a little more in the Australopithecinae. In modern man it is nearly three times as much: about 1450 c.c. for male Europeans of the present day. (We vary as individuals somewhat, but this variation cannot be safely used as a sign of varying intelligence.) How did we achieve this awesome figure? Or why did the ape brain not become human?

In the first place, we should realize that although australopith brains were much of a size with those of living apes, they were probably organized rather differently. Apes have educated front teeth;

they are good nibblers with the incisors and strippers of bark with the canines; and they also do a good deal of investigating and manipulating with their projecting and mobile lips. And they grasp things readily with their feet; altogether, a chimpanzee's equipment for grasping and prying is distributed more broadly over his anatomy than is ours, and this is reflected in his brain. On the other hand, if we know any one thing about *Ramapithecus* it is that his face and his canines were short, and probably used much less like a chimp's. Certainly, at least by the arrival of the Australopithecinae with their small front teeth and their erect posture, manipulation must have become concentrated in the hands, as it is with us. And, since the actual shaping of stone tools began with what seems to have been an advanced australopithecine (see later), we are obliged to believe that, with brains no bigger than apes', the australopiths were already extensive and constant users of random tools of bone, wood and stone. Finally, while we shall never know what they sounded like, if we choose between supposing their sounds and communication were just like apes', or supposing that it was different and somewhat more like ours, we clearly must choose the latter. All this argument is merely by way of insisting that we cannot tell the behavior of the australopiths from their brain size.

We also do not know in what way a larger brain makes us more intelligent. But it clearly has done so. The explanation is not far to seek: natural selection. Given a super-australopithecine with completely developed legs and absolutely emancipated hands, the more skilled making and use of tools would make him an ever more efficient hunter, skinner, and shelter builder. So would the ability to talk, to teach, and to organize his social life better, for greater protection. Obviously, he had burst into a new field, a new environment, in which greater and more flexible intelligence was decidedly adaptive.

With the imperfectly erect posture and the imperfectly free hands of the pongids, their brains are doubtless as large as they can use in their forest life. Perhaps the main remaining question is why both chimpanzees and men seem to have an actual surplus of brain, under the circumstances. Chimpanzees in captivity, put to problems they would certainly never face in the forest, show astonishing abilities. And our own ancestors of a mere fifteen thousand years ago, quite like us in brain and body, were living lives far more primitive than what they certainly were capable of, wasting their intellectual sweetness in the air of a cave. Perhaps natural selection produces plenty of leeway. Perhaps our idea of what constitutes mentality is too naïve. At any rate, it is a useful and necessary thing in science to recognize when you are dealing with an exceptional case, and modern man can certainly be described as an exceptional case.

9. THE PLEISTOCENE:
AGE OF MAN

AFTER ALL that had gone before, modern man strode onto the stage almost abruptly. It took him, to be sure, perhaps a million years, which is the later part of the Pleistocene epoch. The man-apes had lasted into his time, having prepared the way with an upright hominid body, though hardly outdistancing the apes in brain. But in this next period there appeared a succession of true men, in whom brain size was carried all the way from that level to our own, in a threefold expansion. I call them "true men" here, but that is a loose expression. For, on the one hand, the australopiths were true hominids, and on the other the early "men" were, to begin with, certainly very different from ourselves.

In fact, it is somewhat difficult to say what a "true" man is, but all hominids after *Australopithecus* are now generally grouped in the single genus *Homo*. It is even difficult to make clear distinctions from *Australopithecus,* and differences in brain size between the two were not impressive to begin with. It is probably better to say that the new people had achieved a skeleton which cannot be distinguished from our own, as far as we know, and were all about as big in the body as we are. Also, they show a definite reduction in the size of the molar teeth compared to the australopiths, as well as a diminution of the jaw, and so eventually of the face. Certainly, their brains soon became larger. And they were making tools as far back as we can trace them and were surely beginning to speak, as well; we cannot tell if the man-apes had any ability at all to speak.

Onset of the Pleistocene

Wits may allege that speech was invented so that man might talk about the weather. If there could be any justification for such a foolish suggestion, it is that when language was being invented the weather was certainly something to talk about.

During the seventy-odd million years of the Tertiary, the earth's climate had been generally warm and stable, and for many million years before that it had been even warmer. Then began the Pleistocene, a new age of cooler and then of cold weather, marked at the end by major swings between glaciations and warm interglacials.

At its beginning, perhaps three and a half million years ago, there were earth movements and a deterioration in the Tertiary climate. An important group of new mammalian types made its appearance in Europe, Asia, and Africa. This fauna, known as the Villafranchian, included the modern horse genus, *Equus*, which contains horses, donkeys, and zebras but which is distinct from the late Pliocene horse genera such as its own true ancestor, *Pliohippus*, or the three-toed *Hipparion*. The fauna also included genera of the modern elephants and true cattle and, in parts of Asia, true camels. Each continent had its own varieties and local evolution of these, but taken altogether the Villafranchian animals are the identifiers of the long early part of the Pleistocene, which has also come to be referred to as the Villafranchian time phase in itself.

As a matter of fact, fossil animals have always been the best means for broad datings in the time scale. In the Tertiary, when the earth itself provides few clues as to actual period, the animals are absolutely necessary as a guide. The names of the epochs refer to them: Paleocene, ancient recent forms; Eocene, dawn of the recent forms; Oligocene, a few of the recent forms; Miocene, not many of the recent forms; Pliocene, a majority of the recent forms; Pleistocene, most recent forms; and Recent, the living animals of the short time since the Pleistocene. In the same way different periods within the Pleistocene have their characteristic arrays of animal life, which can be used to date the men found with them. This applies, for example, to the man-ape caves in South Africa, where the fairly constant climate makes dating an extremely difficult matter. A higher proportion of extinct species of mammals was found at Sterkfontein and Makapan than was present at Kromdraai and Swartkrans. This indicates, as does other evidence, that these last two deposits, the residences of *Paranthropus*, were later than the homes of *Australopithecus*.

Nor is this all the animals reveal, for they tell a good deal about the climate of the time. If you find the bones of a hippopotamus or a crocodile in a desert this leads you, like a trout in the milk, to suspect the presence of water, in times past, and even of broad rivers and savannas. The quantities of antelope in the man-ape caves assure us that the country roundabout was open, as it is now, and not forested. Animals that love cold or warmth betray the temperature. This can even be fixed rather closely by the finding of mollusk shells in former bays or riverbanks, since the water temperature in which the same varieties live today may be known. Other such inferences may be carried to considerable lengths.

The Ice Begins

Toward the end of the Villafranchian animal phase, the extremes of cold began. There were four of these, and during the last three the ice swelled into continental glaciers; not the kind of ice stream you can see today in Switzerland or Alaska, but enormous blankets like the great cake which now covers most of Greenland, a mile or more thick. Partly forming from fresh snow, and partly moving their grinding weight across the face of the map itself, these vast sheets came down over much of Europe and parts of Asia, and over Canada and the eastern United States, while smaller icecaps formed in the mountains further south. Pushed by the cold and ice, subarctic zones moved down toward the equator. In the tropics the weather was also disturbed, but just how rainy phases matched precipitation toward the poles has never been fully determined.

After each of the cold phases there was a reaction to higher temperatures, and to weather actually warmer than today's. So the Ice Age is to be looked on less as an era of cold than as one of long-term—and somewhat irregular—oscillations between warm and cool. During the three interglacial periods, in fact, the ice sheets melted away entirely, and animals typical of warm places roamed northern Europe and the British Isles. The Second Interglacial in particular seems to have been of great length, and there were moderate recessions within the glacial phases themselves.

Altogether there was at least as much time during the later Pleistocene when the climate was warm as when it was cold. The fourth and final cold phase was quite recent, and remnants of actual continental glaciers linger on in one or two parts of the world, to say nothing of the great ice bodies on Greenland and Antarctica, which may not have changed at all. Even now, the temperature is not as high as it was during the interglacials. No one can say whether climate has settled down to a happy medium, or whether there is more of the Ice Age still in store, after an interglacial period which we may only just have entered. The latter is not at all unlikely.

Nor is it known what caused the Ice Age. It was not the sign of a dying sun, or of the end of the world. It was too sudden a shift, relatively speaking, and besides there have been several other such short periods of glaciation, well back in the earlier life of the earth. While there may have been significant fluctuations in the heat arriving from the sun, the actual trigger was probably the known rise of mountains like the Alps, the Rockies, and the Himalayas, at the close of the Tertiary, to a degree causing a doubling of the average heights of the land surfaces of the continents. This not only produced greater areas of high altitude as cold spots, but also disarranged the pattern of winds and storm cycles moving around the world, and led to greater snowfall in strategic places. The shifts from cold to warm and back would need other causes. One hypothesis is this. As the cold progressed, the oceans of the world cooled off. Then ice choked the north polar sea, the Arctic Ocean, and its outlets. The main source of moisture for snow in the north was thus sealed off, and precipitation stopped. At that same time, while the Arctic Ocean got colder, the other oceans could warm up again from solar heat, unchilled by cold water coursing out of the polar sea. A warm period ensued, and the arctic ice melted; once again the free exchange of waters cooled the oceans generally, making possible the arrival of another glacial phase.

The causes of the Pleistocene glaciations are not important in the annals of mankind. The effects are. We know too little of the life of the times to say much about these effects on the human family itself, but we can judge from other animals. In the capture of the northern continents by sheets of ice, or by an arctic barrenness, species perished by the hundreds (probably including many of the anthropoid apes), so that today Africa is the one place where the large mammals continue to flourish in something like their Tertiary luxuriance. And as zones of climate moved back and forth, the animals adjusted to particular geographic zones must have been herded and driven and shoved around the face of the earth to an exceptional degree.

In addition, all this stimulation probably speeded up small-scale evolution and adaptation in the animals—nothing spectacular, but something like the development, in the Last Glacial phase, of a cold-suited woolly rhino from the usual type—since rapid changes in environment (mere tens of thousands of years, that is) would induce more rapid changes in adjustments of living species. Man himself must have been under the impact of these many things as well, not only from the rigors of nature as the ice drove him south or the warm weather led him north once more, but also because of his dependence to so great an extent on other animals for food.

Animals reflect climate. But the earth registered the effect of ice and water directly. Here the main event was the transfer of water onto the land by snow during the glacial phases, and its return to the sea during the interglacials. Masses of creeping ice scoured the landscape, making gravel out of rocks and mountains, and spreading it in river valleys, or leaving it as a breastwork, a moraine, to mark the

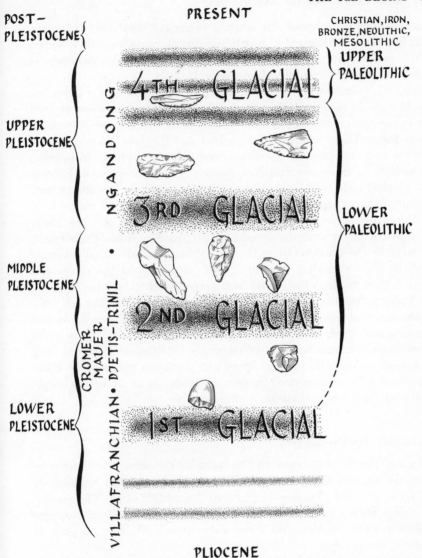

PRESENT

POST—
PLEISTOCENE

CHRISTIAN, IRON,
BRONZE, NEOLITHIC,
MESOLITHIC

UPPER
PALEOLITHIC

4TH GLACIAL

UPPER
PLEISTOCENE

3RD GLACIAL

LOWER
PALEOLITHIC

MIDDLE
PLEISTOCENE

2ND GLACIAL

LOWER
PLEISTOCENE

1ST GLACIAL

NGANDONG

CROMER MAUER DJETIS—TRINIL

VILLAFRANCHIAN

PLIOCENE

A graph of the later Pleistocene. Following the long period of the Villafranchian fauna, there were several minor glaciations followed by four major ones. These each had subdivisions, only those for the 4th Glacial being indicated. The divisions on the left (Lower, Middle, Upper) refer to animal life, and some of the most important faunas are also shown. On the right are archaeological periods, with some tool types suggested by sketches. The time scale is *not* correct: the Second Interglacial was much longer than shown, and the Villafranchian was perhaps twice as long as the entire chart.

glacier's furthest advance. In warmer regions it was rain, not snow, that fell. Big lakes formed in North America and in Africa, their shores a wonderful watering place for man and beast; and thousands of stone tools litter these old shores now.

The incorporation of so much water in the form of ice caused a world-wide lowering of the sea level. Ocean beaches were formed far below the present shore lines where, unfortunately, we cannot inspect them. Then, when the ice melted and the lake levels lowered, the sea rose, this time far above its present limits, so that old beaches lie as high as three hundred feet above those of the present. Indeed, the glaciers today still hold enough water to raise the oceans at least seventy-five, perhaps two hundred feet, if they should all melt.

As sea levels dropped in cold periods, the mouths and the lower channels of rivers were deepened by water rushing down them faster, because of the greater fall to the sea. When the tide of cold turned and the glaciers melted, the rising sea levels slowed the rivers and caused them to drop their sand and gravel in their own beds, silting up in deep deposits. When the cold came back and the seas fell once again, much of this gravel was washed away, but in places banks and terraces remained, as remnants of the old floor plains. Thus many rivers have terraced valleys, with terraces which can be traced long distances, and which can be assigned to a particular phase of the Pleistocene. Any bones contained in such a terrace are of its age, or older; anything lying on it must be younger.

Human Implements

In and about lake shores and terraces lie the stone implements of man, the imperishable remains of his poor worldly goods. No tools go back as far as the Pliocene, but toward the middle of the Pleistocene, at a few places associated with the Villafranchian animals, appear Oldowan tools, pebbles with a few flakes struck off along one side to make a sharp edge.

Trimming the pebble all round, and giving a point to one end, produced the hand-axe, a large, crude, but easily recognized tool, which reigned in Europe and Africa from the end of the First Interglacial onward. This was the beginning of the great Acheulian hand-axe tradition which continued on all the way into the Third Interglacial —longer in Africa—with its point and cutting edge improving by becoming flatter, better flaked, with a straighter and straighter outline. (It was accompanied by some crude flakes as well, and in the Far East it was never present, being replaced by single-edged choppers and chopping-tools.)

Only with the Third Interglacial and Fourth Glacial did new techniques of flaking and new ideas for tools appear. At last, in the middle of the Fourth Glaciation, this long Lower Paleolithic tradition ended, and the Upper Paleolithic of Europe saw the simpler tools replaced by skillfully made flake-blades and points, fashioned into a new variety of implements: knives, chisels, shavers, scrapers, spearheads. As we shall see, they were made by men of our own type. This way of life, with the Mesolithic following the Paleolithic after the departure of the ice, persisted for over 25,000 years, a hunting existence much the same as that of a few primitive peoples of our own time, until it gave way before the invention of agriculture, in the Neolithic.

This last was an important moment. It was not civilization, but it was a prerequisite for civilization, and in fact the vast majority of the so-called primitive peoples of today are "Neolithic" farmers—American Indians, Africans, Melanesians. But the Neolithic, and the succeeding civilizations, fall within the last ten thousand years. And so man lived as a really primitive hunter and gatherer of wild fruits and vegetables for all but about one per cent of his known existence, that is, a fraction of one per cent of the whole of time since the beginning of the Pleistocene. In fact, the high-level hunters of the Upper Paleolithic appeared something less than forty thousand years back, and so well over ninety per cent of man's tool-using past was acted out on an even lowlier plane. Although the hand-axes of the full Acheulian development are well-made and handsome tools, the striking fact is the exceedingly slow development of such tools in the long Lower Paleolithic, and the making of them according to a very limited number of ideas.

Human culture has been picking up speed for as long as we can see it, and one cannot escape the conclusion that the early slowness is because the man in the Lower Paleolithic street was still an underbrained beast. And also, that the using of naturally sharp rocks as cutting implements, which culminated in the appearance of the first recognizable pebble tools, must have gone on for a long while at the hands of very primitive men, quite surely still at the australopithecine stage.

Dart thinks the man-apes used animal jaws, still lined with their teeth, as cutting implements, and we cannot be certain they did not make pebble tools. And Leakey has pointed out what cutting tools, however simple, must have meant to such creatures, whether man or man-ape. It is one thing to catch and kill a meat-bearing animal. If you have blunt, short canines, small front teeth, and no claws, it is quite another thing to eat it. The animal is enclosed in skin—tough, living leather—and opening it up demands something sharper and stronger than your natural equipment. You have no idea, until you have tried, how helpful even a crude flint tool can be in such butchering.

His stone implements, then, are immensely important evidence of man—of human action and of human history. Being indestructible, they survive for us to find, unlike bones, all of which eventually vanish unless, by fortunate circumstances, they become mineralized (fossilized) and thus turn to "stone" themselves. Such a great deal may be learned from stone tools that it is easy to try to learn too much, and it is important to understand what they are and what they are not.

They are not fossils, because they do not obey the same laws of evolution as living animals. Therefore they cannot be used for dating in the same way, since very crude, and seemingly early, kinds of tools may persist among much more advanced forms. In the same way, they will not identify the men who made them. Tools are the product of ideas, and the same idea may be housed in quite different human heads. Furthermore, we still have no safe notion of who the first toolmaker was, nor of the general size of his brain, though evidently this might take us back most, or all, of the distance to the man-apes. But in spite of so much caution, a full knowledge of stonework can give powerful contributing evidence of age. In the later stages when tools had become complex—and rather definite assemblages can be recognized—they can give fairly reliable direct evidence of age as well. We shall note this later, in the case of Rhodesian Man.

Fixing the Date

And every possible scrap of such evidence is welcome and necessary, for dating the past is a fantastically intricate business. It looks dressy enough in a textbook or a diagram, with neat successions of climate phases, replacements of animals, advancements of tools. But, as Broom once said, the fossils are not found with labels on them. Imagine yourself in the middle of nowhere, having had the luck to find evidence of man (a bone, a tool, a piece of charcoal) in the side of a gully. If your eye is trained, perhaps you can discern the deposit in which you have found it and recognize it as glacial gravel, or an old lake bed, or a layer of wind-blown sand. If your eye is the ordinary hominid orb, you will discern almost nothing. But let it be trained. You will then need to examine the whole locality, to see how much of a sequence is present and where, if anywhere, some kind of a connection may be made with the known history of the Pleistocene.

Very likely you will fail and will have to turn to the animal evidence. (I am giving you all the best of it; there may not be any.) You collect from the deposit some fragmentary and badly preserved bones; you take them home and study them with the aid of an expert paleontologist, determining which species they belong to. Then you try to decide whether your bones constitute a little gobbet of a well-known fauna of that part of the world, of which the date has been more or less established.

Sometimes you will be better off, making your find within a long series of deposits which cannot be mistaken for general age. Sometimes you will be worse off. The fact is that the scholars are only now filling in the history of the animal nations of the Ice Age. And they are still trying to find perfectly definite connections between glacial events on one hand and pluvial events on the other: between gravel sheets laid down by ice-fed streams in the cold parts of the world, and shore lines made by rain-fed lakes in the tropics.

All this uncertainty (and hard work) could be avoided if it were possible to write down absolute dates, in years, for human remains. To a slight extent this can be done. In parts of the New World one may use the science of dendrochronology, noting the pattern of dry and wet years recorded in some places by growth rings in trees, cut long ago for houses. But this carries back only to the time of Christ, and in the Old World written history itself goes back much further. In Scandinavia and New England one may also count years in varved clays, "varves" being the yearly zones of silt formed on lake beds from the summer melting of glaciers. But this again goes only back to the decline of the last glacier, a few thousand years of no visible significance in the evolution of our physical bodies.

Fortunately, there have been developed two ways of estimating larger amounts of actual time, in different zones in the past, which depend on radioactivity. One of these is the potassium-argon, or K-A, method. Radioactive potassium-40 decays at a constant rate into the gas argon-40 and calcium-40, and the relative amounts of potassium and argon may be compared. Now, if rock is heated very hot, as in lava or a volcanic explosion, any argon in it is driven off, and on cooling it gets a fresh start at accumulating argon. The method calls for locating places where such rock came to rest in association with animals or sediments to be dated, as it has at Olduvai Gorge. The technique measures broadly for very great ages in the past down to perhaps a quarter of a million years (and possibly much closer), and it is thus that Pleistocene beginnings, once thought to be only a million years back, have lately been shown to be about three times that. Relatively few dates have yet been found by K-A, but they have been very helpful. The age of the early examples of *Homo* are now known to be about 1,000,000 years old, that of "Zinjanthropus" to be about 1.75 million years, and the Kanapoi fragment over 2.6 million. It is worth mentioning that the "Zinjanthropus" date has been well supported by a still newer method, called "fission-track dating," in which the number of tracks in a glassy or crystalline rock caused by spontaneous fission of uranium-238 is the indicator of age. Thus there is growing confidence that the total length of the Pleistocene is indeed at least 3,000,000 years.

The second method covers a much shorter and more recent zone in time, running down to the present and giving rather precise dates when well handled. This is the method of Carbon 14. Carbon is an essential constituent of life, and C14 is a radioactive form of carbon. Like other unstable radioactive elements, it tends to lose an electron from its atom, which then becomes an atom of nitrogen. Radiocarbon, or C14, has a "half life" of 5760 years. This means that, of any amount existing now, half will have decayed at the end of 5760 years, another quarter at the end of double that, another eighth at the end of another such period, and so on, the remainder becoming infinitesimally small. However, C14 is continually recreated in the upper atmosphere by cosmic rays, which cause neutrons to strike nitrogen atoms and make them into radioactive carbon; thus C14 is created anew until it is checked by its own rate of decay, so that a small and fairly constant part of the carbon in the atmosphere is the radioactive form.

This same small proportion enters into the composition of living plants and animals. All have C14, but at death the taking-on process stops and it begins to return to the atmosphere at a known rate. Suppose a living thing dies, but without destruction of its carbon (as when wood or bone burns and becomes charcoal). The ordinary carbon remains, but the radiocarbon begins to disappear. It is measured with great care, in an arrangement of Geiger counters. If you find that just half of the normal amount of C14 remains, you have evidence that just about 5760 years have gone by since that tree or animal died. And any other amount of C14 similarly points to some other actual count of years, an actual date. The residue eventually gets so close to zero that it cannot be measured, but advanced methods of reading small amounts have been reaching back toward an age range beyond 50,000 years.

The F Test and Galley Hill Man

The span of Carbon 14 fortunately embraces all the complicated part of recent human history, but this is only a small fraction of the Pleistocene as a whole. The K-A test is more approximate, and cannot be applied to every find, but only when the right rocks are present. However, it is not essential to have absolute dates for all of the ancient men, but merely to know where they stood in time relative to each other and to the scheme as a whole. For this you need two things: evidence that the deposit concerned belongs to such and such a phase of the Pleistocene; and assurance that your fossil actually comes from that deposit. This last is not a minor point.

There is now at least one chemical method for shedding light on both these matters: the fluorine test. It rests on the fact that the mineral matter of bone has the faculty of picking up the element fluorine from ground water, extremely slowly but rather steadily, so that the fluorine in a fossil may rise from a minute amount in living bone to something more than two per cent in a bone from the Middle Pleistocene.

This must not be confused with either of the radioactivity tests, for, while they furnish an actual clock, the F test is not a true time scale at all. Fluorine can be taken up by a bone only if fluorine is present in the ground water, and the taking-up may be more rapid in some places than others. The really important point is this: any given fossil should have virtually the same proportion of fluorine in its composition as that of other bones lying near it in a deposit, if in fact it has been in that deposit for the same length of time as they. Nevertheless, the test does give evidence of great or small age in a most general way; just remember that it is no clock.

See what this chemical Sherlock Holmes did in its most famous case, that of the man of Galley Hill. A skeleton, of the type of *Homo sapiens* (modern man), was found in gravels of the hundred-foot terrace of the Thames. Let me translate. This particular terrace has its old flood plain a hundred feet above the present river, and its gravels were laid down as the Thames rose during the Second Interglacial period. Therefore the skeleton gave evidence that our own fully modern type of man had already come into existence well back in Pleistocene time.

This is a venerable problem and a most important one which, as we shall see later, is not yet completely resolved. In the second half of the nineteenth century, modern-looking bones had several times been found, under circumstances indicating that they belonged far down in the Pleistocene. This seemed, on the face of it, unlikely, and in fact the evidence of age soon proved dubious in one case after another. But the Galley Hill skeleton looked better. It lay eight feet below the surface of the gravel terrace (too deep, apparently, for a grave). A workman digging gravel, Jack Allsop, exposed it in 1888. He had been collecting stone tools from the gravels for some time on behalf of a Mr. Elliott, a printer and amateur antiquarian. Therefore both of them were experienced at this kind of thing, and both reported that the levels of gravel overlying the skeleton had not been disturbed after the stream had laid them down.

That is to say, the signs were against a grave having been cut through the gravels from above, and in favor of a body having been actually covered by river silt during Second Interglacial times. Another amateur, a schoolmaster named Heys, came along just as the skeleton had been discovered. He also was a collector, but he did not know about Elliott. He rushed away to find a photographer to record the find in the ground, and while he was off on this praiseworthy mission Elliott and Allsop took the bones out. Heys returned, found the dead man gone, suffered a broken heart, and had nothing more to do with the matter until Sir Arthur Keith wrote to him twenty-two years later. Then he gave the same report as the other men.

By now, well on in the twentieth century, the Galley Hill find had assumed crucial importance as the only strong case for the great antiquity of modern man. Other osseous witnesses had collapsed. And many anthropologists refused to believe that the Galley Hill case was airtight. Finding a complete skeleton was almost too good; the running water should have dispersed it, as with all other fossil remains in the vicinity. But Keith now championed it and even discerned certain special points of primitiveness in it (a thick skull, rather heavy brows, a shallower notch atop the mandible's upright part) which would sit well with a vast age. Keith later lost some of his enthusiasm. The poor Galley Hill Man continued on and on in quarantine, his enemies not knowing quite how to give him the quietus and his friends mainly of the fair-weather variety, not quite daring to clasp him strongly to their bosoms.

Then in the sixtieth summer of his resurrection he met disaster. The skeleton was optioned (from its private owner) for examination in 1948, by Dr. Ashley Montagu, who was quite unable to confirm Keith's old marks of primitive status: evidently Keith had overpersuaded himself somewhat. At the same time the F test was applied by Dr. Kenneth Oakley of the British Museum (Natural History), who had lately revived and developed it from the work of earlier experimenters. And Galley Hill Man flunked the test.

Various other fossil animal bones taken from the hundred-foot terrace were shown to have approximately two per cent of fluorine. Bones from the lower, later, fifty-foot terrace yielded figures in the neighborhood of one per cent. But testings from the Galley Hill bones themselves gave only about half of one per cent. This means that the bones cannot claim association with the honest fossils of the hundred-foot terrace; they cannot be of really great age. Later tests have shown that the skeleton is actually rather recent (about 1360 B.C.). But it was the F test which showed that the Galley Hill skeleton was a skeleton fit only for inhabiting closets. This was a momentous conclusion, because it threw out of court once and for all the single remaining claim of Middle Pleistocene antiquity for a specimen of a man who was certainly of the modern variety.

We have now entered the second century of knowledge of fossil men. We are no longer caught up in a riot of confusion by single discoveries, as happened when the Neanderthal Man was found in 1856, or the Java Man in 1891, or the Piltdown remains in 1912. A general framework of undeniable fact and understanding has been put together, and today a new find fills a gap, or sharpens knowledge, or rechannels ideas somewhat, instead of detonating an explosion of wild guesses and violent controversy.

I say this hopefully. I do not think we shall ever see that kind of day again. We have passed gradually out of the kindergarten. And yet I cannot overemphasize how dimly we actually see what we are peering at. We see through a glass, darkly, not face to face; we are like a blind man who is just beginning to find his way pretty well around a house which, a century ago, he did not know was there. Pleistocene dating and the history of human stonecraft are both complicated subjects, but at least the gravels and the stone tools lie before us in great quantity. Not so the human bones, which are preserved very irregularly, and found only by the best of luck.

Fossil Hazards

It is not easy to become a fossil. If a creature dies, its bones may be promptly eaten and digested by hyenas or other animals. Otherwise they will lie on the ground and decay in a few years. They will not last much longer if they are buried in the earth. But if a carnivore drags the bones into a cave, like those in South Africa, where they become impregnated with hard and insoluble mineral salts, or if they fall into a swamp or a lake bed or some other place where they may last a long time until minerals have a chance to replace or join the material of the bone, then you have a fossil. All this counts against fossils of early man. For he was probably a rare animal in the first place and also, on the whole, too clever to fall into swamps or get eaten by a carnivore.

That is only the beginning: a fossil may be destroyed again in the ground by a change in the soil chemistry. For example, the gravels at that particular spot at Galley Hill actually contained no fossils other than the skeleton. Any true fossils had evidently been leached out by acid in the ground, and so if the Galley Hill Man had been really old he should not have been there at all. Forests likewise have acid soils and hold little prospect for fossils, even though ancient stone tools may abound in them. Therefore, whole areas and whole periods, in which we know men were present, are devoid of human bones. We cannot tell what sort of men they were. There is nothing we can do about it but hope.

I began this chapter by talking about the emergence of actual men. For a long time this was the very area in which the lack of fossils and the ignorance of dates was particularly baffling. We knew that the apes were evolving steadily in the late Tertiary, because of the many fossils of *Dryopithecus*. But hominids were not to be seen until Simons showed the real meaning of *Ramapithecus*, and Leakey, at Fort Ternan, produced evidence of the existence of the same ancestor in Kenya. We were aware of the nature of the next hominid stage, in the australopithecines of South Africa. But South Africa is a cul-de-sac, and the richness of the man-ape finds was due to the presence of limestone caves, which were fine fossil traps. We could hardly concentrate on South Africa as the actual scene of man's origin. Then Leakey produced "Zinjanthropus" and showed what everyone suspected: that the australopithecines must have lived widely in the Old World. (A few unsatisfactory finds strongly suggest their presence elsewhere in Africa and Asia.)

Leakey has also lately found much more than the remains of "Zinjanthropus"; the Gorge has yielded a whole group of specimens already celebrated under the name of *Homo habilis*. There has been much controversy over him; let us come back to *Homo habilis* after looking over some men who are better known.

10. JAVA MAN

HERE IS the greatest story of serene confidence I have ever heard. The confidence belonged to Eugene Dubois, who at nineteen began to specialize in anatomy and natural history at the University of Amsterdam in 1877, under such men as Hugo de Vries and Max Fürbringer. A few years later, starting a promising career in teaching as Professor Fürbringer's assistant, he became engrossed with the notion of finding a really primitive and ape-like fossil of man, and he concluded that the East Indies might be the place to search for it.

He tried to get the Netherlands government to give him an expedition. But if you were a Hollander whose official business it was to disburse money on the prospect of finding a purely imaginary creature in the vast islands of the Indies, just because a young professor's-assistant asserted that it would be a likely place to look, you could have but one answer, and that would be "No."

The dauntless Dubois, however, sought and was given a post as army surgeon in the colonial service in the Netherlands Indies. He told his associates in so many words that he was going out to find the missing link and, to their dismay, resigned his Amsterdam appointments. Professor Fürbringer shrugged his shoulders and muttered to another of his assistants: "Hans im Glück." He was thinking of silly Hans, in Grimm's fairy tale, who kept exchanging the thing he owned for something of less worth, until he ended with nothing. But Dubois gave up his nice little job and made one of the greatest discoveries in all the past of man.

He was not being quite as woolly-headed as he seemed. True, a main source of his excitement was the German naturalist Haeckel, who had drawn up a provisional ancestry for man and had put in, as the latest ancestor, a phantasmic missing link for whom he had selected the designation *Pithecanthropus alalus* (Speechless Ape-man). The zoologists have since passed a law against giving Linnaean names to dream creatures. You now must have an actual animal or part of one, and you must provide a description, along with your proposed name, to show wherein it differs from its closest relatives and thus deserves a name of its own. True also, Dubois' project called for twice the assurance of Columbus and for at least as much perseverance, and as much luck, as the man who finds a needle in a haystack.

Nevertheless, Dubois' ideas were clear in his mind, and he wrote them down in an article. He followed Darwin's suggestion that man had probably lost his hairy covering in a hot country. He accepted Wallace's belief that looking for early human remains should be done where apes still lived today. He noted Virchow's remark that vast regions, particularly in the tropics, were totally unknown as far as fossils went. Furthermore, Dubois was aware that suggestive animal remains were coming to light in northern India and that there were caves in Central Sumatra which might also yield the object he was after. So, for the knowledge of the time, he was adding things up pretty well. He had the determination. And he certainly had the luck.

Dubois and Pithecanthropus

He took himself to Sumatra and began poking around in caves in his free time. When the authorities grasped his purpose they freed him for research, and he went at it in earnest. But his only finds were orang teeth, with certain other fossils, which convinced him that the cave material was too recent. At any rate, no men. Here luck made her first entrance: a Mr. van Rietschoten found a fossilized skull at Wadjak in neighboring Java. It was passed on by the Royal Society in Batavia to Dubois, who got permission to include Java in his territory. He went to Wadjak and found another of the same sort himself! They were interesting and like the living natives of Australia in appearance. But they were no missing links—not what he was seeking.

Three years had now gone by, but at last, working in Central Java, he came across a small piece of a human jaw, late in 1890. The next year he found a promising place in the bank of the Solo River, near the small village of Trinil, where a fossil-bearing bed lies close to the present level of the water. In the course of one month he exposed a few ape-like teeth, and then the treasure he was looking for: a brain pan (the top and part of the sides and back of the skull) too large to be that of an ape and too small to be that of a man, but just exactly right to be an "Übergangsform," a "missing link." The next year, forty-five feet away but in precisely the same level, he brought to light the femur, or thighbone, of a man. In 1894 he published a full description of the Java Man. Borrowing Haeckel's old name, he christened him *Pithecanthropus erectus* and put him in a new family, Pithecanthropidae, between the Pongidae and the Hominidae (because he felt the skull so crude as to be still subhuman). Apart from this last gesture, his diagnosis is the one which still prevails, of an upright, human walker with a very primitive cranium. The whole thing was a brilliant feat and an astonishing triumph.

It was, for obvious reasons, a sensation in Europe. The first really primitive kind of man, the being so long talked about in the abstract, had suddenly appeared, if not in the flesh, at least in the bone. And yet his reception was not a glad ovation but a fierce controversy, and indeed during the next forty years *Pithecanthropus* underwent some embarrassing moments. In 1896, Dubois himself assembled the opinions of nineteen other authorities on the find: five of them thought the skull to be an anthropoid ape, seven thought it human, and seven considered it intermediate. To the anti-evolutionists, of course, the whole thing was an illusion, and even those who were willing to gaze upon it at all were able to find at least fifteen grounds on which to quarrel. Some said the skull was that of an idiot, others that it was normal. Some said it was human; others said it was a monkey, a chimpanzee, or a gibbon. The Java Man could speak. The Java Man could not speak. Perhaps the sorest question was whether the skull and the leg bone were actually parts of the same creature, because of the apparently more "human" status of the leg, because of differences in the amount of abrasion the two bones had undergone, and because they were separated, when found, by a distance of forty-five feet.

And *Pithecanthropus* was not the only sufferer. In a strange way, as von Koenigswald has put it, the Java Man became Dubois' own fate. The two brought glory to one another, and then sorrow. Dubois began to feel an identity with the fossil. Its detractors were his own enemies; his anthropological colleagues all became suspect, and Dubois was not at home to them any longer. And at last he withdrew the bones from scientific contact. He took them to his house at Zijlweg 77, Haarlem; he put them in a box; he took up his dining-room floor and buried the box in the ground below it; he put back boards, liner, and carpet; and he ate his meals above the Java Man for many long years. Jealous adversaries, he had come to think, might even steal the precious fossils. For all these years, too, he kept the Wadjak skulls in a glass case, but with newspaper pasted to the inside of the glass, so that the skulls could not see out, and nobody else could see in. Only in the 1920's did he relent and expose the Wadjak crania to science. Later still, he was persuaded to put the remains of *Pithecanthropus* in the museum at Leiden, in a small safe inside a larger safe.

In the meanwhile the original controversy had died away, and Dubois' first judgment had come to be broadly accepted. One voice alone now cried that the Java Man was no near-man at all, but a super-gibbon whose principal occupation was walking about in the trees. A big-brained gibbon, said the voice, whose leg bone showed lines of stress which meant that it was not used like a man's. And here it was that *Pithecanthropus* felt the unkindest cut of all. For the voice was that of Dr. Dubois himself.

This was a strange thing. Dubois, steadfast while others argued, began to vacillate when everyone agreed with him. Shortly after restoring Java Man to society, Dubois changed opinion of his status, making him more human. But he changed again and came to the belief that his beloved fossil was not a sub-man but a super-ape, supporting his bizarre argument by several new fragments of femurs which had turned up in collections made in the year 1900 and also by ingenious hypotheses regarding evolution which found no favor among his colleagues. He changed his mind one last time, admitting a mistake in interpreting the stress lines on the femur, but by now confusion was complete.

Dubois died during the last war, to be forever honored for his brilliance and energy in finding Java Man. Before this time the fossil had been vindicated, and its place was more important than ever. The ancient uproar had been replaced by a peace of unanimity wherein the rest of the world watched apathetically while the elder Dubois broke lances against the younger. At last, any doubts about the association of skull and leg bone (and after all, it had never been necessary to suppose they had come from the same individual, but only from the same kind of being) vanished when the fluorine test eventually showed the femurs and the skull to be of the same—considerable—age.

But for forty years no more of the Java Man had ever come to light. A mighty expedition went out from the Academy of Science in Berlin in 1907 to the Solo River, where it dug hard and systematically; according to von Koenigswald, the scene of its labors is still readily detected by the litter of broken beer bottles. The one result was a collection of mammalian fossils to define the "Trinil fauna"; Dubois' own collections had left much to be desired for exactness. But not a sign of *Pithecanthropus* did it discover, which only goes to emphasize how much Dubois, like Broom, was luck's companion.

Von Koenigswald and More Skulls

When at last Java yielded more pieces of her ape-man, this was due almost entirely to the persistence and the intelligent organization of a newly appeared paleontologist, G. H. R. von Koenigswald. He worked for the Geological Survey of the islands, lost his job in 1935 but made a comeback in 1937, and served as a paleontologist till 1948. He spotted a most likely area in Central Java for useful fossils in 1935, and taught local villagers to collect and keep fossil remains as they washed out of the ground. These he purchased, necessarily at a very low rate per piece. For to get occasional significant pieces, he had to buy vast numbers of unimportant ones, as well as a great deal of plain trash. Just as things were going well, however, he found himself out of a job. He was rescued and sustained by the Carnegie Institution of Washington, when he wrote and described the promising prospects of his work, supported by Father Teilhard de Chardin.

Actually the first new find came by another route. Geological mapping near Surabaya in eastern Java had just disclosed a new layer of the Pleistocene, with a new fauna, the Djetis, older than the Trinil fauna, when an Indonesian collector of the Survey discovered the brain case of a human infant within this same layer, at Modjokerto. Here, because of its youth, was the problem of Dart's young skull from Taung all over again: what did its father look like? Although it was more ancient than Dubois' find, von Koenigswald concluded it must be a *Pithecanthropus*. But he gave it a different name, *Homo modjokertensis*, simply to avoid a wrangle with the elderly Dubois and his imaginary giant gibbon. The maneuver was only partly successful.

This was in 1936. And then von Koenigswald's preparations began to pay off. In 1937 from his most important new locality, Sangiran in Central Java, and apparently from the Djetis bed, came a lower jaw, long, strong, and primitive. Then at last a skull, in pieces. Von Koenigswald himself found one part, and the natives found others. They had begun to appreciate a good thing, and they appreciated their piecework very well; they broke the pieces they found into still smaller pieces, until there were forty of them to be bought and paid for—at ten cents a piece. But the harm was small, financial and otherwise; the breaks of nature and of art were easily repaired. Here was a skull, still baseless and faceless, but much more perfect than the first and almostly exactly like it. Certainly on the night of the great find, forty-six years after Trinil, von Koenigswald decided it was time to pass around rice and salt and have a party, complete with gamelan orchestra and the local dancing girls.

Late in the next year another skull top turned up, that of a young person, and less complete. It was like the first two in shape and came, like them, from the Trinil zone. And in January 1939, this time from the earlier Djetis zone, came the first upper jaw, just as von Koenigswald was going to pay a visit to the laboratory of Dr. Weidenreich in Pekin, where the specimens of Pekin Man were being studied. These two men looked the new fragment over and saw signs of recent breakage. Von Koenigswald sent a message to his collector to search carefully at the place where the jaw had come from, and sure enough the major portions of the back of the skull were discovered, showing signs that the head had been shattered by a heavy blow at or about the time of death. This heavier, cruder individual seems to supply the missing father of the Modjokerto baby.

More than twenty years went by before Indonesian scientists recovered more parts, again at Sangiran and apparently dating from the Trinil zone. A jaw was found in 1962, and then the left side and back of a skull in 1963, with a few face parts which may belong to the same person. A further skull came to light in 1965. It will of course be several years before the new finds can be studied as fully as the earlier ones.

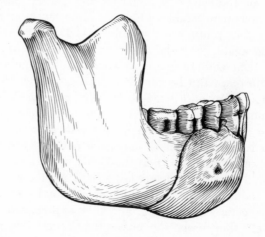

Meganthropus jaw, as restored by von Koenigswald from all specimens. Courtesy of Professor von Koenigswald. Approximately ½ natural size.

Before war interrupted his work, von Koenigswald found a lower jaw fragment in the Djetis zone which was heavier and thicker than any which could be assigned to Java Man, and another such specimen was discovered in 1952. Von Koenigswald named the creature *Meganthropus*. Weidenreich believed it to be a giant form of early man and it was long something of a puzzle. Von Koenigswald has now made a new reconstruction of the jaw, based on all the known parts, and he believes, with Robinson, that it is an australopithecine. We will consider it later.

As to Java Man himself, his several skulls together with a number of jaw pieces, large and small, tell us a good deal. They say the Java

Man was no ape, no freak, no imbecile, but a brutish early human being, and indeed a "hominine" (meaning above the australopithecine level). They say Dubois was right the first time, as von Koenigswald finally tried to suggest to the old man without success. There is some difference, in other words, between an isolated fossil, and a creature known from several individuals, so that one can be certain of the average or typical form. The moral? Do not try to make an ape out of *Pithecanthropus*, or *Pithecanthropus* may make a monkey out of you.

The Nature of Java Man

This most ancient man was about the same size as ourselves, judging from his thighbones. These bones cannot really be distinguished from our own, Dubois to the contrary; and to try finding signs of special primitiveness is probably to run the risk of being fooled, as Keith was fooled by Galley Hill. There is really nothing more to be said. There used to be serious discussion as to whether Java Man was really erect, but now that we know about the australopithecines, we should be more than surprised if he were anything else. His femur shows he walked upright, and his head shows the same, by the position of its base and of the *foramen magnum*.

Nevertheless his neck was stout and strong, with its muscles spread well across and up the back of his skull. And no wonder, for they had work to do. The skull itself was tremendously heavy and thick, in contrast to the australopithecines; and the still-large face and jaw threw the skull forward, much further off balance than in our own head. The jaws, generous in size, contained the largest teeth yet found in the skull of any kind of "man" above the level of the man-apes, and still these teeth were not crowded together but often had slight spaces between them. The dentition was rather more like ours than in the man-apes; the molars were not of such exaggerated size, nor were the incisors by contrast so greatly reduced. And, while the lower molars grew steadily larger from the first to the wisdom tooth (a primitive trait), in the upper jaw the last molar had become relatively diminished in size, as it has in us but not in the australopiths. In the latter, the upper molar size in order is three, two, one; in us it is one, two, three; in *Pithecanthropus* it was two, one, three.

To everyone's astonishment, the front of the upper jaw revealed a diastema, a gap between the canine and incisors like that into which an ape's lower canine fits when he shuts his mouth. It is no illusion—the diastema is the size of an orang's and was found in two different specimens. Java Man is the one and only hominid with such a gap;

none of the australopithecines displayed this mark of the beast, nor did our strange little relative from the Italian Pliocene, *Oreopithecus*.

If this feature of *Pithecanthropus* had been known in the old days much would have been made of its ape-like appearance. But now we had better be restrained. Java Man cannot possibly be closely related to pongid apes, and his canine teeth, though not dainty, are not the strongly projecting kind which need such an open space. Probably he had the space because of the generally broad front of his face and the open nature of his forward tooth row. These are traits in which he is in extreme contrast with the man-apes, whose dental arches were compact forward and much enlarged behind. Probably, also, the gap was a property of males—a sex difference—since some of the pithecanthropi had it and some did not.

Java Man's face was fairly projecting, as the above might suggest, although his lower jaw was long, rather than deep, with its more human, smaller, molar teeth. He could probably chew better than he did most things, for his brain was very small. Its size can only be estimated, since all the skulls were more or less broken. The first (found by Dubois) has been figured to have a volume of 900 cubic centimeters or more; the second 775, possibly less; and the 1963 skull 975, so that the Trinil population averages about 880. The 1939 Djetis skull, however, massive as it is, according to a new restoration made by von Koenigswald enclosed a mere 750 cc. If this be evolution, make the most of it. These figures may be compared with apes at some 500, australopiths at perhaps a little more, and European males

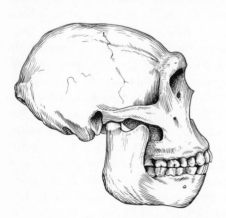 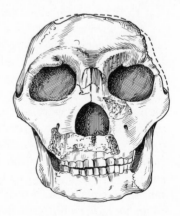

Left: Java Man, from the Djetis zone. From a restoration by von Koenigswald, based on skull IV and mandible B. Courtesy of Professor von Koenigswald. Right, the Lantian skull from Shensi, China (see page 174). ¼ natural size.

today with 1450. That is to say, Java Man at his lowest may have had about 200 cubic centimeters more than an australopithecine, while at his highest he was still some 500 below ourselves. Housed above a long face and a long platform for neck muscles at the rear, this meager tissue of intellect made a poor job of filling out the skull. The skull was widest just above the ears and sloped rapidly in toward a low peak or ridge, leaving no forehead behind the beetling bony brows.

The Age of Java Man

So Java Man was the earliest of humankind—barring the man-apes—about whom we have satisfactory knowledge. And he looks it. We are beginning to know something about his dates, which show that the time span of the known fossils was long, long enough for some evolution to have taken place in his family. His oldest remains were from the beds of the Djetis fauna, and his later (actually the first to be found) from the Trinil zone immediately above. The most recently suggested date (from K-A dating) is about 710,000 years for the *youngest* fossils. The Trinil beds are definitely Middle Pleistocene, and probably correspond to the Second Glacial phase of the north. The Djetis zone is more of a problem: most call it earliest Middle Pleistocene while von Koenigswald thinks it is latest Villafranchian. (Oakley calls this a "paleontologists' battle zone" and sometimes the paleontologists are arguing simply about the animals, not the time period involved.) In any case, the Djetis zone probably corresponds to some part of the First Interglacial of the north, and to lowest part of Bed II at Olduvai Gorge. This suggests that the time span of Java Man as we know him was about 1,000,000 to about 700,000 B.C.

Support for this comes from the fact that the earliest Java men may have coexisted with the australopithecine *Meganthropus*. If this was a *Paranthropus*, as Robinson holds, then we have a repetition of what occurred also in East Africa and South Africa, where *Paranthropus* and more advanced forms surely were present at the same time.

It was Dr. Weidenreich who first claimed that some evolution could be seen here: that the exceptionally thick, low, and heavy skull (number IV, he of the split brain case) from the earlier Djetis level was distinctly more primitive than the other three adult skulls, all of which came from the later Trinil beds. His judgment is being vindicated, in several ways. The time span, we have seen, was longer than we once thought. Von Koenigswald's new restoration of the Djetis skull is even more primitive than Weidenreich's. And just as von Koenigswald finished this restoration, photographs were published of the Lantian skull from China (next chapter). The two are much alike, and are thought to be of the same age. More of this later.

The Solo Cannibals

Pithecanthropus, Meganthropus, and the almost modern Wadjak men were not the only interesting fossils from the opulent island of Java. Above the Trinil beds in many places, and of much later age, lies another set of beds, with another set of animals, the Ngandong fauna. So there is a series: Djetis, Trinil, Ngandong, which is basic to the dating of the Pleistocene of Java.

The discovery of the last fauna came in a great stroke of good fortune. A member of the Geological Survey, ter Haar by name, had lately made his quarters in the village of Ngandong, on the banks of the same Solo River and only six miles from Trinil. One evening he had stepped out to enjoy the sunset when he realized that the river bank here had preserved a distinct terrace remnant, twenty meters above the water, and thus different from the older deposits. His first quick search revealed the horns of a giant water buffalo, and so the Geological Survey fell to work on the terrace in earnest. It turned out to be very rich, with many thousands of animal bones. Not only that; it yielded two shinbones and eleven fragmentary skulls of a new kind of man.

The skulls were found one after another by various workers between September 1931 and November 1932. Von Koenigswald, then young and newly arrived, went with ter Haar to take out the best one, with von Koenigswald doing the photography in such a state of excitement that he underexposed many of his films. These bones have a grisly story to tell. Except for the two leg bones, only heads were found, and these lay in every position, upside down or otherwise. And from each skull a large piece had been knocked out below, usually almost the whole base. From every one the face was missing entirely. Not a vestige, not a jaw, not a tooth ever turned up. In fact, Solo Man was a cannibal, and this was where he had been eating the last, hardest-to-get part, the brain. There are, it is true, various reasons for eating one's own kind. One is to acquire the virtues of the dead, by ingesting the parts where virtue resides—intelligence, the brain; courage, the heart. Another reason is to keep well fed.

You may choose, but in any case we are left with only Solo Man's brain case to inspect. This was massive and heavy, extremely long, and still relatively low and poorly filled out. The brain was much larger than in Java Man, but still rather small; for six of the skulls the estimate of volume runs from 1035 to 1255, with an average of about 1100 cc. So it cannot be said that Solo Man had advanced in brain size beyond Pekin Man of China, who lived much earlier.

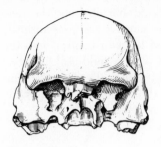
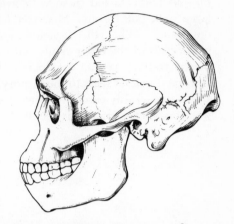

Solo Man. Left, skull XI from Ngandong. Right, side view, with hypothetical restoration of the face by Weidenreich. ¼ natural size. After cast and Weidenreich.

There is, withal, a sort of family resemblance to Java Man. It is this on which Dr. Weidenreich relied, believing that Solo Man was a direct descendant of the Java Man, hundreds of thousands of years later, on the same spot. Evolution, he believed, had gone its own way within this little parish, almost throughout the Pleistocene.

For the late date of the Ngandong fauna is an important matter. The fauna probably inhabited more open country and a cooler climate than the Solo River flows through today. The wide spreading horns of the giant buffalo would have been very poorly adapted to a jungle, and the deposit also contained the bones of a crane which today does not winter south of the Yangtze River in China. So the date is probably the first part of the last, Würm, Glacial phase of the north.

This is a broad and general problem, and we must hold Solo Man over for the time being. His skulls are now in Holland. Von Koenigswald had a complicated and unpleasant time during the war. German-born, but a Dutch national, he was separated from his family and put into a concentration camp by the Japanese, and there were even rumors in the United States that this admired scientist had lost his life. But the fossils did better, even though the Japanese military considered them the property of the expanding Empire and ordered them impounded. They got the Solo skulls, and sent one of them, Number XI, to the Emperor for his birthday. But von Koenigswald hid all the new finds, not yet described and therefore unknown to the conquerors. Swedish and Swiss friends took the *Gigantopithecus* and *Pithecan-*

thropus teeth, mixed them with a lot of others, and buried them in large milk bottles, and Mrs. von Koenigswald herself kept the new upper jaw. What the Japanese got were mostly fakes—beautifully made casts of the older skulls, with dye and brickdust mixed into the plaster so that even an accidentally broken piece would still look like a proper fossil, at least to the visitors. The latter actually showed themselves remarkably careful of their booty, real and bogus, and after the war von Koenigswald was reunited with family and fossil alike.

11. PEKIN MAN

PEKIN MAN was less fortunate. Java Man went into Dubois' locker for a time. But Pekin Man seems to have gone into Davy Jones' locker, and for good. He disappeared, one of the first casualties of the war in the Pacific, half a million years after he had died the first time.

His story will remind you of the South African man-apes more than a little. His remains lay in the same kind of lime-hardened cave fill, and they emerged in the same kind of peekaboo way. Let us go back a few generations, and to the town of Choukoutien, about twenty-seven miles southwest of the present Peking. Here the plain which runs back from the coast gives way to the Western Hills, limestone bluffs laid down in the sea long ago when the fishes were new. During the Pleistocene, water action ate out caves and fissures in the bluffs, at different times. These caves filled up again with earth and fossilized remains, and in some of them, like Locality 1, the large cave used by Pekin Man, the fill became a hard breccia.

In the year 1900 a human tooth (actually not a very ancient one) turned up in a Peking drugstore and drew the attention of paleontologists to the region. A long stream of them started coming to Choukoutien. They worked through the government Geological Survey of China, and the first of them were a Swedish geologist, J. G. Andersson, and an Austrian associate, O. Zdansky, helped by Swedish philanthropy. In 1921 they were led to Locality 1, and immediately they found bits of quartz. Animals do not use quartz, or eat it or wear it, and so it has no business in a cave in limestone and no natural way of getting there. But it is good for making stone tools. According to Roy Chapman Andrews, who was on the scene for much of the early story, Andersson said: "In this spot lies primitive man. All we have to do is to find him!"

Find him they did, bit by bit. Two years later, Zdansky discovered a single human tooth there, and in 1926, after taking a mass of animal fossils back to Upsala in Sweden, he recognized another human tooth in the collections. Enter now Dr. Davidson Black, Professor of Anatomy at the American-instituted Peiping Union Medical College, who, more than anyone else, was responsible for the discoveries to come. Excited by the teeth Zdansky had found, he persuaded the Rockefeller Foundation, backer of his college, to come in on the work and to co-operate with the Geological Survey. An able Swedish paleontologist, Birgir Bohlin, was brought to do the field work. This new phase began in 1927, and after six months of toil Bohlin produced one more tooth. This was enough for Black. After concentrated study of the new tooth he announced the find, and felt justified in alloting it a new human genus and species, *Sinanthropus pekinensis* (Chinese man of Pekin). Black took the tooth on a world tour that winter.

The Skulls Appear

All this intensity of purpose was rewarded. As the old cave was dug into more deeply, and its branchings and crannies were traced out, it began to yield less niggardly portions of Pekin Man. In 1928, Bohlin found fragments of two jaws, parts of skull walls, and a number of teeth. In 1929 a Chinese paleontologist, Pei, became director of the work, and on the very last day of the season, December 2, he himself found the first skull and cut it out still embedded in limestone, with only the top showing. This was what everyone had waited for. Shortly after, Black went to dinner at the British Legation. He scribbled a note about the skull and passed it to Andrews; afterward the initiated gathered from all over the city for a skull viewing, Pekin Man's vernissage, followed by an appropriate beer-and-pig's-knuckles party.

And now Pekin Man made his formal debut in the press. Such was the change which one generation had made, in attitudes toward human fossils, that Pekin Man was greeted with nothing like the Donnybrook which broke out upon the first Java discovery. Rather, he was met with deference, enthusiasm, and immediate acknowledgement of his importance. Only Dr. Dubois remained in character, huffing the skull away, abetted somewhat by our own Dr. Hrdlička of the National Museum, who pronounced the find to be a Chinese Neanderthal, nothing more.

Locality 1, now becoming a really large cavity, continued to give up Pekin men, together with their tools and meat bones. In the next two years other skull parts and jaws were recovered. But in 1934, Dr. Black unfortunately died, the result, it is said, of silicosis caused by dust from drilling on the fossils. This was a setback to operations. However, a celebrated German anatomist, already well known for his studies of the fossil men of Europe, was asked to

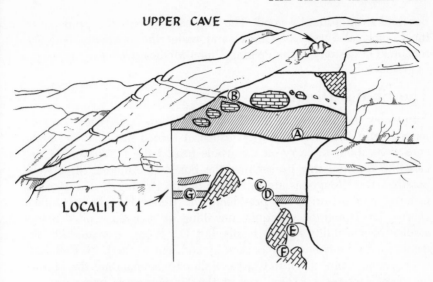

UPPER CAVE

LOCALITY 1

Choukoutien, the site of Pekin Man. The cross section of Locality 1 is from an early stage of the excavations. Shaded bands are zones rich in ashes, tools, and bone. Letters are points where skulls or other bones were found. Limestone blocks (the "brickwork") are partly due to falls from the original cave roof. Position of the Upper Cave is shown above the main section. After Davidson Black.

come to direct the Laboratory at Peiping Union Medical College, and the work at Choukoutien. This was Dr. Franz Weidenreich, and a fortunate choice, as his great monographs on the remains have proved.

Work started afresh, with better results than ever. In 1936 alone major or minor portions of seven skulls were found; and from beginning to end, parts of well over forty different men, women, and children were taken from this brecciated tomb. But now history of another sort began to interfere: the Japanese took over North China in 1937. At first the handicaps to work at Choukoutien were not severe. Once a Japanese general, on his day off, showed up at Locality 1 and announced that he was about to launch his own personal dig. Weidenreich managed to find and pull the right wires to Tokyo at once, however, and the general was not seen again. But difficulties multiplied, and what was worse, the Japanese command showed a mounting interest in the fossils: these, it evidently thought, had become Japanese citizens with the extension of the Empire to North China. At last, convinced that things had become impossible for fruitful work, Dr. Weidenreich in 1941 went to New York, taking with him a set of plaster casts of the skulls, fortunately of Chinese execution and extraordinarily good. The originals, always the property of the Geological Survey of China (and under the Japanese shadow), remained in custody of the Peiping Union Medical College.

The Skulls Disappear

But now the director of the Geological Survey, Dr. Wong, became more fearful—and certainly with justice, it turned out—that the Japanese were about to carry off the whole fossil tribe to Tokyo. He decided to forestall this by sending the bones to America, if it were possible. Dr. Wong was also a trustee of the Peiping Union Medical College, and he urged its president, Dr. Henry Houghton, to take charge. Dr. Houghton was quite unwilling to have the United States assume responsibility for the fossils, but Dr. Wong overcame his objections, and the bones were packed up and sent to the U. S. Embassy.

There they were given to Colonel Ashurst, commanding the Marine detachment at the Embassy, just as the Marines were being ordered to evacuate North China. Colonel Ashurst was told to treat the boxes as "secret" material, to be put with his personal gear. This, and all Marine baggage, equipment, and ammunition, was to be sent on a special train, under the guard of nine Marines, down to the port of Chinwangtao, there to meet the liner *President Harrison*, which was to transport the Marines to the Philippine Islands. So far so good. The train left Peking at five in the morning on December 5, 1941. It arrived in Chinwangtao on December 7.

We know what happened next, to everyone except Pekin Man. We know what happened to the *Harrison:* her crew appraised the situation and grounded her to prevent the Japanese from making immediate use of her; the Japanese refloated her, renamed her *Kachidoki Maru,* and used her as a transport until she was sunk in 1944 by the U. S. submarine *Pampanito.* We know what happened to the nine Marines; they were captured, sent back to Peking, and put in prison camps along with Colonel Ashurst and the rest of his command. We even know what happened to the ammunition and equipment; they were later seen in Japanese possession.

But what happened to the bones is anyone's guess. And it has been almost everyone's guess. That they were actually put on a lighter, which capsized in the harbor. That local Chinese got them and ground them up for medicine. There is even an opium-scented story that they were smuggled safely away by sinister international merchants of the China coast and finally tracked down and purchased by an American medical man who lives in California and guards the hoard like Fafnir, the great worm. At any rate, the press in Japan and in Hong Kong periodically erupted with developments of this tale for some years.

It is quite clear that the Japanese—meaning actual officials—never got the ancient Pekinese. For the Japanese in Peking immediately started looking for the bones, and they went over the United States Embassy "with a fine-toothed comb," according to accounts. They were sufficiently interested, in fact, to lock up and question the business manager of the Medical College, Trevor Bowen, for five days before they were convinced he did not know Pekin Man's whereabouts. Evidently Dr. Wong was a good prophet. The Japanese took to Tokyo the stone tools found at Choukoutien, all carefully and exactly catalogued, where everything was found to be in good order after the war.

So it is evident that the Japanese would have made no bones about the bones. They wanted quite guilelessly to bring them home, and so they must have conducted the most efficient search one could imagine, at Chinwangtao as well as at Peking. There is no reason to suppose they might have hidden the bones away. They did not hide Solo Man, nor did they hide the valuable stone tools. And anyhow, a hidden fossil is no more good to the hider than to the seeker; Dr. Dubois proved that.

It is equally clear that the Chinese have never found them. The government of Communist China is enthusiastic in the pursuit of ancient man. It has opened a museum at Choukoutien, and resumed excavations, of which the results have been a few more teeth and bone fragments. It is totally improbable that anyone in authority in China secretly knows where the bones are.

Certainly they were not sent to the United States. The Chinese government was a party to the guessing game I mentioned, its guess being that the fossils had ended up in the American Museum of Natural History in New York. Pekin Man number XI, it said, had been looted by an American soldier from the Imperial Japanese collection. "In other words," declared the New China News Agency in 1952, "the Japanese imperialists stole it from the American imperialists after the latter had stolen it. It was shipped to Japan and kept in the imperial Japanese collection. After Japan surrendered, the American imperialists stole it again, this time from the Japanese robbers, and put it in the New York Museum."

A fine dish of anti-American propaganda. But strangely enough the story was not made up out of whole cloth. What seems to have happened is this. A distinguished naturalist from over the Atlantic, a man famous in his own specialty and other fields as well, but not closely acquainted with fossil man, came to call on Dr. Weidenreich, before the latter's death in 1948, at the Natural History Museum in New York. He encountered Weidenreich walking down the hall on the floor reserved for staff. "Look at this," said Weidenreich, holding out a primitive-looking human skull with the number XI painted on it. "It's just been brought back from Japan." "This" was Solo XI, the one which had been sent up from Java during the war for the Emperor's birthday. It was recovered by Lieutenant Walter Fairservis and brought back to von Koenigswald, arriving in New York, in September 1946, with the rest of his fossils.

Von Koenigswald was so busy with Java Man that he turned over the Solo skulls to Dr. Weidenreich, orphaned guardian of Pekin Man, to study and describe. That is how Weidenreich came to be walking in the hall with Solo XI in his hands. His visitor paid no great attention to the fossil but, on getting home, came to suppose he had been looking at one of the Pekin skulls—they have a family likeness to Solo. He said as much to some fellow naturalists at tea one day. One of these shortly afterward went behind the Iron Curtain, taking the "news" with him, and thus an innocent little mistake became a big and beautiful piece of propaganda.

So here we have Pekin Man, world traveler, associate of merchant pirates, or pawn of international politics. His weird experiences since 1941 prove, I fear, that fiction is stranger than truth. It is unlikely that he ever left the environs of Chinwangtao. He is, if there is anything left of him, probably there today. The judgment of men who were in China in 1941 is likely to be the right one. Japanese officialdom was hot on the scent of the Pekin bones, but it was not Japanese officials who captured the Marines and looted the train with its secret freight at Chinwangtao. It was ordinary Japanese soldiers. And they doubtless did what ordinary Japanese soldiers, or ordinary American soldiers, would do in a captured train. Expecting something interesting and finding what looked like dog bones, they probably threw the whole lot onto the trash heap or over the dockside. This may be prosaic, but at least it is reasonable. Unfortunately, people have a perverse liking for the improbable and implausible. There were many, for a while, who were certain Hitler had not died in 1945 in Berlin. I think we will see Hitler and Pekin Man again on the same day. Judgment Day.

The Nature of Pekin Man

So, unless and until more skulls are found, we can make no progress with this very important early man. In particular, new ideas, or new chemical tests, can never be applied to the lost material. We are left only with casts and with Dr. Weidenreich's fine descriptions. But this is much better than nothing, because Weidenreich was an extraordinarily gifted describer of fossil man. And such descriptions are all that many anthropologists, unless they are inveterate travelers, usually have at their disposal for their studies of many specimens and types of ancient man.

In fact, though his relics are gone, we actually know more about Pekin Man than about any other fossil hominids, excepting only the australopithecines, because so many specimens were found, and because of Weidenreich's meticulous work. I will describe the Pekin type simply. How simply, or oversimply, you can judge by comparing my few words with more than a thousand large pages published by Weidenreich in the monographs of the Geological Survey of China alone.

Let us say first of all that Pekin Man is Java Man's brainy brother. The two are closely related—very much the same kind of man. Weidenreich said they were merely two races, though most others think this is a slight exaggeration, when it is taken to mean that they differ no more than two of our races of today. Let us say rather that Pekin Man is another edition of Java Man, virtually identical in some respects, but in two very human ways a small advance away from the man-apes and toward ourselves. These two ways are, as you would expect, brains and teeth.

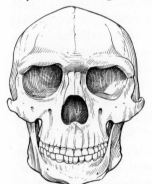 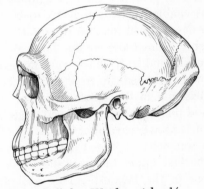

Pekin Man. Restoration of a female skull by Weidenreich. ¼ natural size. After Weidenreich.

The Pekin and Java men did not differ in the skeleton, for both, as far as we know them, had already arrived at a skeleton indistinguishable from our own. Pekin Man, it is true, had rather thick walls to his thighbones, but he showed none of the distinctions in shape seen in the australopithecines.

Nor did they differ in some basic skull specifications. Both skulls were equally thick—very thick for humanity—and both had equally large and beetling bony brows. And in the base, the most fundamental part of the skull—something for the top of the neck, so to speak—they were alike, with the Pekin men only showing signs of a slightly less massive neck attachment at the very back and in the region of the ears.

But above this base plate Pekin Man's brain was larger than Java Man's, by about 200 cubic centimeters, possibly more. The few measurable skulls averaged about 1075 cc., which suggests a figure for males of about 1150 cc., to be compared with modern men having 1450. This is a clear rise above Java Man and must have been close to the value for Solo Man. And the increased volume is evident in the shape of the skulls. Though still slanting sharply inward above the ears, the sides were broader and the central ridge higher; and there was a distinct bump for a forehead, immediately contrasting with the low slope running back from the brows in Java Man. In fact, this greater rise of forehead threw the bony brows into sharper relief, with a deep furrow running across the forehead just behind them. But paradoxically, the primitive look this furrow imparts is actually due to a progressive feature, the angle created by the embryo forehead.

The same degree of progress is seen in the teeth. Robust, and with obvious primitive traits (cingulum, root and cusp arrangements), such as enabled Davidson Black to be sure of his ground in recognizing a new kind of man on three teeth alone, they are nonetheless diminished from those in the Java specimens. And with this, the whole mouth suddenly looks truly human. The dental arch is shorter and more rounded in front, and there is no sign of an opening or diastema in the upper row. The jaw is shorter and more compact, and this is reflected in a real angle at the chin: not a true bony bump such as we have, but not a smooth receding curve either; instead, a somewhat flattened and steeper front. Finally, in the molar teeth, the first upper molar is the largest (the second in the Java Man), but in the lower teeth as well, the third molar—wisdom tooth—is now shorter than the second.

Pekin Man used his teeth on a diet much like our own in essence, a mixture of meat and vegetables. And he had tools to cut his food up with and fire to cook it. So any demand by natural selection for powerful jaws was probably already a thing of the past. All this is known from the fill in the cave in which his bones lay.

Locality 1 and Its Contents

It may not be true that he "lived" in the cave. More likely he "frequented" it, as did bears, hyenas, and many other carnivores, including no less than six members of the cat family, not counting a sabertooth. These frequenters and predators, man among them, are probably responsible for bringing in the bones of many other animals: big horses, big camels, buffaloes, elephants, rhinos, and a very large number of deer, as well as sheep and antelopes. Much of this must have been Pekin Man's own leavings, judging from the other kinds of rubbish he left. There were also quantities of bird cherry seeds, signs of the vegetable side of his diet.

High and low in the fill were layers of ash and burned bones, hearths where the men had sat and cooked. Now this is very early evidence of using fire (which is also just coming to light in Europe), and it is important. Its meaning for early man is not warmth mainly, nor even as a weapon in the rivalry with other beasts for use of the cave. Rather, it is that cooking makes meat more edible and digestible for us. Man is a primate and a descendant of primates, and the higher primates are adjusted to a diet which is very largely vegetable. But there is more energy in the proteins and fats of meat, which their omnivorous systems can use, especially if the meat is partly broken down by heat. So fire and cooking unlocked the door, for man, to greater efficiency and economy of diet, by letting him make a much greater use of meat.

A second factor in the success of developing human life was good stone tools. These Pekin Man had. The Cro Magnons of Europe or the North American Indians would have derided his efforts. But for a man whose brains still lacked thirty or forty per cent of our own advance beyond a chimpanzee, these implements were nothing less than praiseworthy. They were by no means the crudest which are known to archaeologists. The characteristic tool of Pekin Man was a pebble trimmed to make an edged chopper. He also had flake scrapers, and points consisting of a crude beak. And he used animal bones as tools a good deal, although he does not appear to have shaped them before using them.

Locality 1 must have been an odorous place in those days. But Pekin Man was worse than a poor tenant. Last but not least in the inventory of the mess he created in the cave is the state of his own remains. Like Solo Man, Pekin Man was a cannibal. The disorder in which human bones lay was no mere lack of funerary fastidiousness. And there is this guilty statistic: few parts of his trunk or limbs lay within the cave, the vast majority of fossil parts being from the head. Plainly, he did his killing and dying outside and brought only the skulls of his fellows indoors, there to eat the brains by breaking through the base of the cranium. A good many pieces of face and jaw were present, but not affixed to the brain case.

But all this is his affair. What's done is done, and we might as well be thankful that he was unwittingly packing away skulls for future science. If Pekin Man had had any latter-day compunctions about anthropophagy, Dr. Weidenreich would have had far less to dig up and write about.

Those grisly wakes must have gone on for many thousands of years. While Pekin Man picked bones, pecked flint, and dug out his colleagues' brains, the floor of the cave rose higher and higher, until earth and bones had filled its whole great space, over 100 feet high, and as much as 500 feet long in one direction. There was no sign of changes—of different periods of weather, or of animals, or of human types and tools. Nevertheless, the animals are so varied that they do not tell a precise story of either cool times or warm, except that the climate was not glacial. The current estimate of date, based on the fauna at Locality 1, is the warmer break between two parts of the Second Glacial phase. Therefore Pekin Man was either a contemporary of the Trinil Java men, or lived slightly later. The difference in time could hardly have been great enough for significant evolution.

The Lantian Man

Does this signify a little tribe or clan, hanging about the spot, faithful to it for two or three thousand generations? Surely not. It means that, as in the case of South Africa, Locality 1 was a place favorable, during the Middle Pleistocene, for occupation and fossilization, and was in fact probably on the fringes of a much larger sphere populated by Pekin Man. The truth of this has recently become evident.

Years ago von Koenigswald, in his apothecary-shop hunts among the dragon bones where he found Gigantopithecus, also turned up a few teeth which are nearly the same as those from Choukoutien, but slightly larger. He named this relative Sinanthropus officinalis (drugstore Sinanthropus). Since the teeth came from somewhere in South China, this was already a small indication of the wide territory of Pekin Man.

Recently Chinese scientists have found something much more important. In 1963, at Chenchiawo in Lantian District, Shensi Province, they recovered a lower jaw in good shape, and in 1964 on Kungwangling hill (about 20 kilometers away) some face parts, a tooth, and a good skull cap, all of which turned out to be from the same skull. The date at both places is believed to be earlier than that of Pekin Man, and to correspond with the oldest Java specimens.

The correspondence holds for the skull and jaw as well. The jaw is more robust than those of Choukoutien, and the skull in a number of ways recalls the Djetis Java Man, especially as now restored by von Koenigswald. It is low and excessively thick and the brow ridges are massive, although arched near the middle in an unfamiliar way. Dr. Woo has figured the cranial capacity as about 780 cc., close to von Koenigswald's estimate for the Djetis skull.

This is a most satisfying discovery, not least because it fulfills an expectation. We see a contemporary and obviously close relative of Java Man well up in the Chinese mainland; it is fairly clear that only one general kind of man occupied the whole Far East during the Middle Pleistocene. We now have not merely the uncle of Pekin Man, in the earliest of the Java men, but apparently his father as well, in the new Lantian men. We see a small degree of progress between the earlier and the later specimens. Long afterward we find Solo Man on Java, most likely a later development of the same family line again, and in fact showing relatively little advance for the long lapse of time. Possibly the picture is too simple, but this gives us several well known and related forms constituting a major human stock in eastern Asia, apparently throughout the whole Middle Pleistocene and beyond.

12. EUROPE, AFRICA, AND THE RISE OF HOMO

W̲HEN WE TURN to the west of the Old World, and the well-studied continents of Europe and Africa, there is a curious reversal in the nature of our information. In Asia stone tools of man have not been traced back into the Lower Pleistocene, nor even to the hands of Java Man, though there can be no question that he made and used them. In Europe, where the Paleolithic sequence has been intensively studied for decades, tools can be followed back further, and in Africa further still to simply trimmed pebbles, or to many-faceted round implements which may have been used to break up meat bones.

So for the west there is a much richer knowledge of human tools, and a longer story. But there has never been found, for the early Pleistocene, a group of skulls of one population of man to compare with that from Choukoutien or from the Solo River. In fact, before about 1950 the frustrating lack of human remains from these levels was almost complete. But the next fifteen years brought a series of finds, scattered and fragmentary, which help a great deal.

Heidelberg Man

The major exception, the sole early find of *Homo,* was the Heidelberg jaw of 1907. The jaw did not thrust itself forward; it was found because Dr. Otto Schoetensack of Heidelberg University was looking for it and had been looking for twenty years. About seven miles southeast of Heidelberg, at the village of Mauer, a huge sand pit had been dug against the side of a long series of Pleistocene deposits of clay, sand, and gravel. Cut vertically to a great height, this fine ladder of strata, with its fossil animals, was more beautiful to the eye of a geologist than a garden of flowers, and Dr. Schoetensack was one of the professorial bees who buzzed around it. He felt certain that somewhere in the face of the vast exposure the remains of man would sooner or later come to light, and he infected the owner of the

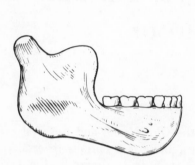
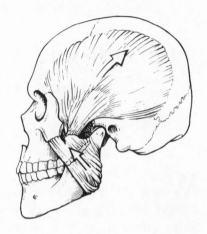

The Heidelberg jaw (left) in profile. After Schoetensack. ¼ natural size. Right, the main muscles of the jaw in biting. From the angle, the *masseter*, partly cut away, which pulls up and slightly forward, being attached to the under edge of the cheek arch (zygomatic arch). From the coronoid process, or forward point of the upright branch, the *temporal* muscle, pulling up and slightly back, being attached to the side of the skull. (Drawing not to scale.)

pit with the same feeling. It finally happened: a big human jaw, quite by itself, was found in the sand, well down at the base of the bank and nearly eighty feet below the top of the deposit.

No convincing stone tools have been found in these beds. The animals at Mauer (archaic horses, a straight-tusked elephant, and the Etruscan rhino, as well as a variety of bears, deer, bison, etc.) are a group which follows on the Villafranchian. So the Heidelberg Man may be about as old as the earlier Java men, overlapping with the last of the man-apes of South Africa. A very ancient man indeed, belonging to the end of the First Interglacial or the beginning of the Second Glacial.

This jaw is well preserved, having most of its teeth in a state of moderate wear, except for four left molars and premolars, broken at the time of discovery and only partly repaired. Before the man-apes and the later finds of Java Man, the jaw was alone in its great size, and it is still impressive. It is perhaps a shade heavier than the jaw known as Pithecanthropus B.

Compared to other human jaws, the most striking thing about its shape is the great breadth of the ascending ramus, or branch. This is the vertical blade which underlies the back part of your cheek and which carries the condyle, or knob for the joint, at its hinder corner. To the forward corner, the coronoid process, there attaches one of the main muscles which close the jaw. This is the temporal muscle, which fans out on the side of the skull. To the outer surface of the lower portion of the ramus there attaches the other main muscle, the masseter, a short broad muscle which runs up to the under edge of the cheek bone. This is easily felt: it stands out sharply when you grit your teeth, and so may be used for dramatic effect as well as for chewing. Therefore, while the width of this ascending ramus may be related in part to the length of the whole jaw, it also suggests jaw muscles of power and efficiency. The Heidelberg jaw is in the class of the great *Paranthropus* jaws from Swartkrans, though not on a par with the larger ones. It is not as high, suggesting a less massive face. While the face was probably projecting (since the jaw is certainly long), its upright and forwardly directed coronoid process suggests that the skull above the face, where the temporal muscle lay, also extended well forward, so the face as a whole probably did not have a markedly protruding mouth region.

Nonetheless, the width of the whole jaw, and the generous expanse of ascending ramus, indicate big muscles, and wide-flaring, strong cheek arches on the vanished skull. All this power is peculiar, because the teeth, the real business edge of the whole machine, are not very large. They are not small, but they are not in proportion with the jawbone, so to speak (the same can be said of the Swartkrans jaws, to a degree). In size the teeth do not approach those of australopithecines. They are in fact nearer to modern man than they are to Java Man; the dental arch is even distinctly smaller than Pekin Man's. The teeth are rather modern in character, as well, though of good size, and with crowns which are robust right down to the base, and with big roots. Their upper surfaces are worn flat. The canines are well reduced in size and have been ground level with the other teeth, as one would expect. And the molars are of recent proportions, with the hindmost being somewhat smaller than the one in front of it.

Beyond guessing that he had a wide, not strongly projecting face, we cannot reconstruct the Heidelberg Man's skull nor get any worthwhile idea as to the size of his brain. As to his relationships with other hominids, this is clearly the jaw of *Homo*. It suggests the australopithecines somewhat, in its breadth, size, and chunky, nonpongid look. The chin region is certainly primitive. It is, however, much inferior to the man-apes in thickness, and in total height. And of course the smaller, modern-looking teeth, set it off sharply from *Australopithecus*.

They also tend to distinguish it from Java and Pekin Man, and the jaw shape would also not be at home among those of the Far East. The amount of primitiveness is about the same, but some kind of a regional difference is suggested.

An Early Hungarian

Almost sixty years went by before the next such fossil came to light in Europe. Dr. László Vértes discovered a place at Vértesszöllös west of Budapest where, during the mild break in the middle of the Second Glacial phase, men had been camping, eating animals of the chase, and making small tools of the "pebble" variety. Their camp-site was a small saucer-like depression, no bigger than an average room, formed earlier by the rising waters of a hot spring. This warm spring itself may have made it an attractive spot in the cold climate. In and around this basin Dr. Vértes collected a very large number of simple stone tools, especially pebble tools—the first to be found in Europe. In 1965 he was using explosive charges here and there like Broom, because of the hardness of the rock, and he had the same kind of luck. Just over the edge of the basin, apparently where ancient refuse had been thrown, one of his charges split the rock just where a piece of bone was embedded. It was an occipital bone, the back of the head, all by itself; no other piece of this skull was found or is likely to be.

This is a very important fossil. Rather thick, and with a well-marked angle and ridge for neck muscles, it is nevertheless far more advanced than Java or Pekin Man, and indeed seems larger and less angled than the same bone in the Rhodesian skull (see Chapter 15). Dr. Andor Thoma, giving the fossil its original description, has estimated the capacity of the whole skull at 1400 cc., a modern figure, and in consequence has named it *Homo sapiens palaeohungaricus*. The important possibilities are: (1) this bone might conceivably be the back of Heidelberg Man's head, and (2) it might also represent a direct forerunner of the Steinheim and Swanscombe people (Chapter 15). Are we here at the origins of *Homo sapiens?*

Ternifine Man

We go now to North Africa and another site belonging to the beginning of the Middle Pleistocene (just after the Villafranchian, about the time of the Second Glacial of Europe, and probably of the later Java men). In Algeria, a little southeast of Oran, when the sea was beginning to fall with the onset of the Second Glacial, there existed a spring-fed pond at Ternifine. Men frequented the pond, and like the people at Choukoutien and Vértesszöllös, they were untidy. They let their tools and meat bones get into their water supply, along with the bones of other beasts of prey. To the springs at Ternifine came zebras, giraffes, and many antelopes; elephants, rhinos, and all the kinds of carnivore; saber-toothed cats and giant wart hogs left over from the Villafranchian; an archaic collection generally. And here and there in the debris in the pond there came to rest Acheulian hand-axes, an early variety of this tradition but well made for their time, better than anything from the hands of the men we have reviewed so far.

Finally, thick beds of sand filled and buried the whole depression. In our own times it came into use as a large sand pit, tools were discovered, and archaeologists dug there in 1931. They stopped work part-way down, however, because of striking water and also from fear of undercutting Moslem graves next to one side of the pit. But the government enabled Professor Camille Arambourg to work in 1954 and 1955, with special equipment and pumps. He made a major excavation: he was able to go fifteen feet lower, down to the clay of the ancient ponds. Part of his reward was three human jaws and a parietal bone, all right at the bottom.

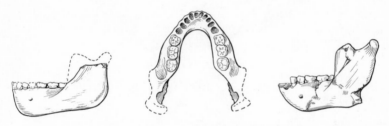

Jaws of *Telanthropus* (left and center) and Ternifine Man. ¼ natural size. After Robinson and Arambourg.

The parietal bone, from a young person, does not tell us much. While not extremely thick, it has features like Pekin Man's, including the pattern of blood vessels on the inside, and suggests a low, poorly filled skull. The jaws, large and thick, are well preserved. In size and shape they match those of Pekin Man, and this appears to hold for traits of the teeth as well (a cingulum or collar of enamel is present on the premolars). But the total size of the molar teeth goes further and matches Java Man. Perhaps the ascending ramus of the jaw was as broad as Heidelberg Man's, but the teeth of the latter appear to be different in nature. Arambourg pointed out the good likeness to the Far Easterners, but believed that the differences were enough to grant Ternifine Man a genus of his own, *Atlanthropus mauritanicus.* Others, however, accept Professor Arambourg's assertion that the Ternifiners are close in form to Pekin and Java Man, and therefore reject his new genus.

East and South Africa

One of Leakey's recent prizes at Olduvai was an excellent skull top, found in the upper part of Bed II in 1960, well above the level of "Zinjanthropus." This part of the bed is Middle Pleistocene, and contains hand-axes, as did the Ternifine pond. In addition, a provisional potassium-argon date places the age of the skull at 500,000 years. It should therefore lie in the same general time zone as the others I have described, particularly Pekin Man and perhaps Vértesszöllös.

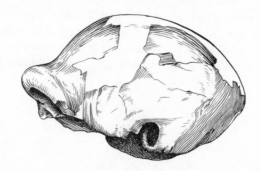

The *Homo erectus* skull cap from upper Bed II, Olduvai. ¼ natural size.

Evaluation of the skull has not been completed, nor a proper description published, although Professor Heberer has named it *Homo leakeyi.* Nevertheless, its most general characteristics are plain enough. Like the Far Easterners, it is thick and low, and somewhat crested along the midline. Its brow ridges are prominent, perhaps even puffier than those of Java Man. Other details will await the slow work of further preparation. This probable brain capacity has been estimated at 1000 cc. which, with its other features, puts it fairly on a level with Pekin Man. It could perfectly well be the skull of Ternifine Man, but obviously this cannot be shown either way just now.

A final early man is constituted by three scraps of lower and upper jaw, found by Broom and Robinson at Swartkrans, in the same deposit as *Paranthropus.* The best of the pieces is a lower jaw, and Broom and Robinson perceived its differences from those of the man-ape, and named the new form *Telanthropus capensis.* Sir Wilfrid Le Gros Clark, always a careful observer, suggested that "Telanthropus" might simply be a female *Paranthropus,* of smaller size; Robinson, however, finds too clear a distinction in tooth size from his many specimens of *Paranthropus,* and it is now generally agreed that "Telanthropus" cannot be an australopithecine. In fact, Robinson himself has abandoned the name "Telanthropus" and transferred the fossil to *Homo.*

The lower jaw resembles the Heidelberg specimen a little, and certain details in the region of the nose and bony upper gum on one fragment point to a face quite different from the man-apes and more vertical. The teeth, as I have indicated, are in the range of *Homo.* Finally, let us note the important fact that some stone tools have also been found in the deposit, so the recognition of both *Homo* and *Paranthropus* at the site is of first importance.

Homo erectus

The net effect of all these later finds is a somewhat new view of man in the early Middle Pleistocene. We see a certain likeness, a sort of stratum of humanity in what now looks like a moderately well-defined time zone. Dating, always difficult, is always subject to revision, but the eight localities we have just reviewed (including Java and China but excluding Solo) now appear to have an age in years running from possibly 1,000,000 to 500,000 or a little later. As to physical likeness, let us admit that a jaw here, an occiput there, is not the most satisfying evidence of homogeneity. Those parts that do match, however, show a rather surprising similarity. The Chinese and North African jaws are the best example, with the Heidelberg jaw seeming the most remote. The Pekin skull as a whole is more refined and larger brained than that from Java, but the latter could be the parent of the former, certainly over such a span of time.

All this has caused anthropologists to recognize these likenesses in naming. Originally, as we have been seeing, almost every new form of man was given his own genus, even in recent years. But a generation ago Le Gros Clark and others pointed out that Pekin Man could not possibly stand as a genus separate from Java Man; Weidenreich in fact considered him no more than racially distinct. At best, it was felt, he might be a different species, and in general practice was therefore renamed *Pithecanthropus pekinensis.* Professor Le Gros Clark proposed that no more than two genera should be recognized for all fossil men (other than australopithecines), namely *Pithecanthropus* and *Homo.*

Professor Ernst Mayr, now Director of the Museum of Comparative

Zoology at Harvard, went even further. Even though Java Man was primitive and small-brained, his whole pattern of adaptation and way of life (fully erect walking, large body size, meat-eating, tool-making) was the same as that of later man, including ourselves. Therefore, by proper zoological practice Java Man could not even be looked on as belonging to a different genus from ourselves, and Mayr included him in *Homo.* After gulping a few times, the anthropologists have followed suit.

Accordingly, Java Man becomes *Homo erectus.* For several reasons, all the other early Middle Pleistocene men go into the same species. The first reason is their general likeness, now so much more apparent. The second reason is the fact that they were contemporaries, broadly speaking. It is most unlikely that two different species of *Homo*— populations unable to interbreed—could have existed at the same time without showing more physical difference. This would now therefore seem to apply even to the somewhat distinct Heidelberg jaw. So at the moment these fossil men, from North China to South Africa, are no more than differing regional populations, perhaps subspecies, perhaps about like our races (although in fact the earlier fossils seem more primitive than the later).

The Vértesszöllös man is a probable exception, and there may be just now an even greater impression of homogeneity in type and time than will eventually prove to be warranted. There is also always the danger of getting a little bit hemmed in by terminology. The general similarities all over the Old World, and the apparent stability of form over perhaps half a million years, are surprising. Nevertheless, that is what we now see, and what we call *Homo erectus.*

Homo habilis?

The next problem is: how did *Homo erectus* arise from *Australopithecus?* We must now assume that he did so, instead of coming from some other, unknown ancestor. *Homo erectus* is established everywhere in the early Middle Pleistocene—there are no other kinds of men. Also, the Pleistocene has now been dramatically stretched out, so to speak, somewhat in the middle but very considerably in the Villafranchian. When the whole Pleistocene was thought to be a million years or less in length, the time allowed for transforming *Australopithecus* into Java Man seemed incredibly short. But now we may think of one or two million years for this gradual process.

As I have said, Robinson has always insisted on the distinction between *Paranthropus* and *Australopithecus*, between a large vegetarian and a small mixed feeder, whose differences in adaptation and anatomy justified a genus for each. The paleontologists, beginning with Oakley, are satisfied that the *Paranthropus* sites were later than those of *Australopithecus*, certainly in South Africa, and that *Paranthropus* probably lived into the Middle Pleistocene. Robinson some time ago suggested that while *Paranthropus* was thus persisting and becoming perhaps more specialized, something more like *Australopithecus* was evolving into *Homo*. The general correctness of this seems to be borne out by finding the jaw of "Zinjanthropus" in Middle Pleistocene deposits at Peninj, demonstrating the definite late survival of *Paranthropus*. The picture is also enlivened, broadened, and complicated by the appearance of *Homo habilis*.

We now go back to Olduvai. I said earlier that the Leakeys found far more there than The Dear Boy. They found, of course, the *Homo erectus* skull cap. But their further finds make Olduvai look like Christmas morning.

These finds began in 1960, shortly after the original "Zinjanthropus." Stone implements turned up at the same level, briefly suggesting that The Dear Boy himself was the artisan. A very small pair of lower leg bones (tibia and fibula) also came to light nearby; if these were to be assigned to "Zinjanthropus," he would have been rather top heavy. But then, somewhat below in Bed I, were found the lower jaw, two partial parietal bones, and bones of the hand of a young creature, much smaller and totally different from "Zinjanthropus." In the next few years, fragmentary remains of a similar nature were recovered, not only in Bed I, below "Zinjanthropus," but also at the same general level, high in Bed I, as well as above, as far as the middle of Bed II, thus carrying up into the Middle Pleistocene (but not into the hand-axe zone). All this evidence, from at least six individuals, is unfortunately broken and meager; nevertheless, it is spread up and down the strata at Olduvai Gorge, so that the time positions of the different finds, relative to one another and to "Zinjanthropus," are all clear. This is one of the wholly exceptional aspects of Leakey's material; elsewhere, only in Java is there any stratigraphic evidence in one place for these early fossils.

This all shows that two quite different hominids were present. One was *Paranthropus*. Who was the other? And were there more than two?

First review of this material, representing at least seven individuals, gave an impression of general similarity. Bones of the skeleton were of small size. The skeleton of a foot, and the two lower leg bones, which are now presumed to belong to the same creature, have been studied by the English anatomists Napier, Day, and Davis. They are pronounced completely adapted for bipedalism of the human kind although, like the *Australopithecus* hipbones from South Africa, they show minor signs of imperfection compared to the same bones today. The foot exhibits fully developed arches and the general proportions across the instep necessary for human walking. Now these parts do not overlap with the South African specimens (no pelvis here, no leg and foot there) and so there is nothing to show that we are not dealing with more small individuals like the Sterkfontein *Australopithecus*.

The skull (or skulls) is a different matter. In the first place, the teeth are somewhat smaller than those of australopithecines, particularly in the breadth. The jaws are not so heavy. But the greatest contrast lies in the brain case, which for two individuals has been partly restored. This is thin—as in *Australopithecus*—with a rounded slope at the rear—also as in *Australopithecus*—but is altogether higher, rounder, and apparently larger. Thus it appears to be decidedly more progressive than *Australopithecus* but to be quite different from the thick, low, angled cranium of *Homo erectus*.

Professor Phillip Tobias (Dart's successor in Johannesburg) has taken the two parietal bones of the 1960 skull, to make a cast of that part of the brain which they would have covered. Proceeding from this to estimate the whole, he arrived at a figure of some 675 to 680 cc. for the brain volume, a figure which, for a young individual of a small-bodied species, seems to be a decided advance over the known australopithecines, and definitely larger than *Paranthropus*. Tobias' effort has been met with scepticism by his colleagues, who say that the supposed brain volume depends largely on how you incline the two parietal bones in or out. But Tobias has an answer. If you hold your two hands up in front of you, and bend the fingers in to touch their tips, you will have a model of the parietal bones. If you separate your wrists, the volume enclosed goes up; if you bring them together, it goes down. But Tobias points out that what you lose at the top you gain at the bottom, because the enclosed space gets deeper as the angle at the top gets narrower, and that the estimate thus comes out about the same in the end.

At any rate, Leakey, Tobias, and Napier felt they had discerned a new hominid species. It was clearly distinct from its bedfellow, *Paranthropus*. It was equally distinct from the larger, crude-skulled *Homo erectus*. It was most like *Australopithecus*, but more advanced, particularly in brain size, and Tobias at least thinks that the association of stone tools with the bones here at Olduvai justifies regarding the species as *Homo*, not *Australopithecus*. Accordingly, in April 1964, the three, using a name suggested by Dart, launched the species in the pages of *Nature* as *Homo habilis*.

Professional indifference, scepticism, or downright hostility are tra-

ditional on these occasions; remember Dart and 1925. Suffice it to
say there has been disagreement in this case, both as to the interpretations placed on the material and as to the procedure in naming
it. This all seems small compared to the great importance of the
material itself and, it must be said, the great promptness with which
Leakey made it available to every colleague who wished to study it.
Full study of such material is a slow process, and solid interpretations
are also blocked by such things as the fact that we do not know the
time relations between East and South Africa as yet, and so some of
the answers must wait for this.

Actually, there appears to be more agreement among various students than they themselves admit. Leakey now finds that one of the
specimens, from the bottom of Bed II, seems more pithecanthropine,
i.e., like *Homo erectus,* than the rest, leading him to suggest the possibility that by Bed II times there were actually three forms at Olduvai:
Paranthropus, habilis, and an early *Homo erectus.* Others, like Robinson, find differences between the Bed I and Bed II *habilis* specimens,
with the former having lower jaws which are thicker and narrower
within, and teeth which he does not believe are really distinguishable
from *Australopithecus.* Similarly, Tobias and von Koenigswald have
together reviewed much of the African and Asiatic material, and believe they can see four stages of an actual evolution running from the
South African *Australopithecus* to *Homo erectus:* between these they
place one step represented by the Bed I specimens plus *Meganthropus*
of Java, and a second step represented by the lower Bed II individuals, and also by "Telanthropus" from Swartkrans and the earliest
specimens of Java Man, from the Djetis zone.

This looks like the reasonable reconstruction for the time being.
We have *Homo erectus* spread out in the Old World, and *Australopithecus* must have been similarly spread out at an earlier time. With
no present evidence of other essentially different hominids, we must
get from one to the other, and we have a million years to work with.
We start with *Australopithecus* as a small-bodied meat eater and
hunter, very likely using the bones and jaws of other animals for his
tools, with a minimum of shaping, as well as naturally broken stones.
He then began actually to fashion tools, perhaps by further work on
shapes already formed in bone, but finally on raw stone having no
more shape than a pebble. Ability and brain size increased, and
Olduvai indicates that this began when body size still was small.
Then body size also increased, and the high round skull changed to
one which was low, thick, and sharply angled at the back. I do not
myself see any difficulty in this shift in head form. If the general mass
of the body, and thus of the skull, were to double, while the brain in-

creased by only 100 cc. or so, this would amount actually to a proportionate decrease in the brain, and the head would be expected to undergo a relative deflation.

This was a continuous evolution. Is it necessary to sandwich a new species, *habilis*, into the line? Robinson would simply include *Australopithecus* in *Homo* and be done with it. Otherwise, the Bed I *Homo habilis* looks anatomically like an extension of *Australopithecus*, and the change from bone-tool using to stone-tool making as the criterion putting him in a new genus is not entirely satisfactory.

As for *Paranthropus*, this vegetable-chewing "hominid gorilla" left tool-making severely alone. He did not compete with *Australopithecus* or *Homo*, being a different kind of animal, and he shows no signs of evolution. He may have lasted over a very long part of the Villafranchian; he survived into the Middle Pleistocene, like the big ground-ape *Gigantopithecus* in China, and then disappeared.

13. THE NEANDERTHALS

WE HAVE got up to *Homo erectus;* now we must get beyond "him." If Olduvai Gorge—and this is the only evidence we have—gives us the clue to events, this stage of man had been developing slowly from nearly 2,000,000 to perhaps 1,000,000 years ago. He was an early contemporary of *Paranthropus* at Olduvai, but apparently a later intruder in South Africa at Swartkrans. This need not mean he was doing his evolving in East Africa. Over so long a time, bands of the *Homo habilis* stages would have been moving back and forth across the Old World. So *Homo erectus* need have had no single home and no single spread outward from one single place, for all the homogeneity he seems to show. Dr. Bernard Campbell has suggested recognizing the several kinds of *Homo erectus* (as described by 1965) as subspecies, with appropriate names, so that, for example, the original Java Man of the Trinil beds becomes *Homo erectus erectus.* He puts them into this table.

Homo erectus

Grade	Europe	N. Africa	E. Africa	S. Africa	E. Asia	S. E. Asia
3	*heidel-bergensis*	*mauri-tanicus*	*leakeyi*		*pekinensis*	
2						*erectus*
1			*habilis*	*capensis*		*modjokertensis*

This not only saves some of the old names, as the reader will recognize, using them in more appropriate fashion, but also suggests some change or evolutionary progress, a continuation of what Tobias and von Koenigswald see in *habilis,* and what Weidenreich saw happening in Java Man. More broadly, however, we discern a stage of man, much the same everywhere, between about 1,000,000 and 500,000 years ago coming down to the end of the Second or Mindel Glaciation. Then, unfortunately, instead of getting better the evidence becomes much worse for about 400,000 years, until the last glacial phase, the Würm, is under way. During this another well-known assemblage of men, the Neanderthals, were succeeded by a final form, man of today. We have no Olduvai Gorge to give us sequences. We have simply the problem of Neanderthal Man, his coming and his going, a problem to which everyone has his own answers. Before we try to find the still-puzzling connections, let us take a march-past of the Neanderthals[1] and the men who followed them.

In spite of the problems they raise, the Neanderthal men are a welcome sight. There are so many fossils of them: burials, cannibals' remnants, skulls washed into river banks, isolated jaws, natural casts of brains and limb bones, and even footprints in grottoes. Nor are they from a few spots, but from all over Europe (excepting Britain and the northern countries), from North Africa, and on eastward into the Near East, Iraq, and Central Asia itself. And they range as broadly in time as in space. They first appear in the Third or Last Interglacial, carrying on more numerously into the first (fairly long) stage of the Fourth Glaciation. Then they come to an abrupt end, in the mild phase which followed, being replaced everywhere by men like ourselves. This replacement actually took many centuries. Seen against their history of perhaps a hundred thousand years, however, the disappearance of the Neanderthals is such that they might as well have been herded together and pushed over a cliff.

Neanderthal Portrait

Although it can be overemphasized, as for any human population, the Neanderthals generally show considerable similarity in the possession of a special character of skull and skeleton. What is more, the first Neanderthals to be discovered were all in Western Europe, and are rather extreme in this special character, so that they seem to depart furthest from their successors, *Homo sapiens*. For these reasons the westerners have usually and conveniently been referred to as the "classic" Neanderthals. Describing them will give us both the strongest contrast and the best point of departure.

If we look at a sort of composite of the many fossils, this is what we see: a fellow with a big face, a low but large skull, and heavy

---

[1] The "Neanderthals" have been so variously defined by different students of ancient man as to lead to serious confusion. Some writers automatically include the Steinheim and Mount Carmel specimens, described in a later chapter. Some, adding terms like "Neanderthaloid" and "Neanderthalian," have even included the Rhodesian and Solo men, thus meaning a stage of development, or a group, called by Weidenreich the "Paleoanthropinae." In reaction to this, Sergi limits "Neanderthal" strictly to the fossils of the Fourth Glacial phase of Europe. By the Neanderthals, I mean a group of fossil men connected in geography, time, and physique, the men described in this chapter, and them only.

bony brows. Brains, it is quite clear, had become essentially as large as those of today, but crania were still crude. Apart from this, Neanderthal skulls are not hard to recognize. They were low, without the elevation of the mid-line seen in most other types of man. Probably to counterbalance the large face, the skull projected in the back in the fashion called bun-shaped or wedge-shaped, being drawn out into a projecting occiput, with a well-marked but smooth ridge across it for the neck muscles. And it had a highly characteristic rounding or bulging of the sides, this bulging being further back

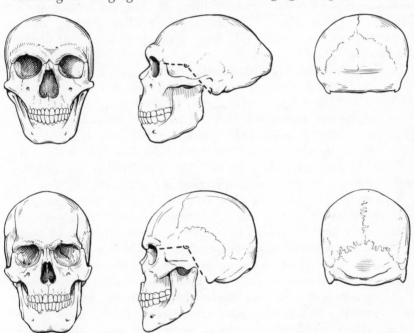

A comparison of the skulls of Neanderthal Man and *Homo sapiens* (not drawn to scale). These features of Neanderthal Man may be noted: lowness and breadth of the skull, form of the brow arches, large nasal aperture, marked forward and backward projection of the skull, wider angle at the base of the brain case, poorly developed mastoid processes.

than the widest part of our own heads, which is usually above our ears. This is a Neanderthal family feature, as is their style of brow, which curved upward over each eye and is typically seen to be of an even thickness all the way across.

More than anything, the structure of his face betrays the Neanderthaler. This face was a projecting one, but not primarily in the mouth region; in fact, the bony gum was distinctly vertical. Rather, his whole mid-face was carried forward, as though someone had seized his skull, while it was still soft, by the bridge of the nose, and pulled. This would have given him a rather high nose, which he had. It would have lengthened the whole fore part of his cranium, lowering his forehead and unbending the base of the skull, where it forms an angle under the forebrain and behind the face. This same moving of the eyes and nose forward, and further away from the ears, would have flattened the side of the face, making the cheekbones slope back smoothly from the region of the nose, with no angling at the sides (no "high cheekbones" like ours), and no hollow ("canine fossa") in the front of the cheek. This sum of effects is what you find in the cranium of a Neanderthal.

Lower jaws reflect a similar situation, being, at least in some cases, rather long (natural in a face which is set well forward on the skull). It is hard to give these jaws a single description, but, compared to modern mandibles, they all have the following features. They are "chinless," meaning that the fore part is receding, and such suggestion as they give of an actual bony development on the chin is slight. Also, the ascending ramus is broad and rather low, and the angle at the corner of the jaw is near a right angle, so that the bottom of the jaw does not slope downward to the chin, like ours.

As to the skeleton, this was stranger still, having traits not seen in any other kind of man. The Neanderthals must have been short in stature, but powerful and bear-like, dangerous to face in a wrestling match. The men stood just over five feet, the women just under. They were barrel-chested, and their limb bones tended to be heavy, short, somewhat bowed, and above all large in the joint. (To be quite accurate, individuals varied considerably in heaviness of the actual shafts of the long bones: some really very heavy, others much less so.) The forearm was especially short. This in itself made it a somewhat more effective lever, for sheer strength, than our own forearm. In addition, the two bones of this member, the radius and the ulna, straight and slender in us, were also slender but curved apart somewhat in the mid-sections, suggesting even heavier muscles and also making the arm effective in twisting motions as well. Neanderthal Man may have been both powerful and skillful in the use of his arms. As to his legs, he has often been pictured as walking with a "primitive" bent knee and even with a slightly separated great toe and a tendency to walk more on the outside of his foot. These assumptions do not now stand inspection, though it is true that the joint surface of his tibia, or lower leg bone, usually did slant backward at the knee to a degree only rarely seen in modern man.

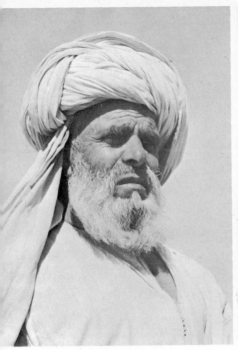

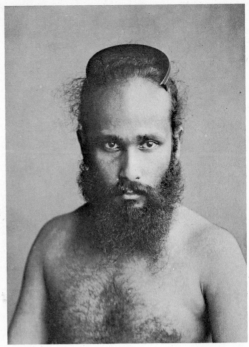

an of Baluchistan, West Pakistan

Sinhalese man, Ceylon

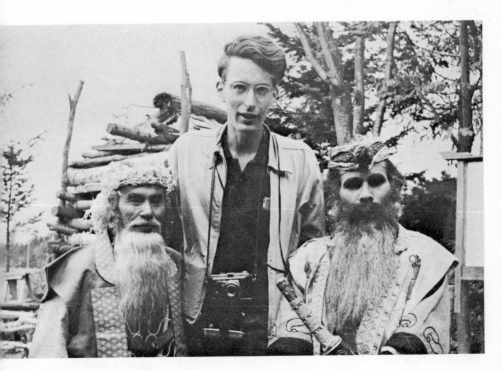

. Nordic between two Ainus of Japan

WHITES AND OFF-WHITES: VARIATIONS ON A THEME   PLATE I

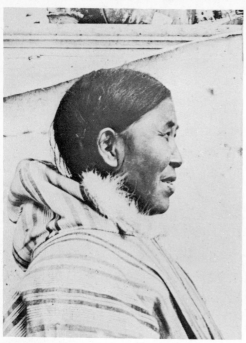

Alaskan Eskimo woman
COURTESY PEABODY MUSEUM

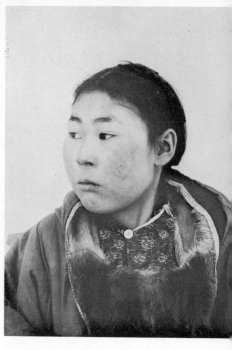

Siberian woman
COURTESY AMERICAN MUSEUM OF NATURAL HISTORY

FACES OF SIBERIANS, ESKIMOS, AMERICAN INDIANS

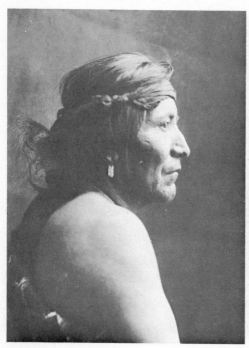

Navaho Indian man
COURTESY PEABODY MUSEUM

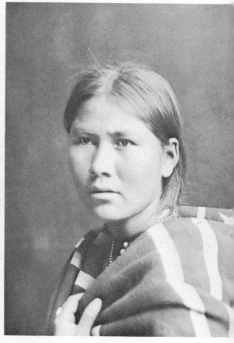

Navaho Indian woman
COURTESY PEABODY MUSEUM

PLATE II

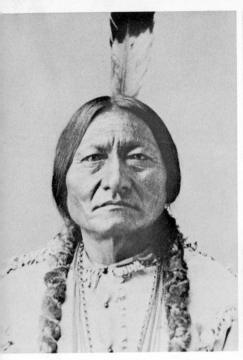

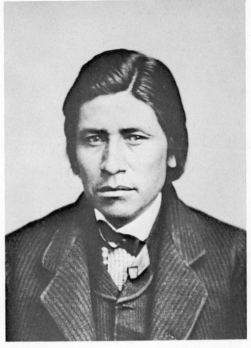

Sitting Bull, a Dakota Sioux
COURTESY PEABODY MUSEUM

A Dakota Sioux
COURTESY PEABODY MUSEUM

VARIETY IN AMERICAN INDIANS

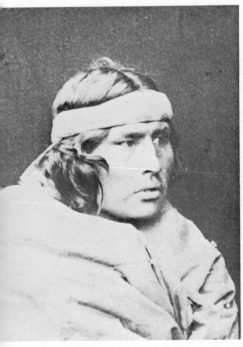

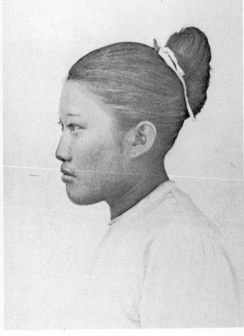

Araucanian Indian, Chile
COURTESY PEABODY MUSEUM

Arawak Indian woman, northern South America
COURTESY PEABODY MUSEUM

PLATE III

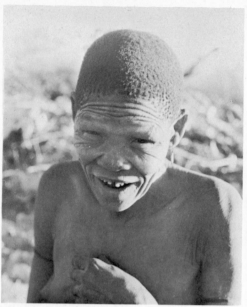

A Bush woman, Southwest Africa
COURTESY LAURENCE K. MARSHALL

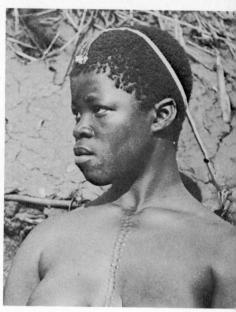

South African Bantu woman
COURTESY PEABODY MUSEUM

AFRICAN FACES AND SHAPES

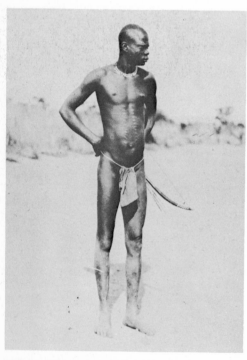

Nilotic Negro, Lungwari tribe
COURTESY PEABODY MUSEUM

PLATE IV

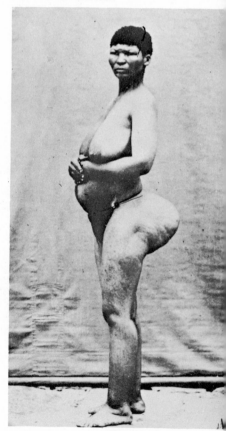

Hottentot woman with steatopygia
COURTESY PEABODY MUSEUM

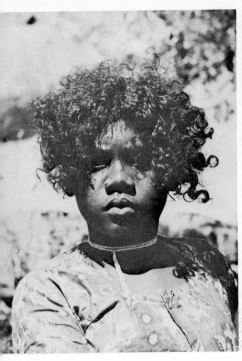

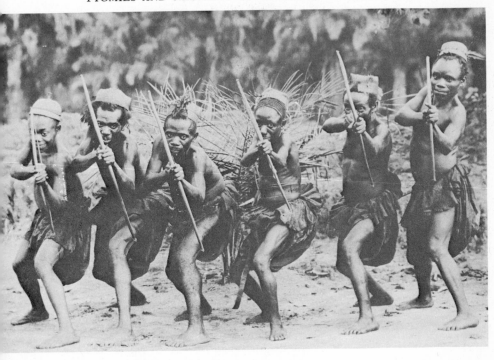

Kadar woman, southern India
COURTESY CARLETON COON

Negrito of Bataan, Luzon, Philippines
COURTESY PEABODY MUSEUM

PYGMIES AND NEGRITOS OF AFRICA AND THE EAST

Pygmies of the Congo forest, Africa
COURTESY THE AMERICAN MUSEUM OF NATURAL HISTORY

PLATE V

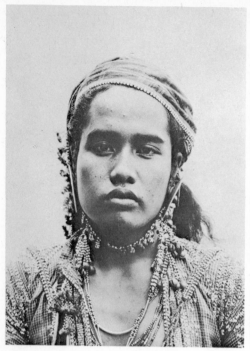

Bagobo man of Davao, Philippines
COURTESY PEABODY MUSEUM

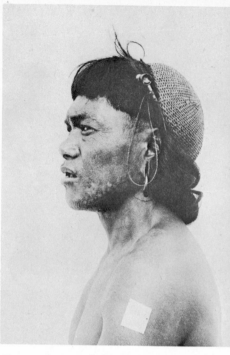

Bontoc Igorot of the Philippines
COURTESY PEABODY MUSEUM

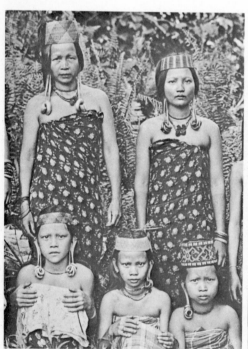

Kayan woman and girls, Borneo
COURTESY PEABODY MUSEUM

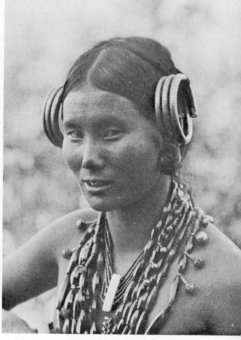

Naga woman, Assam, India
COURTESY PEABODY MUSEUM

PLATE VI — SOUTHEAST ASIA, A MELTING POT

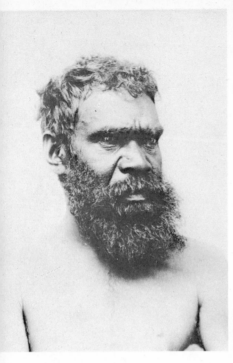

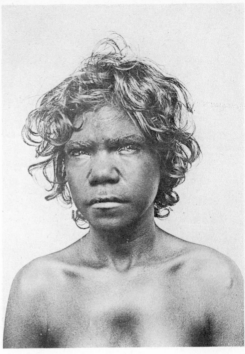

an from South Australia

Girl from Northern Australia

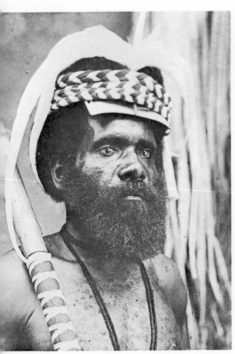

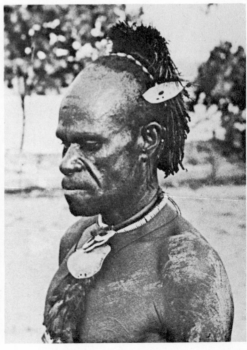

an from New Caledonia

New Guinea man, Sepik River

THE AUSTRALIAN ABORIGINES, AND MELANESIANS
WHO LOOK LIKE THEM   PLATE VII

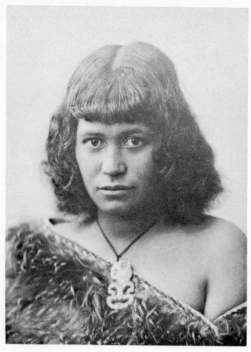

Maori woman, New Zealand
COURTESY PEABODY MUSEUM

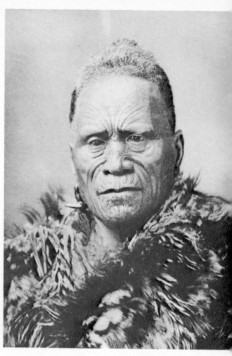

Maori man with face carving, New Zealan
COURTESY PEABODY MUSEUM

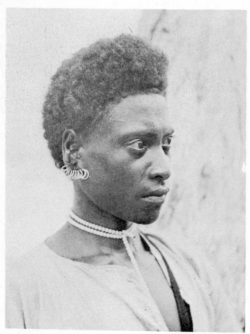

Solomon Islands man suggesting Negro type
COURTESY PEABODY MUSEUM

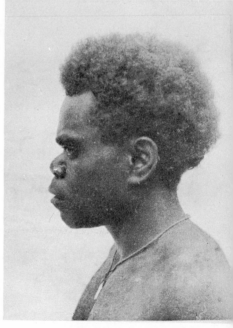

Solomon Islands man suggesting Negrito t
COURTESY DOUGLAS OLIVER

PLATE VIII   POLYNESIANS AND MELANESIANS

Also, although the shape of his neck bones has also been grossly misinterpreted in the past, it seems safe to conclude that the Neanderthals were rather bull-necked, with strong muscles at the back to balance the long head with its pulled-forward face.

The Early Neanderthals

The earliest Neanderthals lived in the warm times of the Last Interglacial. These first ones are known from Saccopastore on the Aniene River just outside Rome, and from Ehringsdorf near Weimar in Germany. Unfortunately the specimens are not in good condition. However, they seem to suggest a somewhat milder version of the portrait of the later ones, and they may not have been so heavily built. In some, the skull base was well bent behind the eyes, as is the case with us too. And in some the back of the head did not stick out in such a point but was more gently rounded from crown to back of neck, once more like ourselves. However, it would be a mistake to think that all the later Neanderthals subscribed closely to that portrait; some of them also departed from it, in lacking a pointed back to the head, or the very specific form of brow ridge. None of them, however, can be classed as anything but Neanderthal. The family look, like the Hapsburg jaw, is there, both in the face and in the peculiar flat top and bulging sides of the brain case.

Add one important find, made in 1949, to the early Neanderthals: the Montmaurin mandible. It came from a filled-up cave near Toulouse in southern France, together with warmth-loving animals of the Third Interglacial (conceivably, as Vallois believes, of the Second Interglacial). It is not at all like modern man. It is more bulky and primitive than Neanderthal jaws in general, with some features like the Heidelberg Man (thick and sloping chin region, for example). At the least, Vallois points out, it certifies the early establishment of rather definite Neanderthal characters. At the most, it makes a link by which the ancestry of the Neanderthals points back toward the Heidelberg Man himself, not the first time this ancestry has been suggested.

During the Third Interglacial in Europe, hand-axes and the older kinds of flake implements were petering out and giving way to reduced and special forms. In particular, new methods of flake striking and edge chipping had arrived, making for more efficient knives, scrapers, or small points. The Neanderthals were evidently taking part in the development of these things, and by the beginning of the Fourth Glacial period a definite set of tools, traditionally called the Mousterian culture of Europe, can be recognized as the handiwork of the Neanderthal men of that time. In fact, the men themselves are often referred to as the Mousterians. But this custom is not applauded by the archaeologists, who say that tools are tools and bones are bones, and that sources of confusion between them should be avoided. In addition, there were several distinct Mousterian traditions, not one only, and the question of whether different kinds of Neanderthal men were involved is under consideration. All the same, this does not prevent us from using the Mousterian culture, in the broad sense, as the spoor of the Neanderthals, since whenever a skeleton has been found with that culture in Europe, it has been a Neanderthal skeleton. Elsewhere a certain caution is the word.

A Change in the Weather

With the onset of the Fourth Glacial a new, very definite phase of history began for the Neanderthals. They became arctic explorers, so to speak, while staying in the same place. Ice descended on the British Isles and on the northern edge of Europe from Scandinavia, and came down out of the Alps as well. This turned Central Europe into an arctic province. South of the ice the ground froze, and the Mediterranean-like climate of interglacial times gave way to tundra, cold steppe, and plain. The rewards for facing so much unpleasant weather were, probably, that game continued to be plentiful and even, in certain places, more accessible. For there now appeared cold-weather versions of certain animals we think of today as tropical —elephants, rhinos, horses—which flourished handsomely on the forage of this climate. In Italy, moreover, some of the warmth-loving animals of the interglacial (hippopotamus and Merck's rhinoceros) managed to hang on into the first part of the new cold.

Though using them earlier, the Neanderthals now found caves a vital refuge, and signs of their occupation are everywhere. They got the upper hand of the cave bears, doubtless with the help of fire, and in doing so they showed both their prowess as hunters and their concern with religious ideas. In several caves in Switzerland, dating either from the first of the colder weather or even from the end of the Third Interglacial, Neanderthal men left the heads or skulls of bears, arranged in some definite way—once in a sort of vault made of blocks of stone. These bear collections might be nothing more than Neanderthal trophy rooms. But they could have had other trophies. And the bear, their dreaded enemy, would be a good candidate for serious religious concern. Further, we know of actual animal cults among living tribes: the Ainus of Japan go in for bear sacrifices, as do various Siberian aboriginals.

Religion is the likely bet for another reason: the Neanderthals were the first people known to have buried their own dead. True, they were also given to toying with loose heads, because such disembodied crania were left in several caves, on Gibraltar, in Italy, and in Greece. But judging from their positions, even these skulls were likely laid down with pious intent. And there is no doubt about the complete bodies which were put in graves made in the floors of caves during the early Fourth Glacial: they were true burials, religiously conceived. For the departed were supplied with tools of stone and sometimes other goods.

Now this might signify nothing more than the South African Bushman custom: they inter all a dead man's possessions with him, simply to get rid of them, contaminated as these are felt to be by death. But one Neanderthal boy was buried in Soviet Central Asia in a grave partly lined with goat horns, and this, like the bear skulls in Swiss caves, suggests more complicated spiritual ideas. Probably the stone tools were meant to help the soul against the bears and the other problems of the afterlife.

At any rate, it is because of these cave burials that the "Mousterian" Neanderthals were the first fossil men, not of our own type, to be discovered, over a century ago. This was an odd turn of fate for our understanding, because these late Neanderthals were more peculiar in their physical form—with short, heavy limbs, to say nothing of an exaggerated kind of cranium—and so they gave the search for "missing links" a slightly crooked start.

The Man from Neander's Valley

The very first was a child's skull taken from a cave at Engis near Liège, Belgium, in 1829; it fell to pieces and went unrecognized for what it was for more than a hundred years. The next was a woman's skull from Gibraltar. Somebody found it in 1848 in Forbes' Quarry and brought it around to the Gibraltar Scientific Society. But except for desultory mentions of a curious skull which did not identify it as Neanderthal, it escaped examination. Eventually it got to England, but even there nobody noticed it until 1906. Darwin evidently never heard of it.

Darwin did hear of the original Neanderthal Man, who made his appearance in August 1856, causing an immediate sensation. He came by his clumsy name in a roundabout way. In the seventeenth century there lived in Düsseldorf a poet, composer of hymns, and a headmaster of a school, Joachim Neumann. He liked to be known by a Greek translation of his name (New Man): Neander. He also liked to seek solitude in a wild, pretty little valley some distance from the city. Here, east of the Rhine where the land begins gradually to rise, there is a special elevated area cut right through the middle by the narrow valley of a small stream, the Düssel. The citizens of Düsseldorf in time paid Neander the bucolic honor of naming the gorge after him, calling it the "Neanderthal," and a pretty spot it must have been, with steep sides containing several caves.

But it is no longer the narrow defile it was from Mousterian times until the nineteenth century. Its flanks were formed to a great extent by limestone, and this began to be quarried away, broadening the ravine to the wider valley of today. In 1856 workers emptied one of the caves, the Feldhofer Grotto, and found bones in it. They took the bones for an animal's and threw them down. Luckily, the owner of the place, a Mr. Beckershoff, saved them at the last moment. We shall never know much about the finding; the cave, of course, is no more. How many of the bones got lost at the time we cannot tell, but bones of arms and thighs, the skull top, and part of the pelvis were kept.

These surviving fragments were given to J. C. Fuhlrott, founder of the Natural Science Society of nearby Elberfeld and teacher in the *Realschule* there. This time the low skull with its massive brows and the bowed limbs—including an ulna of the lower arm with an injury on it which prevented bending the elbow more than halfway—did not go unnoticed. Fossil discoveries need the right discoverer, and Fuhlrott was a member of this all too small band. He saw the singular nature of the specimen, and he came to the conclusion that it was definitely "antediluvian," like other cave fossils; that it was a real fossil man who had got washed into the cave by the Flood itself. Now this was the time, of course, when interest in evolution was everywhere and also a time when there was still a confusion, in scientific minds, between the Biblical Flood and the new knowledge of the late Ice Age. So Fuhlrott's opinion, in the language of the day, would correspond to our recognizing the Neanderthal find as "Pleistocene man."

Fuhlrott turned the bones over to Professor Schaaffhausen, anatomist at Bonn, for description. The latter also showed commendable judgment; he pointed out that the actual circumstances of the find were not sufficient to show that the skull was "diluvial," but that its form showed it must be old, older than such "ancient" inhabitants of Europe as the Celts and the Germans. Then everyone had his say about the Man. The evolutionists were pleased, naturally; and the anti-evolutionists, naturally, held the skeleton to be a freak. Virchow, the great German pathologist, said it was pathological, a victim of

disease, and he clung to this decision for over thirty years. Huxley
scouted such an idea and refused to go even that far afield, though
evolution never had a greater advocate than he. Huxley regarded
the skeleton as one of modern man, extreme in its features but still
Homo sapiens. The discreet Darwin said nothing, preferring to stick
to what he knew about at first hand—one of his secrets of success.
Only William King of Galway gave it as his belief at the time that
a human species, normal in its own way but different from ourselves, had come to light, and he named it *Homo neanderthalensis.*

These are among the more sensible conclusions. Look what one
German anatomist proffered as the explanation for the man from the
Neanderthal cave. The fellow must have had rickets, he said, looking at the bowed limb bones. This and the bad elbow caused the
poor man such pain that his brows were puckered in constant an-
guish; naturally the massive bony ridges grew out in response to the
muscular effort, going the Elephant Child's trunk one better. Further,
the bowed legs indicated a horseman, and the skull looked like
that of a Mongol, he said (actually, it would almost be easier to

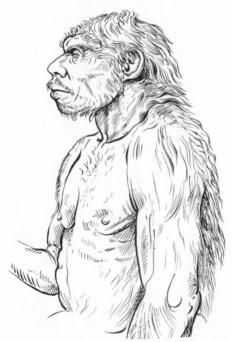

A restoration of the appearance of a Neanderthal Man, redrawn
from Z. Burian. Hair, and exact facial features such as lips, are
conjectural, but the anatomical impression is probably good.

mistake a Mongol skull for a cannon ball than for the Neanderthal specimen). Hence the remains were probably those of a Cossack of the Russian forces pursuing Napoleon west in 1814, who had been overcome by his illnesses and had crawled into the cave to die. But this misinformed guesswork sounds like the wisdom of Solomon compared to the effort of an English colleague. Wrote he, "*It may have been* one of those wild men, half-crazed, half-idiotic, cruel and strong, who are always *more or less* to be found living on the outskirts of barbarous tribes, and who *now and then* appear in civilized communities to be consigned *perhaps* to the penitentiary or the gallows, when their murderous propensities manifest themselves."[2] (Italics mine.)

While everyone was still suffering from inflammation of the imagination, a jaw was found in 1866 in the cave of La Naulette, in Belgium, accompanied by Mousterian implements and the bones of rhino, mammoth, and bear, thè first tangible evidence of the true

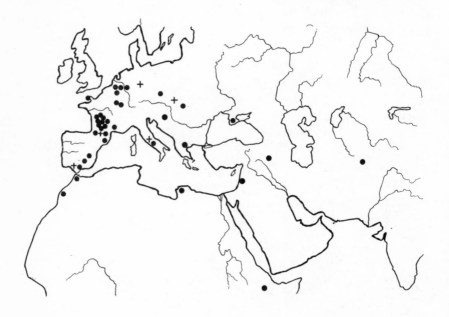

Distribution of the Neanderthal men, from the principal finds. Dots: known and probable Fourth Glacial specimens. Crosses: known and possible (e.g., Gibraltar I) Third Interglacial specimens.

[2] Quoted by Loren Eiseley, in *Darwin's Century* (New York: Doubleday, 1958), p. 274.

age of the Neanderthalers.[3] Coming in the midst of the excitement, and the guesses as to what a missing link should be like, the La Naulette jaw was generally described or referred to in publication as extremely ape-like, with huge projecting canine teeth. Even the careful Darwin cited this description in his first reference to the Neanderthals in 1871, in the *Descent of Man*. But as a matter of fact, the jaw had no teeth left in it at all. It is a good workaday Neanderthal jaw, nothing more.

Of course this is amusing now, but we should be fair and remember that these anatomists were among the best men of their day. If you have the skeleton of that first Neanderthal Man before you, and at the same time try to imagine yourself a hundred years back, it is easier to comprehend the disagreements. For the skeleton is quite incomplete, above all in lacking a face. And in some ways, I think, it does not show forth as pronounced a "Neanderthal" character as some of the others we have in hand today. Thus it is scarcely odd that the mid-nineteenth century did not jump right away to the well-defined views of the mid-twentieth.

The fog of uncertainty and conjecture began to dissipate only when further finds were made. The year 1886 produced two skeletons, much like the original one, from the cave of Spy, near Namur, again in Belgium. Now talk of freaks was outlawed. The few years just before the First World War saw a number of discoveries now famous, mostly from the Dordogne region of southwestern France: La Chapelle-aux-Saints, Le Moustier, La Ferrassie, La Quina. Other finds have followed, major or minor, from Spain, from Italy—none in England, but a possible tooth from the island of Jersey—and from southeastern Europe, Russia, Israel, and Iraq. The cave Neanderthals of Europe soon became a well-known variety of man. The great French student of them, Marcellin Boule, was able to describe the type in great detail, and to point to it as a highly uniform, highly specialized kind of man. Although fifty years ago there was every excuse, it is now plain that Boule overdid this. For example, in restoring the important La Chapelle skeleton, he appears to have erred in making the skull too long and forward-hanging, and in making the spines of the neck stand up like a gorilla's.

[3] Note that the 1856 Neanderthal Man is assigned to the late group only by presumption, since there is no real evidence now of his age. The Gibraltar Woman likewise is undated; physically she is rather more like the early lot.

Neanderthals in Africa and Asia

We have so far been doing a biography of the Neanderthals of Europe, particularly Western Europe. The cave people extended from the middle of the Fourth Glacial phase, about 35,000 B.C., back to the beginning of the Würm; and the Third Interglacial Neanderthals reach still further into the past, for no one knows how many thousands of years. Certainly a long history. What about other Neanderthals, outside of Europe?

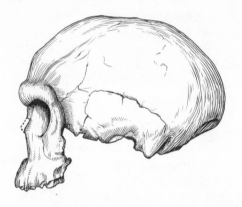

Jebel Irhoud skull. ¼ natural size.

In Morocco, two skulls were found, in 1962 and 1963, at Jebel Irhoud in the filling of a rock fissure along with tools of an African version of Mousterian and animals corresponding in time to the early Würm of Europe. From descriptions published so far, the skull vaults can be recognized as approximating the classic group, but the face of at least one lacks the marked forward projection of the Neanderthals and instead has the features of modern man, though

Opposite:
A page of Neanderthals. In the center is a restoration of the type of the "classic" Neanderthals, based on Monte Circeo, the best preserved, with jaw and teeth added from other specimens. Top left, Saccopastore I (with breakage, including brow ridges). Top right, Ehringsdorf, after Kleinschmidt's reconstruction. Second row, Krapina fragments, after Gorjanovic-Kramberger. Bottom left, Shanidar skull as reconstructed by T. D. Stewart. Bottom right, Teshik-Tash boy (right side reversed). All ¼ natural size.

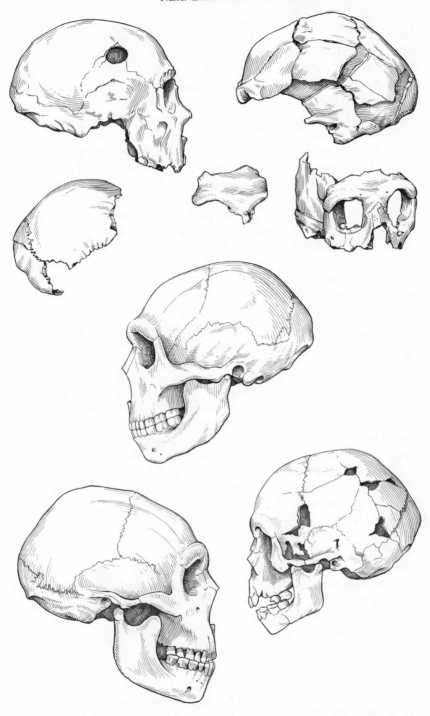

they are considerably larger; the face is also reported to lack a canine fossa, or depression in the cheekbone, like other Neanderthals. Elsewhere, Neanderthal remains from Africa are scrappy: a piece of upper jaw, from Tangier, and fragments of mandible, two being from the Haua Fteah Cave in Cyrenaica and one from Porcupine Cave, Diredawa, Ethiopia. They are unsatisfactory specimens, but they cover a big stretch of territory, from the Strait of Gibraltar along the Mediterranean and down the Red Sea to the Horn of Africa. The first two finds, at least, belong to the same general period as the cave Neanderthals in Europe, a probable date for the Haua Fteah jaws being 40,000 B.C. One of these is a fairly good fragment, of recognizable Neanderthal form, but none of the mandibles really tell what kind of Neanderthals they represent. The Diredawa specimen may be later and is especially dubious in any event.

In the Near East things have been better. On Mount Carmel, in Israel, a cave (Mugharet et-Tabūn) yielded a large male lower jaw, and the skeleton of a woman, a palpable Neanderthal. She had the low skull, arched brows, and broad mouth of her European Neanderthal relatives. The back of her head, however, was rounded, not pointed. Also, she was rather delicately built, perhaps out of mere femininity. The large male jaw has a rather good chin for a Neanderthal.

The Tabūn Woman was found in 1931. In 1961 a Japanese excavation in Israel found another good skeleton nearby in the Amud Cave. In the mountains of northern Iraq, Dr. Ralph Solecki of the Smithsonian Institution and his party excavated in the huge Shanidar Cave, where some forty feet of fill go down from modern times through the Neolithic and late Paleolithic into Mousterian remains. In these last, Solecki in 1953 found the bones of an infant Neanderthal, eventually followed by six more of his kind. In 1957 he laid bare the skeletons of three adults, all of whom had been killed, buried, and unfortunately well smashed, by rock falls from the cave roof. The varying depths and spots where they lay suggest (with the potent help of C_{14}) that these accidents took place at various times from 50,000 B.C. back to perhaps 70,000 B.C. The least smashed of the Shanidar men was a strange cripple, with a withered right arm, the lower part of which had eventually been amputated.

The Tabūn Woman and the Amud Man apparently lived in the same time span. They also seem to have shared a degree of kinship with the Shanidar cripple, judging from their features. Though all immediately strike one as Neanderthals, each had a somewhat rounder back to the head than is typical of the Europeans, and the men seem to have been of larger size. The Shanidar and Amud skeletons suggest individuals of about five feet seven or eight inches and the

Amud Man had a head which was enormous, bigger than the European Neanderthalers, whose heads were certainly big. Both men shared a peculiar deepening of the nasal cavity inside the nose, not seen in *Homo sapiens;* and the Shanidar Man and the Tabūn Woman had an unusual attenuation of the pubic bone of the pelvis, also not seen in *Homo sapiens* (this part of the skeleton is very seldom recovered and so it cannot be said how widespread the feature was among Neanderthals). These skeletons therefore suggest a well-defined Neanderthal population allied to, but slightly distinct from, that of Europe.

From further east came the Teshik-Tash boy, he of the goat-horn sepulchre, found in Uzbekistan, Soviet Central Asia, in 1938. Although this child was only eight or nine years old when he died, he showed rather clear signs of developing into an adult of the classic type of Neanderthal, with a pointed back to his head, large teeth, and a flat cheekbone lacking a canine fossa. He already had a big brain (1490 cc.), so that he was on his way toward a brain volume distinctly over modern Europeans.[4] He had a few "advanced" particulars, however, especially in a greater height to his skull than would be typical for classic Neanderthals.

A Greek Exception

No Neanderthal bone had ever been found in Greece before 1960, when two Greek archaeologists found a lone skull in the Petralona Cave southeast of Thessaloníki, along with animal bones which suggest that it is of Last Glacial date. Like the Monte Circeo skull in Italy, the face was encrusted with lime from drip water, but it is in excellent condition and, in spite of the limey mask, obviously of a general Neanderthal type. However, it shows marked individual features, not reflecting the classic form. It is large, low, and long, but instead of having the round outline in back view, it is very broad at the base, rather steep-sided, and slightly crested along the top. Both the brows and the eye sockets are more squared off. In other ways also, he suggests non-Neanderthals such as the Broken Hill skull of Rhodesia (which we come to later) or the Solo men. Is he simply an unusual Neanderthal? Or is he suggesting that in

---

[4] It may be noted that other juvenile specimens also show the distinct Neanderthal traits early in life, such as the brows, the protruding back, and the bulging sides. This is particularly true of the fine Engis skull, in Brussels, a child about seven years of age. The fact is a strong argument in favor of the distinctiveness of the Neanderthal line and against close community with our recent ancestry. This is especially so if one appeals to "pedomorphism," a principle of evolution in which descendants express the juvenile form of ancestors, since the skull of modern man is not that of a young Neanderthal.

this southward direction, where we otherwise have only African scraps, there was a definite trend of departure in form from the classics of Europe?

A Chinese Neanderthal?

Other parts of the world are very poorly known for this period and in fact for all the Upper and the later Middle Pleistocene. An important piece is therefore the upper face and fore part of a skull found in a limestone cave at Mapa, in Kwangtung Province, China,

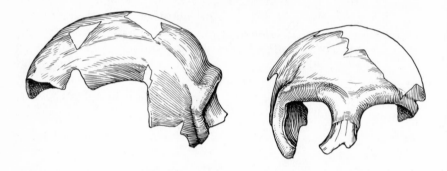

The Mapa skull cap from China. ¼ natural size.

in 1958. Unfortunately its date is quite vague: it might be contemporaneous with the Neanderthals and it might be considerably earlier. Its partial state also makes for vagueness. It does not appear as strikingly Neanderthal on first glance, though it strongly suggests a man of the same grade of evolutionary advance. It certainly has a far better-filled skull than that of Pekin Man.

In such details as can be picked out it seems to agree again and again with the Neanderthals, even though the total impression is not clear. The eye sockets are round, the brow ridges are also rounded and fairly thick near their mid-portions; the skull is evidently long, low, and broad far back, without a mid-line crest. It could be a faraway Neanderthal: that is to say, it could be a sole representative, the only one found so far, of the most eastern of a series of populations starting with the classic Neanderthals of Western Europe, going through the slightly different one of the Near East, and through several other such on out to the Orient. With its unknown date the skull says all too little; nevertheless, it seems quite different from the Solo men, the only other known candidates for ruler of the Far East in the later Pleistocene.

14. HOMO SAPIENS ARRIVES

It IS TIME to meet the Cro Magnons. In Europe the cave Neander-thals came to a relatively quick end, and their place was taken by a different kind of man, who was entirely like ourselves. This is one of the clearest events of human history.

After its first assault on Europe, known as the Early Würm or Würm I, the Fourth Glacial phase ameliorated somewhat; according to C14 this was between 42,000 B.C. and 30,000 B.C., with the mildest point about 35,000 B.C.[1] Forests once more grew northward from the Mediterranean shore. During this interval new ideas in the making of stone tools came to fruition. The ideas developed, it is true, on the basis of existing techniques, but they constitute so distinct a for-ward step that they are taken to mark the opening of a new chapter in stoneworking: the Upper Paleolithic, the last part of the Old Stone Age. Tool styles and types were not the same all over Europe, any more than among the different American Indian tribes. But the new stonework rested on a few broad inventions in the flaking of flint, so that all the tools have a family resemblance. An amateur can recognize them and distinguish them from the tools made earlier (many of which, by the way, continued to be made).

Above all, the makers of the new tools could strike off a flake from

[1] There will be considerable reference to this date of 35,000 B.C. in what follows. I wish to explain now that it is not meant to be a precise date (there continues to be some uncertainty about exact figures) but rather symbolizes a short period of time before which there were Neanderthals in Europe and after which there were modern men. At the moment, Mousterian culture in France can be dated as late as 36,000 B.C., and possibly almost to 33,000 B.C., while deposits with Upper Paleolithic culture (Aurignacian, not the earliest known!) have been dated as older than 32,000 B.C. Elsewhere, as we shall see, it is possible that Rhodesian Man survived well beyond this chosen date of 35,000 B.C., while the Niah Cave boy of Borneo, a representative of modern man, may have lived well before it; again, however, these ages are thought to be good estimates but not precise dates. This whole matter of dating is just the one which will be undergoing constant refinement and adjustment everywhere. But in the meantime I need a reference point, and so I say 35,000 B.C. as one might say "12 o'clock noon" to mean the middle of the day, more or less. It may well turn out that such a dividing date should actually be somewhat later as far as Western Europe is concerned.

a core in such a way as to get a knife-like blade. Such a blade may be trimmed further into a number of special tools or weapons: knife; spear point; awl for making holes in skin, wood, or bone; scraper for fleshing the inside of animal skin to make leather; shaver for trimming lance shafts; and so on. Bone work became important, and their coarse· needles show that they were sewing themselves skin garments.

Now all this does not mean that the Neanderthals shivered helplessly in the cold; on the contrary, their tools were evidently used on skin also. But the Upper Paleolithic people had more and better, with a greater variety. They lived the same life as the Neanderthals, using the same caves and hunting the same animals, for almost thirty thousand years. The glaciers finally began to thin and shrink, and the woolly rhinoceros and the hairy mammoth disappeared, leaving horses, bison, and, above all, reindeer as the chief food animals of the late Pleistocene and after. Indeed, the Upper Paleolithic men hunted the same choice valleys used by Neanderthal Man, and in cave after cave the remains they left lie just above the Mousterian levels. But they were special and skillful hunters: at Solutré in France, they killed a hundred thousand horses, and at Předmost in Czechoslovakia, a thousand mammoths (over a long period of time, to be sure). The Neanderthals were surely able and valiant in the chase, but they left no such massive bone yards as this.

The new people were good artists as well as good hunters. They began drawing the animals they hunted on cave walls, first in black outlines, and later filling them with earth colors, to produce the magnificent galleries at the Font de Gaume at Les Eyzies, at Lascaux near Montignac, and at Altamira near Santander on the north coast of Spain. These graceful, lively works of assured artistry have now been awarded their just recognition by the modern art world. They are the more wonderful because they caught, from life, animals which no man has seen since the end of the Ice Age. That they were done by accomplished artists is emphasized by the fact that only a very few of the many paintings could have been made by amateurs and dabblers, who were probably not allowed to deface the walls.

It would be flattering, of course, to think that the high art and better stone tools mean that a new level of intelligence had arrived with the new kind—our kind—of man. But that would be unfair to the Neanderthals. Furthermore, we have no license to think so. What can we tell from art? For all we know, the Neanderthals may have brought choral singing to a higher plane than has ever been reached since; with their big noses they probably had fine resonant voices. As for the stonework, the Neanderthals were as competent as anyone of their time. How can we tell they would not also have advanced here? The work of the Upper Paleolithic was, after all, simply the latest in the long series of improvements and inventions made during the Pleistocene. Finally, for sheer brain size, we have not yet outdistanced the Neanderthals. One of the skulls from La Ferrassie had a cranial capacity of 1640 cc., and the Amud Man from Israel had about 1800, a figure seldom attained by individuals today.

As a matter of fact it cannot be said just how the new tools and the new men were connected; the archaeology at present is far from clear. In central France, whence so many of the skeletons, Neanderthal and Upper Paleolithic, have come, the first culture of the Upper Paleolithic (Perigordian) has various connections in tool types and techniques with parts of the Mousterian complex, and in fact looks to some students like a purely local transition. The next culture (Aurignacian, to which the Cro Magnons belong), and in fact the first to appear in parts of France, Spain, and Italy, is in a different tradition, and clearly an invader, though from where is not known. Neither culture seems to be a simple immigrant from the Near East. Furthermore the first Upper Paleolithic culture of central Europe was different from both and earlier than either, as was apparently the beginning of the Upper Paleolithic in North Africa. Dates in the Near East are not clear, but Professor Dorothy Garrod and others have found a sort of forerunner of the Aurignacian in Syria and the Lebanon, very much earlier, dating back to the end of the Third Interglacial but then succeeded by a culture of the Mousterian family. At the moment we can only say that this whole great region saw cultural changes around 35,000 B.C. which were rapid by Stone Age standards, and that in Western Europe we behold an abrupt change in the population—there must have been an immigration into Europe from somewhere, of a new kind of man too different from the local Neanderthals to have sprung from their loins in lineal descent.

Skeletons at Cro Magnon

The first of these cave men, dug up early in the nineteenth century, was brushed aside both by laymen and by men of science. With few exceptions, all refused to believe that the skeletons could have lain there since "before the flood," mingled though they were among bones of mammoths and other extinct animals. It was in 1868 that Louis Lartet found the Old Man of Cro Magnon and four other skeletons under an overhanging cliff, right in the village of Les Eyzies, and recognized them as true Ice Age men of our kind.

The Cro Magnons, however, were not the very first of the new faces

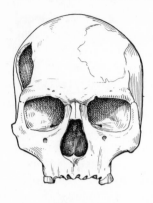 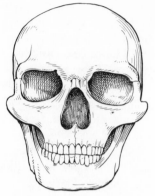

Upper Paleolithic skulls. Left, Lautsch I, after a photograph. Right, skull of Cro Magnon type from Grotte des Enfants, after Verneau. ¼ natural size.

in Europe. Among the earliest are believed to be the Combe Capelle skeleton of the same district (a great Neanderthal center as well) and skulls and skeletons from a cave near Lautsch (Mladeč), Czechoslovakia. These firstcomers had long, high, and narrow heads, especially Combe Capelle, who also had a long face and a strong jaw. They seem to have been of medium to small body size. They are the people who arrived in the warmer interval after the first period of the Würm cold.

On the other hand, the people found in the Cro Magnon rock shelter lived a few thousand years later, after the cold had come back, and probably just about 30,000 B.C. Their faces were broader—distinctly broad—and their heads not so very narrow. Certainly they were tall in stature and powerfully built. Many other European skeletons of this same time resemble them, so that the "Cro Magnon type" has been long used to cover them as a group.

These differences are interesting but not especially important. In the generation before us, the distinction between the Combe Capelle man and the Old Man of Cro Magnon was warmly insisted on (and as warmly denied). But the distinction is not as great as this suggests, and the Lautsch skulls fall in between, lessening the gap. I think it is fair to say that the two types probably differed about as much as an Irishman and an Austrian of today, or less.

Such a statement is truthful in another way; these people were Europeans, the forerunners, and at least partly the ancestors, of the people who live there today. There can be no doubt that they were members of the White, or Caucasoid, racial stock, because the features of their skulls and facial skeletons all have that stamp. The one actual painting of a man so far known, a small bas-relief at Angles-sur-Anglin, gives us a White man (actually a lightish purple, but the effect is "white") with black hair and a black beard.

A Look in the Mirror

But this is getting a little ahead of the story, before we are quite done with the Neanderthals. We can deal with these details in a moment. The important thing we are viewing in the Combe Capelle men, about the year 35,000 B.C., is the grand entrance of *Homo sapiens*. Who is he? He is modern man; all living men are of this single kind. All equally, moreover, and none more than any other. For the skeleton is much the same in every race of man; and as for the rest, it must be borne in mind that it is no more typical of the species to be white of skin than to be black, for a Siamese cat is not more of a cat than a tabby, nor is a great Dane more profoundly and movingly a dog than is a dachshund.

Let us have a good look at *Homo sapiens*. His skeleton has nothing new in it, compared, let us say, to Rhodesian Man, although perhaps his neck has a little less work to do and may be smaller. For his skull is lighter than was typical for any of the men we have reviewed. He is the only man with a really domed head and high forehead, with vertical sides and a rounded back to his brain case. And he is the only man with so thin-walled a skull and so light-boned a face.

This face is extremely delicate in structure, and well pulled in below the forehead, throwing the nose into relief. Here we differ somewhat from race to race, with the skeleton of the nose bridge tending to reflect how far the upper face is pulled in. When a modern face projects, it does so mainly in the region of the teeth and gums. So sunken is the middle portion (except for some very full-faced types like Eskimos) that there are canine fossae in the mid-cheek, over the sinuses, on either side of the nose. These hollows accentuate the angles of the cheekbones at the corners, and they are absent in the Rhodesian skull and the typical Neanderthals. Our teeth are much reduced in some races, but not in all; there are no great distinctions. But the bony chin sitting on the front of the jaw is a good badge of *Homo sapiens*, although it is less a sign of intelligence and determination than of a pushed-in face and a puny mandible.

The most important and characteristic difference we know between sapiens man and his cousins is the collapse of his brows. These ridges, forming a massive bar in *Homo erectus*, as well as in the much later Rhodesian or Solo men, and a double-humped arch over the eyes of the Neanderthals, early and late, have become true vestiges, mere

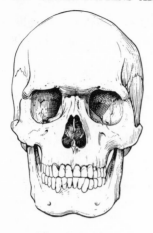 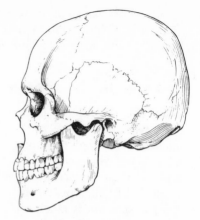

The skull of *Homo sapiens*. This is drawn from the skull of a
native of Fiji where the population probably represents a blend
of the main races of modern man; consequently it demonstrates
a general male human skull, medium in almost every respect,
rather than a particular human stock. If unusual at all, it is
rather strongly built, e.g., in the brow region. ¼ natural size.

adornments of the forehead itself, in ourselves and our late Pleistocene
forebears. The sinuses, or flat cavities within the frontal bone, are
also fairly small; but here it should be remarked that there is no very
strong connection in size between sinus and ridge.

It is the bony brows themselves which have subsided so definitely,
and in doing so they have separated into two portions over each eye.
These you can feel yourself with your fingers, if you are neither
excessively young nor excessively feminine, in which case your forehead may be smooth as an egg. The main brow element is a short
oblong mound slanting upward and away from the mid-line, on either
side, so that the two sides together tend to form a V, in the middle,
overlying only the inner part of each eye socket. (These have no
correspondence with your everyday "eyebrows" or supercilia, but lie
above them.) In addition, at the outer upper corner of the socket on
each side there is a more modest swelling or none at all. This is separated from the central part by a groove running inward over the
edge of the orbit. And it is this groove which makes a good distinguishing mark of sapiens man, for such a separation is absent in
the continuous brow overhanging the eyes of every other member of
the human family.

There you have *Homo sapiens*. And there you have the men of the
present, and the men of the Upper Paleolithic. Some of the latter, like
the Předmost skulls, had rather strong brow ridges, it is true, but

these are more an accentuation of the form seen in modern man and there are equally "primitive" men today. And the Cro Magnon people had just the brows one would find in a large robust man of the present. Although it is easy here to fall into the error of thinking we ourselves are perfect, or that evolution clearly had us in mind all the time, it is not unfair to say that *Homo sapiens* seems to have finished up all the unfinished business of human progress in the Pleistocene.

For example, although we have very few parts of the skeleton other than skulls, it seems that *Homo erectus* had passed beyond the australopithecine uncertainty as to some details of the skeleton and had perfected the upright posture, establishing the same skeleton that we have today. They had, however, small brains and still powerful jaws —the trend to brain increase had only just started. In the middle range the Neanderthals and the Rhodesians (actually very recent) had arrived essentially at a brain to meet the needs of a man, a brain about as large as ours. But they had only just begun to remodel the skull and to let teeth, jaws, and face fall back to the more modest size which is all that is needed in an animal who can cut his meat and cook it. Finally, although the new styling is suggested in the early Neanderthals, it really remained for sapient man to contain the enlarged brain in a more economical envelope: higher, thinner, more globular by virtue of a rising forehead and rounded back, and altogether more simply balanced on the spine. At the same time the lesser demands of chewing had allowed the face to be pulled back under the smoother brow and forehead about as far as is anatomically possible. All the little traits I have mentioned throughout only express these trends and stages.

A Little Variety

At any rate, *Homo sapiens* represents, I believe, the emergence of a well-defined type, the establishment of a distinct strain. He should be considered in this light. He does not now overlap the main groups of other men or reproduce, in individuals or tribes, their distinguishing traits. Certainly he is widely different from the curious cave Neanderthals of the Fourth Glacial, even if he has some slight likenesses to their Third Interglacial forerunners. But his physical distinctiveness does not in itself say how long ago he came into existence as we know him. That will be our next problem.

Back to the caves, and a general look at the Europeans of the time. Tall or short, they all shared a kind of ruggedness and large size of the skull, a size which is matched nowhere by whole populations and is approached only by the Scandinavians, or the Irish, or the original Anglo-Saxon invaders of England. What does this ruggedness mean? A Neanderthal legacy? It has been argued that some, at least, of the Upper Paleolithic men evolved straight out of the Neanderthals in Europe and that the Predmost type was transitional (with its short stature and well-marked brows), the Cro Magnon specimens being a later and more fully modern stage. Others, however, thought rather that the earliest invaders bore the brunt of contact with the Neanderthals and so had some actual mixture with them. This is opposed by the facts: the Lautsch skulls are entirely non-Neanderthal. So I doubt both possibilities. The truth is that all the new people are perfectly good specimens of *Homo sapiens* as I have defined him. They do not look part Neanderthal, as you might expect from such propositions as I have mentioned. Nor do the new people even show much variation. Surprisingly homogeneous, most of the many skulls are close in type to the "Cro Magnon," with a minority forming the long-skulled, narrow-faced Combe Capelle lot.

But there are also a couple of possible oddities. One is the Chancelade skeleton of France, belonging to a late Upper Paleolithic stage, the Magdalenian. Against the background of half-frozen Europe, his tools and way of life originally gave a faint suggestion of the life of the much later Eskimo of the Arctic. And the skull of this man, who was short in stature, suggested an Eskimo also, and thus the arrival of members of the Mongoloid stock. Once made, the suggestion became a rolling snowball. Like an Eskimo's, the skull is long, narrow, and pitched to a high keel in the middle; the face is broad and the nose is narrow; the jaw is broad and strong and is furnished on its inner surface, below the cheek teeth, with lumps of extra bone, common in Eskimos and believed to be a response to long-continued heavy chewing. List all these things on paper, and you have an Eskimo. Look at the skull itself, and you have no such thing. With all these features it still looks like a European, albeit one with broad cheeks. So strike this "Eskimo" from the list of possible foreigners.

A more puzzling case is another pair of skeletons, probably mother and teen-age son, found buried together in the Grotte des Enfants, one of the Grimaldi caves on the Riviera just at the Italian border of France. The skeletons have been called the "Grimaldi Negroids" because, while also showing a strong family likeness to one another, both have a Negroid appearance and Negro skull traits. Without getting ahead of things, I may say that it is quite inexplicable how an isolated pair of Negroes might have got to this place at this time. The whole matter is probably a coincidence. For one thing, it is believed that the Negroid look of the mid-face is due to breakage and inept reconstruction, which has never been corrected. But this does not explain the other Negro traits: upright, rather bulbous foreheads, large teeth, low and rather receding chins. To an eye familiar with the crania of different races, these, and general appearances, are striking. Another striking fact: a complicated statistical analysis (a discriminant function) to distinguish between the skulls of modern Negroes and Whites stamps the Grimaldi woman as Negro. This again may have been affected by the reconstruction made. It is unwise to brush away these "Negroes" simply because they may be inconvenient, and the solution is less obvious than the "Eskimo" Chancelade Man, but they are best put on the dubious shelf. Doubtful cases of fossil man have had a way of resolving themselves in favor of the less fantastic probabilities, as we shall see again. It pays to be conservative.

And the conservative position is to view the Upper Paleolithic people as Whites, coming in and dispossessing Neanderthals. Of course, this eviction did not happen overnight. Nor do we know how it happened, and whether we may imagine the two kinds of man doing battle to the death. But almost certainly they did not. The newcomers might, in fact, have extinguished the Mousterians simply by more successful hunting, getting the game first. But the two might have met, even peaceably, and with some slight interbreeding; however, in Europe at least, the probabilities are against more than this. For they would have been naturally hostile competitors, having different ideas and speaking different languages, like the Navahos and the Pueblos, or the Iroquois and Algonquin—and we should not suppose that such tribes were any more open-minded about foreign competition than we are. Furthermore, there were probably important spots, avenues of game, or critical passes, such as the meeting of valleys at Les Eyzies. There must have been real rivalry for command of these, just as bands of Australian aborigines view infringement of their rights to water holes as a fighting matter.

You could write a novel about this, and people have done so. But these must remain novels. We only know that, in Europe, *Homo sapiens* came to stay and the Neanderthals vanished.

15. UNFINISHED BUSINESS

WHERE DID the usurpers come from? How long had they existed? I am not simply asking where Combe Capelle Man was in 35,001 B.C. Rather, we now enter the whole question of the origins of *Homo sapiens*, already touched on in connection with the now-dismissed Galley Hill skeleton.

It is the worst present problem in our evolution. Of course we have other gaps to face, but here it is not a question of lack of fossils. For the late Pleistocene we have all the Neanderthals and all the men of the Upper Paleolithic and a number of other finds, just about to be introduced. Yet the problem obstinately remains unsolved. Who are we—us, ourselves—and what have we to do with Neanderthals? What are the connections of the two kinds of man? Here the anthropologists divide.

The problem cannot be seen, much less solved, simply from what I have related in the last two chapters. There I described in broad and fairly simple outline the two great human groups of Europe, the men of the Upper Paleolithic and those I have chosen to define as Neanderthal. The latter, we saw, makes its appearance in the Third Interglacial, and flourishes in Europe with obvious representatives in North Africa and Asia for perhaps half of the Würm or last Glacial phase. About 35,000 B.C., the crucial date, it gives way rapidly to *Homo sapiens* in Europe. After this point in time, we do not know positively of any other kind of humanity surviving elsewhere in the world. If we took just this picture, and overlooked the rapidity of the process, we could assume that the Neanderthals evolved directly, and in Europe, to their successors. This simplified explanation, in fact, has had its followers from the beginning right down to the present.

But we face complications. This chapter is about a whole series of facts and finds which have to be woven around and through the homely fabric I have so far presented. Some of the finds are of outstanding importance, and all of them must sooner or later be explained before the main problem is answered. They change the picture from simple to complex. But, then, we should never have expected our history to be a primer for children. On the whole, these further fossils tend to bracket the Neanderthals, some falling earlier in time, and others in the critical later days shortly before Neanderthal Man disappeared; that is, those relatively few millennia in which he must have given rise to *Homo sapiens*, if that is what he did.

In addition, we are now considering the entire Old World, and not simply its northwestern quadrant. The central question is this: is there evidence that *Homo sapiens* was present, or was evolving, at a time well before his Fourth Glacial entrance in Europe? Do the fossils show that he is actually a strain distinct from the Neander-thals I have described? You will remember, from Chapter 9, that in the nineteenth and early twentieth centuries there was a procession of false witnesses to the great antiquity of *Homo sapiens* and that the last of them, the Galley Hill Man, collapsed some time ago in a cloud of fluorine ions. The long and heated argument over them in those days was due to everyone's realization of their crucial nature: if legitimate, they would have proved that a fully devel-oped line of modern man existed at the same time as the Neanderthal or even Solo Man, or earlier still, and that this line was therefore not directly descended from any such but reached far back into the past.

This idea, in its pristine simplicity, has been abandoned along with the "fossils" on which it rested. The wide distribution of *Homo erectus,* more recently discovered, urges that nothing more advanced existed before the end of the Second Glacial phase. But the fossils to which we now turn cast doubt on any such uniformity of grade during the time of the Neanderthals.

Mount Carmel: The Oven and the Kids

I have described the Neanderthals from Israel: the Amud Man, and the woman from et-Tabūn (Cave of the Oven) on Mount Car-mel. It is an interesting and important region. Plentiful stone work shows a long succession of Levalloiso-Mousterian remains, of a gen-eral kinship to the European Mousterian. But this basic culture is interrupted by layers carrying what seems like a too-late Acheulian hand-axe culture, and by others with a too-early Upper Paleolithic, "Pre-Aurignacian" blade industry, all these cultures overlapping in most unorthodox fashion. And the fairly plentiful human bones are also strangely intermediate between Neanderthals and men of our own kind, reaching almost from one to the other.

A joint British-American expedition dug the Tabūn cave and an-

other. The Cave of the Kids, Mugharet es-Skhūl, was one of anthropology's great finds: it contained ten buried skeletons, in different
states of repair and in a densely cemented matrix, difficult to work.
These people lived subsequent to the Tabūn Woman and her companion with the big jaw; distinctly later (10,000 years has been
suggested), and following some kind of climatic interval which saw
the disappearance of hippopotamus and rhinoceros from the area,
along with some other animals, and the new appearance of others
still. The people themselves were of a different kind, approaching
closely to *Homo sapiens* as we already know him. Skeletally they
were tall, strongly built but straight-limbed, and so quite unlike their
hulking contemporaries of the cold northwest. There were faint suggestions of skeletal relationship to Neanderthals, such as relatively
short forearms with somewhat bowed radius and ulna, but it would
not be safe to look on these as something out of the range of modern
man.

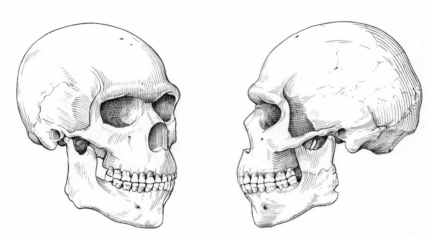

Skhūl V, best preserved of the skulls from the Skhūl cave on
Mount Carmel. Reconstruction by Charles E. Snow. Drawn from
the original. ¼ natural size.

Their brain case was like ours in size and shape; high, flat-sided;
and round, not projecting, in the rear. But the fore part of the skull
wears a Neanderthal look. The brows are marked, and slightly Neanderthal, though differing in being more like a pronounced shelf, not
as heavy or bulbous as in Neanderthal men. The forehead, in one, is
rather low and sloping; in another, of respectable height. In one, at
least, the nose and mouth are full and somewhat projecting, in a sort
of imitation-Neanderthal form; however, the malar bones and the

cheek arches are like ours, well angled and with a canine fossa along-side the nose. The jaw is intermediate as well. It has an abrupt angle, but one not resembling the Neanderthals, and it has some forward pro-jection of the teeth, but also a definite chin.

It is hard to assess these people accurately. They are surely closer to us than to an average Neanderthal, just as the Tabūn Woman is the opposite. They are separated from us by the size and nature of their brows and by their remaining facial projection, and that is about all.

These are not the only such Near Eastern remains from the early part of the Würm. The Galilee skull, a frontal bone from Zuttiyeh, a cave on the Sea of Galilee, is more or less Neanderthal-looking, but its brows bunch more toward the mid-line, so that it is aberrant in this way. (It is probably pre-Würm and pre-Mousterian, and associated with the Jabrudian culture, containing late Acheulian and "pre-Aurignacian" elements.) Another Galilee cave, Jebel Kafzeh, pro-duced more bones, including one very good skull. These people recall the Skhūl tribe. The skull, however, from published photographs, shows possible Neanderthal affinities only in its strong brows, the face being completely retracted like our own, and the vault departing from that of Homo sapiens in no visible particular.

Now, what are all these Near Easterners trying to tell us? This is difficult and important evidence. At the present, it is believed that the Tabūn Neanderthal Woman lived about 39,000 B.C., and that the Skhūl cave was inhabited substantially—several thousand years at least—later on. In other words we have, in fairly late times, a Nean-derthal population (Tabūn, Amud) giving way to almost-sapiens.

In the past, when the date of these people was supposed to be con-siderably earlier in time, interpretations were two. One, that in these fossils we are witnessing the actual evolution of sapiens from Nean-derthal Man, before his grand entrance into Europe. Two, that the Skhūl people represent a mixture of the two kinds of man, so that we are witnessing the arrival of Homo sapiens, already developed, from somewhere else. However, if the date is as late as now inferred from C_{14} dating, the Skhūl people crowd to Cro Magnons in time. The latter could hardly have developed from the Tabūn Neanderthals and migrated to Europe in a mere ten thousand years. So the idea of replacement and absorption is more appealing. We might consider that the Cro Magnons replaced the Western Neanderthals while mix-ing with them very little, whereas the Near Eastern sapiens immi-grants acquired more genes from their predecessors, who were in any case not so extreme in form as the cave Neanderthals of the West.

Such an interpretation means that *Homo sapiens* must already have existed elsewhere, but would not make him much older than the Europeans. It also requires that he developed in some place outside of Europe and the Near East. We may remember that archaeology has shown strange breaks in the succession. At some points a late Acheulian suddenly intrudes; at others a seemingly too early Upper Paleolithic, a Pre-Aurignacian stone culture, appears and disappears again without continuing. These distinctions and replacements cannot be related to the several skeletons. But, at the best, they give signs of quite different populations coming into contact here in the late Pleistocene. At the least, they show that the Near East itself was a zone exposed, if not to constant migrations, then to culture intrusions from different directions, which certainly implies contacts of some sort.

Steinheim and Swanscombe

In the Skhūl people we find a brain case of modern appearance. For signs of the early existence of this form of brain case let us turn to the two oldest examples of it ever found in Europe, the skulls of the important women of Swanscombe and Steinheim. They are, in fact, the only human fossils of consequence in the early part of the long span between the end of the Second Glacial and the beginning of the Fourth. They are clearly dated to the later part of the Second Interglacial phase and must have lived at very much the same time, one in England and one in Germany; the detailed similarity of the fossil mammals found with the two has been termed quite remarkable. The age might be as much as 400,000 years.

Steinheim is north of Stuttgart, in western Germany. The skull was by itself, with no lower jaw and no other bones. Badly damaged behind the left eye, it also had a sizable hole in the base—brain eaters again. It came from twenty feet down in a gravel pit near this town, in 1933, following a twenty-year vigil by Dr. Berckhemer, like the vigil of Schoetensack at Mauer.

Could this Steinheim Woman be a grandmother of Neanderthal and sapiens together? She looks in both directions. Her skull was low, and various estimates of her brain size average something like 1150 cubic centimeters—small by modern standards, but not extraordinarily so for a woman of no great bodily bulk. At the same time, her brain case had contours reminiscent of ours: flattish on the sides and gently rounded in the profile of the back, with an honest forehead in front. Here is an impression of modernity quite different from either the Neanderthals or such thick-skulled creatures as the men of Pekin.

But she was obviously Miss Middle Pleistocene in other ways. Although she is missing her front teeth, these seem to have been of generous size, and the conformation of her upper jaw as a whole, especially in the fore part, has a Neanderthal look. But her back teeth appear modern, and they do not suggest a heavy lower jaw.

Her nose was broad. And her brows were large and heavy. Still, these brows lacked the clear double-arched type which is such a character of the Neanderthals; they were slightly separated over the nose and thickest at their outermost portions. Also, her face has not the forward thrust of the Neanderthals, one of their most notable features.

How do you score her? Fairly evenly as between sapiens and Neanderthal, but not specifically like either and rather more primitive than both. Take her as a common ancestress, if you wish, but remember that she goes back a tremendous number of generations. While she may resemble the Neanderthals by having primitive features, it is perhaps surprising that she is not more primitive than she is.

The Swanscombe Woman was more perfectly dated but less perfectly preserved. If you want to go to Galley Hill, you take a train from London down the Thames beyond Dartford, and get off at Swanscombe Halt. Here the river dropped a long and complicated series of gravels, as it rose level a hundred feet above today's stream in the later part of the Second Interglacial. The Barnfield gravel pit exposed a wall of these gravels forty feet high. This pit has yielded hand-axes of the Acheulian variety, showing several stages of their long development, in successive layers in the gravel. In fact, here is a classic example of the neat labeling and storing of man-made tools which geology is sometimes good enough to provide. The place has long been infested with archaeologists, both professional and amateur, and it was one of the latter, A. T. Marston, a dentist, who first found the Swanscombe skull.

Geologically speaking, this is probably one of the best dated skulls in history. Mr. Marston, by keeping an eye on the Barnfield pit, recovered an occipital bone in June 1935. It was in excellent condition, but separated from the rest of the vault. Evidently the skull of a young woman, only just adult, had come apart along its sutures, or seams, as it washed down the Thames not long after the death of its owner. Marston found the bone in the lowest of seven distinct layers of the Upper Middle gravels, a layer from which have regularly come hand-axes of the Acheulian III stage. Removal of gravel went on, with Mr. Marston never far away, and in March of the next year, from a spot eight yards away in the very same seam, there came to light the left parietal bone—the left side wall and top—of the same skull, also well

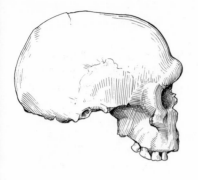
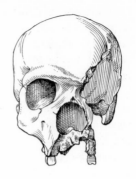
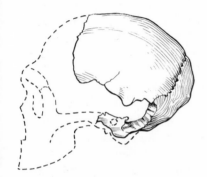
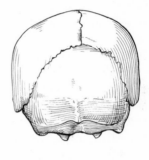

The Steinheim and Swanscombe skulls. Above, Steinheim. Below, the Swanscombe bones assembled in side and rear views. The profile shows Breitinger's restoration of the missing parts. (The temporal bones of the Swanscombe skull are not present, so that the parietal bones appear to overhang the occipital on either side.) From casts and photographs, also following Breitinger. ¼ natural size.

preserved and fitting the occipital bone neatly along their common edge. From then on, the remaining gravel at this locality, bearing the important seam, was reserved from commercial use, to be examined only by professionals and qualified amateurs. After twenty years Mr. J. Wymer and Mr. A. Gibson found the parietal bone of the other side, in July 1955—again in the same level. Now nobody needs three birth certificates to prove her age, but that is the kind of certification in depth which we have for the woman of Swanscombe.

Aside from being such a true-blue early Englishwoman—the earliest, and the only one prior to Upper Paleolithic times—what are her particular attractions? They are her suggestive resemblances to ourselves, as far as one can tell from the back half of a skull, without frontal or temporal bones: vertical and moderately high sides, with a well-marked higher mid-line, and a rounder occiput. In spite of the incompleteness, there is no confusing her with the other non-sapiens men.

But this back half of the skull is also that part of the big-browed Steinheim specimen which seems most "modern." And it was recognized long ago that the two could not be definitely distinguished from one another. In the Swanscombe skull the likeness to sapient man is perhaps even more emphatic than in the case of Steinheim. The brain size (uncertain without the forehead) would have been about 1300 cubic centimeters, close to modern female figures. There are nevertheless primitive features, in a certain lowness of the vault, with thicker bones and an unusual breadth across the back. And Dr. T. D. Stewart detected a certain dropping down of the lateral edges of the occipital bone relative to the middle, which is a trait of Neanderthal Man and not of sapiens. In addition, Drs. J. S. Weiner and B. G. Campbell conducted a complex statistical analysis of all the measurements they were able to take on the Swanscombe bones, for comparison with a large group of modern skulls from the Iron Age of Israel. By this means they were able to show that, in size and shape, the back of the head in Swanscombe and Steinheim was somewhat less like modern man than in the best Skhūl skull, but more so than in several of the "classic" Neanderthal men of Europe. The missing Swanscombe forehead, of course, would tell much of the story. In fact, recovering the second parietal bone of the skull in 1955 was something of a disappointment; what everybody prayed for was the frontal bone. That bone must be, or must have been, somewhere in the gravels, and its finding is devoutly to be wished. Was Miss Swanscombe large-browed, like Fräulein Steinheim, or was she small-browed, like us?

This was long and fervently discussed. Her strongly sapiens-like look, from back and side, always suggested to the eye a modern-looking forehead profile and brow ridge. Also, the Steinheim skull was at one time mistakenly supposed to be much later in time, and therefore more closely related to the Neanderthals. Yet, in the first study made of the skull and published in 1938, Le Gros Clark and Morant thought that the fore part might have been massively developed and that the skull was sufficiently similar to Steinheim so that the two might represent the same human population. Dr. Breitinger of Vienna, in a most painstaking comparative analysis of form and measurements, has likewise concluded that a large brow is far more likely for Swanscombe than a small one. So, after a generation of talk we seem to be back at this conclusion as the reasonable one. The skulls are much alike and they are contemporaries.

Together, they proclaim the emergence of a brain case with the basic contours of *Homo sapiens,* in the Second Interglacial, at a time probably much closer to *Homo erectus* than to ourselves. Human development during the last half million years seems to have arrived at key stages: final enlargement of the brain, in the Neanderthals, and a lightening up of the structure and face in *Homo sapiens.* But here we have brain cases of nearly modern size and shape in the Middle Pleistocene. And that, as long as her face escapes us, is the main meaning of the Swanscombe Woman.

The Fragments from Fontéchevade

If we move on into the Upper Pleistocene (meaning the Third Glacial and later), we come to signs of skulls with more sapient features still. One bone, of probably Third Interglacial date, but possibly older, was found at Quinzano, near Verona. It is a lone occipital—the back and base of the skull only—which recalls the Swanscombe skull in its breadth and thickness and in its non-Neanderthal appearance. The same likeness recurs in two other important fragments from the Fontéchevade Cave in central France (Charente), fragments which also demonstrate that early skulls do not have to have big brows.

This, like other French caves, was used in the Fourth Glacial by a whole series of occupants, up to Magdalenian times, the final phase of the Upper Paleolithic, and back to the Neanderthals, whose Mousterian implements lay just above the cave floor. Or rather what seemed to be the floor; it was a hard stalagmite base running from the cave out over the slope in front of the cave mouth as well. But Mlle. Germaine Henri-Martin, an archaeologist and the daughter of an archaeologist, decided that this apparent "floor" would bear looking under. In 1947 she succeeded in getting through it, to find seven more meters of deposits, containing tools of the Tayacian industry and the bones of warm-weather animals, especially Merck's rhinoceros. This material is of Third Interglacial date, and not late either. And embedded in the same deposit were parts of two skulls: a patch from the brows of one, about the size of a silver dollar; and most of the top of another, this one showing signs of having been burned in a fire.

There is enough of the second skull to tell a good deal. The brain was probably over the 1450 cubic-centimeter mark, that is to say, above the average of European men of today (the sex of the owner cannot be told). In its outlines the vault of this skull is indistinguishable from modern man, although it is definitely thick and is particu-

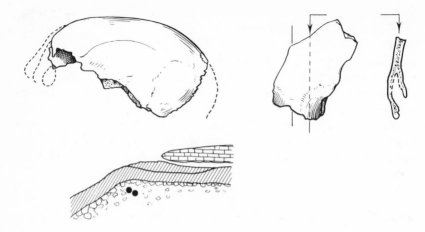

The Fontéchevade finds. Left, the skull cap of Fontéchevade II. This shows how the position of the frontal sinus can be told. This would be in an impossible position (too far back) if the forehead were reconstructed like Neanderthal Man's (outer dashed line), but is in appropriate position for a forehead of modern shape (inner dashed line). ¼ natural size.

Right, the forehead fragment of Fontéchevade I, half natural size. In the front view (left), the vertical line is the mid-line; the dashed line shows where the cross section (right) was drawn, 1 centimeter to the side, near the inner corner of the eye. This is where the brow ridge is normally most projecting, and the cross section shows both the slight development of the brow and the fully developed sinus inside. Below, a diagram of the Fontéchevade Cave. The shaded area is the Mousterian and Upper Paleolithic levels, above the stalagmitic floor. Dots show the position of the skull parts, in Tayacian cultural remains below the floor. All after Vallois.

larly broad across the back, just where it is broken. It quite surely had the same rounded posterior profile that we have, with no heavy ridge for the neck muscles—but this would apply to the Steinheim skull. In the front the forehead is broken halfway down, but fortunately there appears, in the broken edge, the very top of the hollow of the frontal sinus. This shows the direction the lower profile must have taken, and this profile could not have ended in a brow of the typical Neanderthal style.

But we need not depend on this skull for such information, because the other individual shows exactly what the brows were like. This bone, too, is thick, though less so than the other skull, and midway between the thickness of modern skulls and those of Neanderthals.

The brow ridge is clear to see: it is slight and just about what would be typical for a woman of today.

Now this is sensational evidence. If there is one constant feature of the Neanderthals early and late, it is the heavy curving brow, and the Fontéchevade skulls certainly lack it. They are therefore damaging to the hypothesis that *Homo sapiens* had no forerunners other than the Neanderthals as we know them. How damaging they are is seen from doubts that have been voiced about them. It has been wondered whether there might have been some mistake in the digging or in the date. But Mlle. Henri-Martin is no amateur digger, and the bones have been given the F test. Their content of fluorine is of the order of the animal bones in the lower layers where they were found, and greater than that of bones from above the stalagmite floor which sealed them over. (In any event, in the spot where Mlle. Henri-Martin was digging, outside the present cave roof, all the layers above the stalagmite had been removed long before by earlier diggers, so that there was nothing higher up to get accidentally mixed with the layer below.) Thus there can be no doubt as to the age of the animals and tools below that floor, and hence no real doubt about the skulls.

It has also been charged that the evidence of the brows is not conclusive. The brow region is missing, after all, on the larger skull. As to the smaller fragment, it has been asserted to be, not from a full-grown, modern-looking woman, but only from a young individual, still immature, in whom the characteristic Neanderthal brows might later have developed. But Dr. Vallois of the Musée de l'Homme, who has the bones in his care and has written a monograph on them, rejects this whole interpretation completely. This is mainly because, moderate in thickness though it is, the frontal fragment has a well-developed frontal sinus, which would not yet be present in a young child. Even this important evidence is hardly necessary, for the Neanderthal skulls show that their distinctive brow began to develop early in life, since it can be recognized for what it is in boys like the one from Teshik-Tash. And so it will take something quite extraordinary and unexpected to dislodge the Fontéchevade pair from their position as people of basically sapient skull form, present in Europe as early as the first Neanderthals, and probably before.

This is not to say that the Fontéchevade fragments are indistinguishable in all ways from modern man. I have mentioned the thickness and the breadth across the back, both characteristic of Swanscombe. Drs. Weiner and Campbell were able to make use of the bones in their mathematical analysis, and found that the Fontéchevade skull top was no nearer to the modern series chosen than Steinheim or Swanscombe, and certainly less so than Skhūl V, but nevertheless always closer than the western Neanderthals.

Kanjera Man

We have further evidence of this same general kind from Africa. The Kanjera skulls, though badly broken, have occiputs, brows and faces. Kanjera is on the eastern shore of Lake Victoria. Early in his career (1932) but already making important finds, Dr. Leakey picked up a number of fragments of four skulls which had washed out of the ground (and been trampled by cattle), fortunately finding some pieces still embedded in the soil. Leakey at the time believed them to be Middle Pleistocene, from the associated animals, and drew attention to their importance. For they are unquestionably entirely like modern man, except for being a little thick: the brow parts, present in two of them, and the canine fossa, or depression in the cheek, present in one, as well as the whole form of the skull, are in each case perfectly "sapiens," with no resemblance at all to other forms of man, and with no suggestion whatever of Neanderthal relations.

When these skulls were tossed into the ancient debate about the antiquity of *Homo sapiens,* instant doubts were voiced as to their authenticity. Perhaps Leakey was wrong, and later man and earlier animals had washed out together from different deposits. An actual visit was made to the site but, principally because of rapid erosion, the exact spot of the finds could not be located, and the investigators placed the Kanjera fossils in the dubious category.

Since that time, however, it has become apparent that Leakey was right as to the bones' validity. The skull parts are in precisely the same state as the fossil animals found at Kanjera. That is, they are densely fossilized and heavy (although fossilization would have been rapid here in any case) and with the same materials adhering to them. Furthermore, Oakley has tested all the fossils by the method of uranium estimation, finding no discrepancy between the human and the animal bones. Finally, there is only one deposit at the spot, not several of different periods; and so there is no real reason to suppose that the human remains got washed in somehow from a younger deposit lying higher up.

The situation, therefore, is this. There can be little serious doubt that the Kanjera skulls are true fossils of the deposit. The remaining question is simply the age of the deposit itself. The animals have a Middle Pleistocene look to them, with giant baboons, giant sheep, giant wart hogs, and straight-tusked elephants. The rather primitive hand-axes also look early. The beds themselves are lake deposits of the Kanjeran Pluvial of Africa, which has not yet been satisfactorily related to the glacial phases of Europe. However, the best estimates in round years are an age of not less than 60,000 to 70,000. So we have really modern man in East Africa going back deep into the time of the Neanderthals of the north. Sooner or later, the true age of the Kanjera deposit will be known.

Rhodesian Man

We have been considering men of advanced appearance but of early date. Elsewhere in Africa we come to the opposite: men of recent date but primitive appearance. In North Africa, jaw fragments have been found in three places on the Atlantic coast of Morocco (Casablanca, Rabat, and Temara) datable probably to the earlier part of the Upper Pleistocene (Third Glacial and Third Interglacial). These jaws, with their teeth, are less primitive than the Ternifine examples, but they have various characteristics which recall the latter and, beyond them, the Far Eastern fossils. Remnants of a primitive cingulum are developed on the molar teeth, but on the premolars only of the Rabat specimen. Patterns of the cusps are like the Ternifiners. All in all, they suggest a later and less crude stage of the Ternifine family with the specimen youngest in time, that from Temara, apparently the least crude of the lot.

The jaws do not tell us a great deal. Much more important is the Rhodesian Man, a later citizen of Africa and perhaps a contemporary of Solo Man of Java. Evidently he lived throughout southern Africa. At any rate, he certainly inhabited or used a cave in what is now Zambia, not very far north of the Zambesi River. This was a long, tunnel-like affair running into a kopje, or small hill, standing above the generally flattish country. This cave started at the base of the kopje and sloped gently into its middle, a hundred and twenty feet away. The kopje itself consisted of limestone richly impregnated with ores of lead, zinc, and vanadium.

At some time it appears that ground water deep below, leaching out the soil, caused the kopje's peak to subside, leaving a saddle-like depression at the top and making the innermost end of the cave take a sudden steep dip, to a final point ninety feet below the level of the entrance. The cave, long though it was, filled up in a relatively short period with earth containing bones and stone tools. Among the animal species represented some are extinct, but the majority are still living, which shows the comparative recency of the group. The tools belong to a recognized set of rather late, smallish cutting and scraping tools, the "Rhodesian Proto-Still Bay" culture. This is the first phase of the Middle Stone Age of Africa, known to have flourished here in the latter part of the Upper Pleistocene. Far back in the cave were a few random bones of human beings, including an upper jaw. Down at the very bottom of the last slope, where it had rolled or been thrown, was a skull.

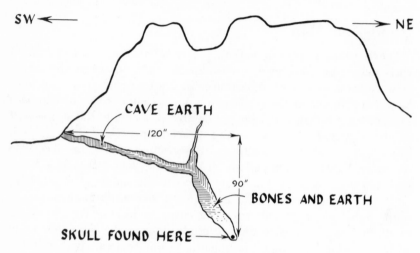

The cave at Broken Hill, in cross section. After J. D. Clark.

A ninety-foot grave should have made a good hiding place, after the cave had filled and its entrance was no longer to be seen. Nonetheless, the skull came back into the light. For the hill itself, being made of ores, became useful to man when civilization arrived. The Europeans appeared, founded a mine and a town, and named them both Broken Hill after a famous mine in Australia. They dug away at the kopje, until now there is only a colossal crater in the ground where the hill stood, and the mining has moved a mile or so away to another part of the lode.

In 1921 the miners had come unknowingly to the deep part of the lost cave. One day a Swiss miner named Zwigelaar and his African "boys" were working here. Mr. Zwigelaar loosened some ore with a small explosive charge, and when the dust cleared, there was the skull, sitting all by itself on a little shelf in the cut, right side up and looking Zwigelaar in the eye. The Africans ran off and did not come back that afternoon; and Zwigelaar was so pleased with the little drama that he stuck the skull on a pole for a day or so to awe the boys further. Then it was taken to the mine office and came into the hands of the doctor, who saw its importance. Also, general curiosity had led to a search of the mine dumps for other remains, which produced several arm, leg, and pelvic bones and another upper jaw. Luckily, collections had and have been made of animal bones and tools as well.

The same year the bones were sent off to London to the British Museum (Natural History), where Rhodesian Man was gladly welcomed as an important new member of the then short list of fossil ancestors. At that time even Pekin Man was unknown. The skull is still a source of pride to the people of Broken Hill, who have given it a place of honor on the city's coat of arms. However, far away from home, absurd fables for some reason began to attach to Rhodesian Man, especially about his discovery. By one account, an entire body had been found, preserved even to the skin by natural embalming in zinc salts. But it was thrown into the smelter except for the skull and a few bones, because it was considered worth more as ore than as anthropology. And a staff member of the Museum (actually more of a popular writer than a scientist) looked at the pelvic bones and conceived the bizarre idea that Rhodesian Man had walked about with a stoop, and so he christened the fossil *Cyphanthropus* (Bent-over Man). Other fictions were picked up around the mine by different visitors, until more than thirty years had gone by, when Oakley and J. D. Clark thought it worth while to look up Mr. Zwigelaar, still living in Lusaka, to ask him for the simple facts. The above is his story,[1] by courtesy of Drs. Oakley and Clark.

The Rhodesian men may have had to stoop in their cave, but out in the daylight they stood as straight as any hominid. There is nothing to say about the skeleton bones except that they can be distinguished in no particular from ours. As to the skull, it is a fine specimen, excellently preserved except for a break the size of your palm low behind the right ear, and for the teeth, which in life were all badly worn, decayed, abcessed, or lost. It is a low skull, though not like the older Far Eastern men. Actually, it is rather large, with a bigger and much more primitive face than ours, though not a very projecting one. The Rhodesian Man must have had a lower jaw verging in width on the one from Heidelberg, though not as large altogether, and higher in its ascending ramus.

But he was a new kind of man. His brain size was about 1300 c.c., still below the modern average but at the level of some living races of today. Furthermore, the skull has none of the thickness of those of Java and Pekin or of the Solo Man. His actual primitive traits were

[1] In 1925, Zwigelaar gave Hrdlička a slightly different version: he exposed the skull with his pick, not a dynamite charge, and he conscientiously took it straight to the mine officials, with no interlude for horseplay.

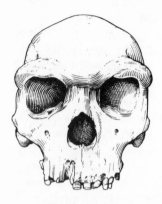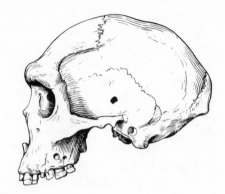

Rhodesian Man. The Broken Hill skull. ¼ natural size. From cast and photographs.

his enormous bony brow ridges above his eyes—a really spectacular development—and his large dental arch and teeth. Even these last were not primitive, the arch being very broad and the wisdom tooth much reduced in size. Also, the second upper jaw found is smaller than that on the skull, suggesting that the average size may have been less impressive than the skull suggests.

For many years this was the only discovery of Rhodesian Man. He was long something of a mystery. In the first place, nothing was known about Rhodesian archaeology when he was found, and no one had the least idea where he belonged in time, until recent years and the further development of knowledge. Secondly, because the skull was an only find there were mutterings of "pathology," meaning that disease might have been responsible for the great brows and large face, as in pituitary giantism. Java Man, you will remember, was also considered by some to be a freak. But as in Java Man's case, another Rhodesian skull was eventually found, and it was seen to be entirely like the first.

Some eighty miles north of Cape Town, west of the town of Hopefield, there is a sandy plain along the coast of Saldanha Bay, part of it with scrub growth and part of it mere desert and dunes. In the sand are the remains of a rich fauna, from a prosperous part of the Ice Age, together with a series of human tools from the latest times back toward the Middle Pleistocene. When the wind moves the sands along, the heavier fossils are left sitting on the surface. Here Dr. Ronald Singer and Mr. Keith Jolly of Cape Town University found, by great good luck, a human skull top in twenty-seven small pieces,

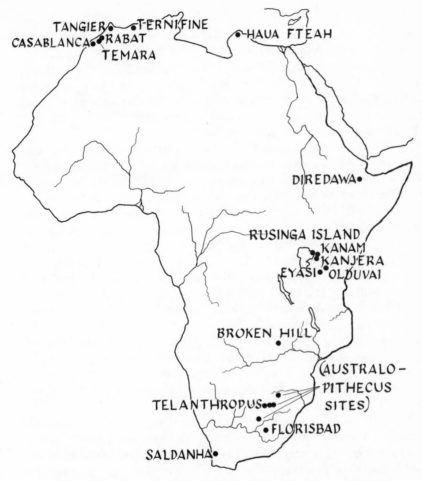

Africa: sites of the fossil men. The *Australopithecus* sites are
included for reference, also that of *Proconsul* (Rusinga Island),
and of probable Neanderthal specimens (Tangier, Haua Fteah,
Diredawa).

picking these up on more than one visit as the wind exposed them. The
pieces fit nicely together to make a skull differing in only slight ways
from the Broken Hill specimen. Somewhat smaller in size, it may be
female. The ridge for neck muscles at the back differs, but not impressively, since the ridge varies somewhat in all populations. The
skull is thicker, a more interesting distinction.

A Lesson in Dating

This find is evidence that Rhodesian Man, like Pekin Man, is not the relic of a one-cave band, but belonged to a definite population covering a wide continental space. Did he also stretch over a good span of time? A little while ago a blown-out skull like the Saldanha fragments would have been at loose ends, giving small possibility of telling what fossils or tools it went with. But the fossil hunters are not so helpless now, and the picture seems bright, with what they already know and what they can find out.

Very exact examination of the Saldanha (Hopefield) site shows that the main fossil animals all belong to a single layer of deposition, which contains late hand-axes and which can only fit into the onset of the Gamblian, the last great rainy phase (supposedly the time of the Fourth Glacial in the north). And Oakley, with fluorine tests and with newer tests for radioactive uranium based on the same principle of accumulation, proves that the Saldanha skull goes with the animals and thus with the hand-axes. Later men at the same place left tools of the next culture stage above the hand-axes, called the Still Bay.

Now we know the Broken Hill Man had Proto-Still Bay tools in his cave, but no hand-axes. We also know that the Still Bay sequence followed right on the end of the hand-axes, and the Broken Hill specimens belong to the early phase of that sequence. Other things being equal, this would make the Broken Hill people just later in time than the Saldanha individual. However, one more adjustment is needed, because the Still Bay culture appeared somewhat earlier north of the Zambesi than in South Africa.

Kenneth Oakley has estimated ages of about 40,000 years for the Saldanha Man and 30,000 for Broken Hill. Desmond Clark, however, thinks Broken Hill may have been earlier, 40,000 years or more, which would be less surprising than the later date. At all events the two are fairly close together. At the least, we can conclude with some confidence that the human beings who lived in southern Africa contemporary with the very last Neanderthals of Europe and possibly later—the men who were changing from the use of hand-axes to the smaller tools of the Middle Stone Age—were the big-browed kind we know from Broken Hill and Saldanha. This is a great improvement; as late as 1949 Professor Zeuner, an authority on dating, could still write that the Broken Hill bones could not even be placed within one of the main divisions of the Pleistocene.

Perhaps we can stretch things even further. In 1935 and 1938, Kohl-Larsen found a large number of small pieces of at least three human skulls near Lake Eyasi. This is up near the northern border of Tanganyika in East Africa and about nine hundred miles as the crow flies from Broken Hill, in the direction opposite to Cape Town. Some of the pieces were pasted up into a very primitive looking "skull," which was baptized *Africanthropus* and believed to be a cousin of the Java and Pekin people. Few anthropologists have exhibited any enthusiasm for this restoration. The individual scraps look more like the Rhodesian type (with the kind of sharp crest for the neck muscles which graces the Broken Hill skull) than like anything else. And other material found at the sites seems to agree in date with the Rhodesian remains found further south. We cannot presume that this is find number three of the Rhodesian type, but we certainly cannot presume the contrary.

All this is a little dry and complicated. But it is really well worth attending to as a fine example of how small facts, and a few skulls, can be put together and, by persistent detective work and new methods of study, be made to say something definite and important to human history.

The Skull from Floris' Spa

Florisbad Man is another skull of unusual importance. It might be contrasted several ways with the Swanscombe skull, as being very late in Lower Paleolithic times instead of very early, as presenting just those parts which are missing in the Swanscombe skull, as being different in "racial" type, and as belonging to the far south rather than the far north. It came to light in 1932, at a place thirty miles northwest of the city of Bloemfontein in the Orange Free State, South Africa. Florisbad, a spa, has a lithium spring which for a long time has been bringing warm mineral water from far down, drying up for periods, and then coming to life and producing springs and geysers, forming new eyes and leaving old ones dead.

The deposits it has laid down are complicated. Its lower layers have yielded extinct animals, stone tools, and a skull. There are four layers in particular, dark in color and consisting of clay or sand which must have accumulated at different times when the spring was in less active moods. Other evidence in the soils shows dry and wet periods in the general region, though study has not yet made clear whether these represent the end of the Pleistocene, or come after. However, the latest Carbon 14 datings of the dark layers give them increasing ages from above down, with the lowest at 35,000 B.C.

In this layer occurs a rather baffling stone industry: it looks like the end of the "Earlier Stone Age" (suggesting a time just about like the

"Rhodesian" Saldanha skull), though nobody has identified it properly yet. Just under this layer was the skull. It lay in a pocket to one side of an extinct eye of the spring, and so it must have tumbled in somehow and been washed around, but there seems to be no doubt that this happened before the critical layer had formed. So the specimen seems to be not younger than the earliest sapient men of the Upper Paleolithic of Europe, and in fact is probably several thousand years older.

At first glance the skull looks primitive, because of its heavy brows. And yet it can only be classed as *Homo sapiens.* Large though they

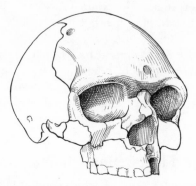

The Florisbad skull. The back part of the skull and the upper jaw are restored, but the region of the nose and cheek show the form of the face. After a cast and photographs. ¼ natural size.

are, the bony brows have that specific character, so different from Neanderthal Man, with a slight notching over the nose, and the division on each side into inner and outer parts, by a barely detectable cleft. In this, and in general appearance, the brow region might be described as just what you might expect if you could command this region to become bigger and more expanded on a modern skull, until it went beyond the limits of anything seen today, or elsewhere in the Upper Paleolithic. This primitivizing does not produce a Neanderthal man, but only a particularly primitive sapiens, judging by appearances.

In its other parts the specimen is less unusual. The face, though broad, is like other sapient men, lacking the large rounded eye sockets and big nose opening of Neanderthal or Rhodesian, and having instead a marked canine fossa and the remnants of a relatively high nose. It seems to have had a non-receding nasal root at the start of the bridge, and it is known to have had a large nasal spine, to support the base of the nose, before this got broken off and lost while it was being examined by an eminent anthropologist, now deceased.

The brain case was relatively low, and probably broad, though the whole back and most of the sides are missing. It was not, at any rate, like Swanscombe, or Kanjera, or the European Neanderthals. Altogether this child of the spring water is not easy to interpret, all by itself. But it does seem to give us a member of *Homo sapiens* who is positively as ancient as any of the Cro Magnon people—and apparently as ancient as the Broken Hill Man too—and who lived far away from the scene of Neanderthal development.

The Boy from Borneo

Although I described them much earlier, along with Java Man, the Solo men, like Rhodesian Man, lived late in the Pleistocene. It is too bad we cannot give them a better date, or say how late they lived, since it would be important to know whether they overlapped with *Homo sapiens*, or Neanderthal Man, or both.

They might well have been contemporary with quite a different kind of man in Borneo. Here, on the northern shore of Sarawak, Tom Harrisson, the energetic head of the museum in Kuching, has been digging in the dust of the enormous Niah Cave, which has only Shanidar for a rival in size. It is full of recent and late Stone Age burials; as one goes down through the floor stone implements of earlier cultures are found. Bones, unfortunately, do not fossilize, but simply disintegrate very gradually indeed. Luckily, just over eight feet down, Harrisson in 1958 found the better part of the skull of an adolescent boy, apparently protected from agencies of disintegration by a rock just above it. Equally important, he found tools of a Paleolithic type (chopping tools), and enough charcoal to get a C14 date of about 40,000 years.

The skull is most decidedly that of *Homo sapiens*, and no greater contrast with Solo Man could be found. The forehead is vertical and rounded, with very little in the way of brow development. The skull has the outlines of a modern skull and the facial fragment shows that while the mouth region projected the rest of the face was tucked under the brain case in modern fashion. Dr. Brothwell of the British Museum, who examined it, thinks that its closest recent parallel may be the natives of Tasmania, now extinct. It is even less primitive in appearance than the skull of an aboriginal of Australia. The remains, though far from perfectly preserved, are quite good enough to make all this clear.

After three chapters of dates and skulls, the significance of the Niah Cave boy should be evident. If there are no errors in the find—and none have been imputed to it—we have exhumed a young man for whom travel would have been broadening. By going to the neighboring island of Java, he might perhaps have been able to see Solo men eating each other. He could apparently have got to South Africa in plenty of time to visit the last of the Rhodesian men. Had he gone to Europe, he could have told the Neanderthals that there was indeed another kind of man to the eastward, who was only waiting for warmer weather to invade. If he was, and is, truthful, he has a lot to say.

16. THE SEARCH FOR
HOMO SAPIENS

FINDING AND STUDYING fossil men is something like a detective story. Not entirely. A story writer can go on to the end, pin the crime on Winters, the butler, and wind the whole thing up with every clever little clue elucidated. But elucidating human fossils is rather exasperating; our hands are tied until we find the fossils to answer our questions, and none of us is likely to live long enough to have a really good view of our Pleistocene history.

In fact, we must realize that the finding of early man is still only in its early stages. Caves in many parts of the world have been industriously looted, especially in Europe. The gravels of ancient river valleys are now unfortunately dug by machine instead of by hand, but we may hope that they will from time to time yield important specimens like Swanscombe. And vast areas of lake shore once used by man now lie deeply buried in many places, occasionally giving up prize fossils by the fortunes of erosion, above all at Olduvai, but also the Kanjera finds, or the Midland, Minnesota, or Tepexpan skeletons in North America. There is nothing to do but be patient, and to understand how very spotty the album of the past now is.

Spotty but at the same time not blank. Like a junior stamp collector who is neither rich nor assiduous, but who at least has an uncle living in Barbados, we can point to a few handsome pages: all the australopithecines of the Lower Pleistocene; Europe and Western Asia in the later Pleistocene, populated by the Neanderthals; and the Far East in the early Middle Pleistocene, with the very satisfactory Java-Pekin branch of humanity. And the pace of finding is speeding up, not slowing down; since the first edition of this book was written in 1958, the number and significance of new finds has been remarkable.

Always subject to correction, we now behold an australopithecine stage within which one line began making tools and changing to a hominine grade. This grade became established in the Middle Pleistocene with considerable uniformity from Europe to the Far

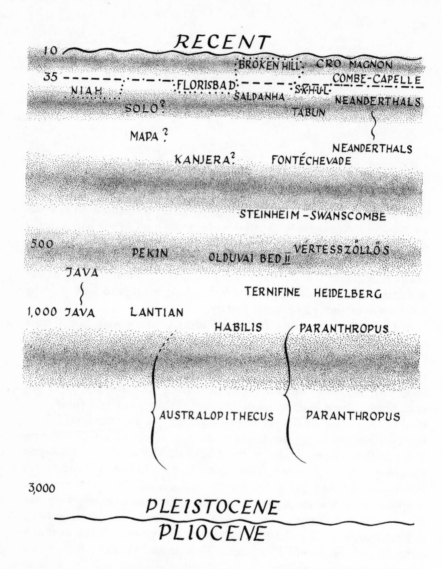

The fossil men plotted on a chart of the Pleistocene. The four cold periods are shown as dotted areas (only the subdivision of the last being suggested). Not drawn to scale: approximate lengths of time in the past are shown at a few points on the left-hand side, in thousands of years. At top, the dashed line represents 35,000 B.C.; the dotted lines the first known appearances in this general period of *Homo sapiens*.

East, although the men of Heidelberg and Olduvai may have differed somewhat from the easterners. Then come the Dark Ages, broken only by unsatisfactory glimmerings; in the late Pleistocene the degree of differentiation seems greater, in the Neanderthals, the Rhodesians and Solo Man. At the end these are all followed by the more uniform population of today. Importantly, it seems clear that some stages overlapped in time: early *Homo erectus* with *Paranthropus*, primitive Solo at least with Swanscombe and Steinheim, and probably *Homo sapiens* and the Rhodesian men. There were, clearly, regional differences, and in some areas progress was early, in some late. We cannot now explain the differences and the changes. We know that culture and the ability to use it was progressing; surely language was becoming more intricate, expressive, and better as a vehicle of thought; climates varied even more radically than today; but we cannot demonstrate how these might have affected the shapes of heads and faces.

Names and Their Meanings

This is a chapter of controversy. It is one thing to review the fossils as I have been doing. It is quite another to put them together in a scheme of evolution and arrive at modern man. Since this is the crucial aspect, I would call it the sapiens problem; others (unless they think they have solved it) call it the Neanderthal problem. Part of the problem, in fact, may be in using the right names, or at least in not using the wrong ones.

Men of today are one single, indubitable good species, *Homo sapiens*, recognized as such since Linnaeus first looked about him. Fossil men used to be honored, on their appearance, with Linnaean names of their own, to give them imposing-sounding labels or to pay tribute to their discoverers, with little or no attention to what this might suggest as to the actual relationships of the fossil. For example, Black named Pekin Man *Sinanthropus pekinensis* on nothing more than three of his teeth, giving him a genus name, *Sinanthropus*, different from the genus *Pithecanthropus* of Java Man. Thus Black was implying that these two might be animals as different as dog and fox, and more different than mountain lion and pussycat (both of which are *Felis*). Later knowledge of the two men made it clear that they were closely allied. This is a mild example. Not counting the australopithecines (or Piltdown Man) fossil men have been put into a new *genus* not less than fifteen times and the number of alleged species is very much greater. Indeed, the literature has become a junk yard of such names and there has been a general abandonment of their serious use.

In fact, it is now considered by most that since the time of *Homo erectus* there can have been only one new species, namely *Homo sapiens*. Or to put it better, since *Homo sapiens* is the senior species, the living one and the one we know about, we must go back to the early Middle Pleistocene before the differences merit recognizing another species, *Homo erectus*. And, although it is more properly a measure of contemporary species difference, we cannot say whether it would have been possible (repulsive as the idea may strike you) for *Homo sapiens* and *Homo erectus* to interbreed. The chances are that they could.

This is doubtless a correct view, but correcting the terminology appropriately makes a few difficulties. The first Neanderthal was quite properly called *Homo neanderthalensis*, that is, he was made a species. If only two species in all are to be accepted, he must be reclassified. In spite of his skeleton, his nearness in time and type to modern man indicates he should be classed with us, not with *Homo erectus:* consequently he becomes *Homo sapiens neanderthalensis*, and we on the other hand for the sake of distinction become *Homo sapiens sapiens*. These are, that is to say, two subspecies. But what about our friends *Homo rhodesiensis* and *Homo soloensis*, to give them their customary names? We should not keep the old names, and we cannot give them new ones, since we are not yet ready to say where they go. Also, what about *Homo sapiens neanderthalensis?* We are not prepared to use a line of type every time we want to speak of him, and at the same time we wish to keep in view the possibly different kinds of Neanderthal instead of covering them with one blanket. Worse yet, different people use the word "Neanderthal" or else Neanderthalian or Neanderthaloid, to include different things. In spite of their distinguishing features, many people have referred to the Rhodesian and Solo men (and of course the Skhūl population) as Neanderthals; for Weidenreich, Rhodesian Man was a Neanderthal, Solo Man was not. Thus it is possible to hide significant distinctions by being too correct or by being too vague. In this book I will use *Homo sapiens*, as I have done heretofore, for living men only, and for the kind of skull they possess. *Homo erectus* means that early group only. In between these two, the other fossils may be called by more familiar names, and moved around to make whatever pattern one likes best.

Skulls and Their Schools

The truth is that almost everyone likes a different pattern. I think it is important to say again that, from the shortage of fossils and the ignorance of causes, we cannot judge conclusively what happened. I

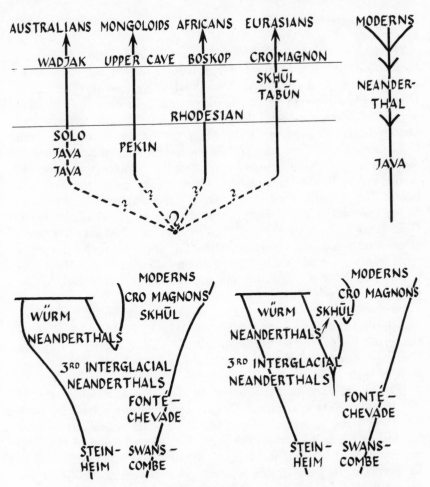

Graphic representations of different theories of human descent. Left, above, the Polyphyletic or Candelabra School, modified (and exaggerated) from Weidenreich. Right, above, the Unilinear or Hat-rack School. Below, the likenesses and differences of the Preneanderthal and Presapiens Schools in interpreting Neanderthal and *Homo sapiens*. These use the same evidence differently. Some "Presapiens" adherents might split the trunk much further down, i.e., leaving Steinheim on the Neanderthal line, instead of taking it as a common base, with Swanscombe, for upper branches, or even as a sapiens ancestor.

will try to spell out some of the difficulties by reviewing some interpretations. They are endlessly varied, of course, and controversial, and I regret to say that they sometimes generate more heat than light.

But they tend to fall into types, and there is often considerable agreement.

The first is the Hat-rack Theory, of unilinear evolution. This goes back to a time when only a few fossils were known and dates were not too clear. A single stem of mankind progressed directly up to *Homo sapiens* through a few simple stages: Java Man, Neanderthal Man, Cro Magnon. There were no extensive side branchings, and nobody became extinct, with Cro Magnon Man arising directly from the Neanderthals of the caves. This underwent some modifications as discoveries continued, such as broadening the "Neanderthal" stage to accommodate Rhodesian and Solo. Dr. Hrdlička was a principal adherent. But it could not face the complications introduced by many recent finds and some time ago was abandoned. However, Professor C. L. Brace of the University of California (Santa Barbara) has lately taken it up again in a vigorous article; this serves to probe the weak spots in other hypotheses but only demonstrates again that the thesis is too simple to account for any of the things catalogued in the previous chapter of this book.

Two others, which have a good deal in common, are the Preneanderthal and Presapiens Schools (to take Vallois' terms). Both of them split the main stem further back in time, to a point before the Würm Neanderthals, who are recognized as a dead end. Just how far back is their point of disagreement.

The Presapiens School is actually an ancient one, which originally saw *Homo sapiens* in substantially his present form reaching far back into the Pleistocene as an independent branch. Its main advocate was Sir Arthur Keith, who abandoned it when the evidence of the day, principally Galley Hill Man (and also the Piltdown skull) turned out to be worthless. Its later version is sustained by Professor Vallois of the Musée de l'Homme in Paris, Professor Heberer of the University of Göttingen, and Professor Gieseler of the University of Tübingen. They insist on the importance of Fontéchevade and on a long separate ancestry for sapiens. They disagree in some details, principally as to how far down the Pleistocene they would like to keep the two human lines unzipped. Vallois would push this well back: he would make the Neanderthals a present of Steinheim and cleave only to Swanscombe, viewing this young woman as a true early sapiens, a line already separate. Gieseler, on the other hand, takes Steinheim as a "Wurzelform," as a probable common parent for both lines if not in fact a possible primitive sapiens.

Adherents of the Preneanderthal School have been Professors Le Gros Clark of Oxford, Clark Howell of Chicago, Breitinger of Vienna, and Sergi of Rome, certainly a formidable phalanx. They view Steinheim and Swanscombe as leading to another, Third Interglacial stem, of a basically Neanderthal nature, which was then parental both to the cold Mousterians and, to the eastward, to sapiens. Such a broad and varying population of the western Old World would gradually have segregated into two stocks. One, isolated in Europe as the cold of the Würm came on, responded adaptively through the extreme form of the cave people; the other, in the Near East, progressed from a more general ancestor through stages manifested by Shanidar and Skhūl to the fully evolved sapiens men who then invaded Europe.

These last two views have their satisfying aspects. The slow spread of discoveries suggests that modern man has no really vast antiquity; the Presapiens hypothesis is probably stretching a point. The Preneanderthal view accommodates much of the evidence. There is no reason why the later Neanderthals of the West should not have undergone a kind of coarsening (not really a regression—their brains expanded); and everything from Steinheim on makes an orderly sequence in the alleged main line. One flaw is the lack of brows in Fontéchevade and their return in the Near Easterners. A bigger flaw, in all the views I have covered, is their enchantment with Europe and the Near East to the neglect of the rest of the world. They each refer to "*Homo sapiens*" but implicitly they seem to mean by this the Caucasoids of the West. If other kinds of *Homo sapiens* are meant, this is not made clear; if they are not meant, the hypotheses are inadequate.

The Problem of Races

This is repaired by the Spectrum, or Funnel Theory of Weiner and Campbell. They envisage a funnel, or several touching funnels, with *Homo erectus* near the narrow end. Above this is "a radial deployment of forms which is reticulate throughout." That is to say, there are tendencies, though not strongly isolated ones, in the general directions of Solo, Rhodesian, Neanderthal, and modern man; Steinheim and Swanscombe are in the funnel area of the latter. This is a looser and expanded version of the Preneanderthal theory, emphasizing overlapping even in the latest stages.

A final hypothesis, which emphasizes separation rather than overlapping, is the Candelabra or Polyphyletic Theory of Weidenreich and Coon. For Weidenreich, human evolution progressed in each major part of the world, essentially apart from what was happening in the other parts. In each case the end result was an advanced form, recognized now as one of the living races of modern man. For example, in Java *Meganthropus* was the first recognizable stage, followed by the rugged Java Man of the Djetis beds and his somewhat less rugged descendant of the Trinil zone. Much later in time, but in direct descent, was Solo Man, whose modern progeny is to be found in the aborigines of Australia. Between these two lies Wadjak Man, whose skulls were obtained in Java by Dubois. These are Upper Paleolithic or later (probably later), and much like the skulls of living Australian natives, though distinctly larger, just as the Cro Magnons were larger-skulled than living Europeans.

Similarly, Pekin Man, away in North China, led eventually to the Mongoloids of Asia. Rhodesian Man was parent to the "Africans," and the Tabūn-Skhūl group was parental to the "Eurasins," i.e., the Whites.

Now Dr. Weidenreich allowed for various adjustments and correctives in this scheme. He granted that the late, Fourth Glacial, cave Neanderthals were directly parental to no one. He believed that evolution in some centers was faster, in some slower. He also suggested that mixture and migration among the regional stocks took place to some extent; and that throughout the Pleistocene man always formed a single species. But his central idea, which he expressed in a diagram of parallel vertical lines, is the one I have described, of parallel evolution. It is a reasonable one. We remember mammal-like reptiles crossing the line into mammalhood at several different points. We remember different orders of mammals separately developing larger size and larger brains. In such a light, the idea that several different lines of man responded separately to the opportunities of natural selection, and progressed to bigger brains independently, does not seem strange. And it puts all the major fossils into the scheme, somewhere at their appropriate grade, instead of viewing most of them, as was often done, as side branches from a sapiens stem, extinct without issue. In fact, it makes almost no allowance for lines becoming extinct, which is, I think, too good to be true. It also makes very great demands on evolutionary convergence. Living races are much alike in tooth and skull— the only things in which we can compare them to the fossils. But Dr. Weidenreich had at least four different evolving human varieties, living far apart, moving ahead by fits and starts, producing their own special peculiarities of form, until they were decidedly more distinct than our races of today. Yet these several careers at last converged to produce the same kind of man everywhere. And all, miraculously enough, breasted the tape at the same time, regardless of how much of a late burst of speed this might call for from Rhodesian or Solo Man.

In fact, to put the argument in strongest terms, we might expect such a pattern as Weidenreich's to have led to more deep-seated and more obvious differences than we can find in modern men. Divergence should have continued. Teeth alone, for example, should exhibit greater differences than they do today. I consider Weidenreich's kind of pattern more applicable, in fact, to the idea of Neanderthal and sapiens separately arriving at large brains, while also arriving at divergent skull and body forms.

Carleton Coon has lately come to the support of Weidenreich in his *The Origin of Races*, incorporating further ideas and all the new material. It is a much more detailed study, though the framework is the same. Five separate lines of man (Australoid, Mongoloid, Caucasoid, Congoid—for African Negroes—and Capoid—for South African Bushmen) began as subspecies of *Homo erectus* and independently evolved to become subspecies of *Homo sapiens*, without losing their community as a single species. Five different geographic zones, then, preserved their racial individuality from the erectus stage. However, while this looks like strict parallel evolution, Coon, more than Weidenreich, sees contact and mixture as an important factor. Progress was not dependent solely on local evolution, but was bucked along by the occasional introduction of genetic material from another line already more advanced, so that by natural selection progressive features would replace older, more primitive features by the advantages they bestowed. At the same time, regional distinctions were not obliterated.

Coon finds a boundary between *Homo sapiens* and *Homo erectus* in terms of brain size (just above that of Pekin Man), tooth size, and flatness of forehead and bulge of occiput. Solo Man is safely erectus. So also (though I think this is wrong) is Rhodesian Man. Steinheim, however, ancestress of the Caucasoids, is clearly sapiens, implying that the Caucasoid subspecies made the grade in the Middle Pleistocene, while the Australoids and the Congoids crossed the line much later.

All this has involved Coon in a lot of controversy, one of the comments pertinent here being whether, if you had two species of man after Steinheim had appeared, you could reunite them in a single one afterwards. But this is probably more a matter of definition than of actual biology. The main question is whether Coon, with his reworking of Weidenreich, has provided the most useful framework for history.

It is certainly comprehensive, and systematically developed. I see in it the same drawbacks as in Weidenreich's version. Furthermore, it is probably too comprehensive for the present state of our knowledge. Much of the material is too little studied, and some of it has been mistakenly described or reported, though I can detect only a few examples of this in Coon's argument from my own experience. A considerable part of the argument lies in tracing connections between *Homo erectus* and races of *Homo sapiens*. For example, Coon quotes (with some amplification) a long list of specific details of the skull found by Weidenreich both in Pekin Man and in modern Mongoloids. At the same time he brings into evidence some important late Pleistocene skulls from China (Liukiang, Tzeyang, Upper Cave) to fill the gap, these having been judged by the authors who originally described them to be ancestors of the modern Chinese. But Dr. Andor Thoma of Hungary has analyzed these same skulls in detail, using measurements and careful appraisal of morphological features. He finds that they have no affinity with the Chinese or with any Mongoloids, resembling primarily the Cro Magnons of Europe and the Ainus of Japan (a non-Mongoloid, European-looking people; see Chapter 19). Instead, Thoma traces the basic Mongoloids of Siberia, by the same methods, to the Near Eastern and early Neanderthals. These are the same people who are supposed by others to have given rise to the Caucasoids; Thoma finds that these Neanderthals and the Siberians resemble each other distinctly more closely than either resembles the Cro Magnons.

This seems to place two queries against the direct descent, in China, of the Chinese from Pekin Man. But these are details. I am saying rather that, in addition to fossil finds, there is still to be done a great deal of intensive work of analysis and comparison, by many people, to pin broad generalizations down with.

An Interim View

If we are being broad, however, I should incline toward a Synthetic Theory, depending neither on too much extinction nor on too much parallelism, with a consciousness of how what we do not know relates to what we do know. This would probably be closer to the Spectrum view of Weiner and Campbell than any other.

As usual, we must start with *Homo sapiens*. Great antiquity for modern man is not now apparent; thus the Presapiens theory in pure form seems unacceptable. On the other hand, there are reasons for thinking that he made his eventual appearance on a line of his own, as part of a radiation also producing Neanderthals and Rhodesian Man, rather than as a simultaneous termination of different lines. It should not be forgotten that *Homo sapiens* is actually distinctive in form of skull and face, which continues to suggest that he rose from one principal root. As to time, we may admit that the Fontéchevade skulls, the Kanjera skulls, and the Niah Cave boy are still rather fragmentary evidence; nevertheless, the closeness of contact in time of *Homo sapiens* with both Neanderthals and Rhodesian Man suggests a real overlap with them. Whether *Homo sapiens* could have risen entirely from a Neanderthal stock (the Preneanderthal theory) is a question, but there seems to be no chance of any modern men evolving right out of the European Neanderthals. If that is so, there is no necessary reason for their having evolved directly out of Rhodesian Man, in whole or in any part. But sapiens must have evolved out of somebody. Where? That is the sticky question. We know the Neanderthals occupied Europe and much of Asia north of the mountains during the critical period, while we assume that Rhodesian men were in possession of much of southern Africa. We have the Kanjera skulls in East Africa. But we will probably not get a good answer one way or the other until skeletons are found in India.

The Coon-Weidenreich answer to the question Where? is: Everywhere! But if *Homo sapiens* had a home of his own, say India, we could still explain some of the same phenomena. Mixture would account both for the survival of some local features, and for the assimilation of all regional variants toward a more common form. We see early signs of *Homo sapiens* on the fringes of southern Asia, in the Niah Cave boy and the Skhūl population. As I have suggested, the Skhūl people are likely to be a Neanderthal-sapiens mixture, to a greater degree than took place when sapiens reached Europe, though of course it is perfectly possible that some degree of mixture took place there as well.

In South Africa, the Florisbad skull might reflect the absorption—"extinction"—of the population of Rhodesian type. More definitely, the Australian aboriginals have always been striking by reason of their rather low and primitive skull, and their large brow ridges. This is of course why Weidenreich and Coon argue that he is the end of the Java-Solo-Wadjak line. But the alternative is that a more regular sapiens population entered Java in the late Pleistocene when Solo Man was still present, that extinction by absorption took place, and that the Australian and Australian-like groups found in the Pacific result from such a survival of Solo genes. Otherwise, in fact, it is a little difficult to understand why the Solo people, after having undergone almost no forward evolution since the time of Java Man, should suddenly have accelerated so late to take rank as *Homo sapiens* by the end of the Pleistocene.

If this general explanation, of hybridity rather than parallel evolution, is valid, then it argues that the sapiens form, prior to migration and mixing, would have been even more homogeneous. This is probably too much of a good thing. In fact, I do not wish to stress this possibility of hybridity too strongly. The whole problem of a home for *Homo sapiens* remains, and I am only repeating my conviction that, within such differentiation as took place among human populations of the later Pleistocene, *Homo sapiens* went through a process of separation from something like a Preneanderthal form, departing from that form about as much as did the cave Neanderthals of Europe.

17. PILTDOWN MAN:
HIS RISE AND FALL

"SEVERAL YEARS ago I was walking along a farm-road close to Piltdown Common, Fletching (Sussex), when I noticed that the road had been mended with some peculiar brown flints not usual in the district. On enquiry I was astonished to learn that they were dug from a gravel-bed on the farm, and shortly afterwards I visited the place, where two labourers were at work digging the gravel for small repairs to the roads. As this excavation was situated about 4 miles north of the limit where the occurrence of flints overlying the Wealdean strata is recorded, I was much interested, and made a close examination of the bed. I asked the workmen if they had found bones or other fossils there. As they did not appear to have noticed anything of the sort, I urged them to preserve anything that they might find. Upon one of my subsequent visits to the pit, one of the men handed to me a small portion of an unusually thick human parietal bone. I immediately made a search, but could find nothing more, nor had the men noticed anything else. The bed is full of tabular pieces of iron-stone closely resembling this piece of skull in colour and thickness; and, although I made many subsequent searches, I could not hear of any further find nor discover anything—in fact, the bed seemed to be quite unfossiliferous.

"It was not until some years later, in the autumn of 1911, on a visit to the spot, that I picked up, among the rain-washed spoil-heaps of the gravel-pit, another and larger piece belonging to the frontal region of the same skull, including a portion of the left superciliary ridge. As I had examined a cast of the Heidelberg jaw, it occurred to me that the proportions of this skull were similar to those of that specimen. I accordingly took it to Dr. A. Smith Woodward at the British Museum (Natural History) for comparison and determination. He was immediately impressed with the importance of the discovery, and we decided to employ labour and to make a systematic search among the spoil-heaps and gravel, as soon as the floods had abated; for the gravel-pit is more or less under water during five or six months of the year. We accordingly gave up as much time as we could spare since last spring (1912), and completely turned over and sifted what spoil-material remained; we also dug up and sifted such portions of the gravel as had been left undisturbed by the workmen.

"Considering the amount of material excavated and sifted by us, the specimens discovered were numerically small and localized.

"Apparently the whole or greater portion of the human skull had been shattered by the workmen, who had thrown away the pieces unnoticed. Of these we recovered, from the spoil-heaps, as many fragments as possible. In a somewhat deeper depression of the undisturbed gravel I found the right half of a human mandible. So far as I could judge, guiding myself by the position of a tree 3 or 4 yards away, the spot was identical with that upon which the men were at work when the first portion of the cranium was found several years ago. Dr. Woodward also dug up a small portion of the occipital bone of the skull from within a yard of the point where the jaw was discovered, and at precisely the same level. The jaw appeared to have been broken at the symphysis and abraded, perhaps when it lay fixed in the gravel, and before its complete deposition.

"Besides the human remains, we found two small broken pieces of a molar tooth of a rather early Pliocene type of elephant, also a much-rolled cusp of a molar of *Mastodon,* portions of two teeth of *Hippopotamus,* and two molar teeth of a Pleistocene beaver. In the adjacent field to the west, on the surface close to the hedge dividing it from the gravel-bed, we found portions of a red deer's antler and the tooth of a Pleistocene horse . . . All the specimens are highly mineralized with iron oxide."[1]

These are the words of Mr. Charles Dawson, a lawyer of Uckfield, Sussex, and an antiquarian of varied tastes. He pronounced them on December 18, 1912, when he and Dr. Smith Woodward introduced Piltdown Man to the Geological Society of London. Present at this meeting were famous men: Sir Ray Lankester, Doctor Duckworth of Cambridge, Professor Arthur Keith of the Royal College of Surgeons, and Professor G. Elliot Smith, then of the University of Manchester (Smith Woodward, Keith, and Elliot Smith all later knighted). There was great excitement over the new fossil since, except for the Heidelberg jaw, the only non-sapiens men then known were the Neanderthals and the first skull of Java Man.

[1] *Quarterly Journal of the Geological Society of London,* vol. 69, 1913.

First Discussions

And Piltdown Man was vastly different from both of them. To anyone's first glance, he had the skull of modern man combined with the jaw of an ape: a skull with a high brain case and a vertical forehead with slight brow ridges, and a jaw with a simian shelf, exactly as in an orang or a chimpanzee. A strange combination. Nevertheless all the bones had been picked out of gravels from the same pit, and all shared the dark brown color of the gravel of lowest stratum and of other bones from the same layer. Furthermore, the skull was rather small in size, as restored, and the bones were extraordinarily thick—apparently primitive, and therefore, one might conclude, ancient. And the only teeth in the jaw, the first two molars, were ground quite flat, in hominid fashion, suggesting that the mandible had worked like man's, from side to side, not impeded like an ape's by interlocking canines at the front. The same kind of jaw action was suggested by the glenoid fossa, the socket for the condyle or joint of the jaw just in front of the ear. But alas, the condyle itself was broken off and missing, so that proof as to how skull and jaw fitted together was lacking.

There was, as I said, great excitement at the meeting. The incongruity between brain case and mandible was noted at once by some, and doubts were expressed as to whether the find represented a real fossil man, or simply the accidental combination of a fossil human skull and a fossil ape jaw. But these remarks evidently reflected plain astonishment rather than deep doubts, and most of the men present agreed that Dawson and Woodward were correct. Elliot Smith said that the apparent paradox of the association of a simian jaw and a human brain was not surprising to anyone familiar with recent research on the evolution of man, stating that the growth of the brain had preceded other human traits in development. (How wrong: but Elliot Smith was a brain specialist, and this was 1912.)

Smith Woodward gave it as his belief that, if the canine tooth had been found, it would have proved to be intermediate, larger than a man's but not protruding like an ape's, not sticking up in such a way as to prevent rotary chewing and the flat wear of the molar teeth. Smith Woodward even exhibited a model canine tooth he had made, to show what might be expected. Keith seems to have been bothered by certain features, especially the flat tooth wear, which made him think the suggested reconstruction of Piltdown Man was too ape-like. Keith did not actually demur to the validity of Piltdown Man, although in all the years which followed he continued to regard it as an enigma. Not so Smith Woodward, who had no qualms about the combination, which he named *Eoanthropus dawsoni* (Dawson's dawn man).

Thus, in spite of the genuine and well-grounded surprise of the anthropologists, the Piltdown remains were quickly accepted as an important new kind of ancient man. This acceptance was fortified in the next few years by certain further developments. The following summer, in 1913, Smith Woodward and Dawson returned to the Piltdown pit to look for more of the skull, aided briefly by Father Teihard de Chardin. This Jesuit Father later became a renowned paleontologist, particularly in working with Davidson Black at Choukoutien and with Roy Chapman Andrews in Mongolia, but in those years he was a young priest staying at a Jesuit College at Ore, Hastings, and collecting fossil plants in the district. He had become a friend of Dawson's, working with him and Smith Woodward at Piltdown the first year, before the discovery was announced.

Dawson and Smith Woodward had little luck that second summer, although Dawson made a truly extraordinary find, right in the gravel: the small bones of the nasal bridge and, apparently still in place behind them, remains of one of the extremely delicate filagree-form turbinal bones which support the mucuous membrane inside the nasal cavity. This fell apart on finding, but the parts, carefully saved, were glued together again with feminine deftness by Mrs. Smith Woodward. Later, one hot day in August, Father Teilhard worked so zealously in his black clothes that he had to be persuaded to rest. He was sitting on one of the dump heaps beside the pit, running his fingers through the gravel, when he found, of all things, a canine tooth. Sure enough, as Smith Woodward had predicted, it was smaller than an ape's but distinctly larger than a man's and well worn into the bargain.

When this was presented to the Geological Society, Keith expressed further surprise. He thought the canine tooth was still rather large for a jaw used in human fashion, which would produce level wear on the other teeth. Also, he considered it odd that this tooth should be so worn, as in an older man, when certain aspects of the jaw looked youthful—for example, he believed that the missing wisdom tooth, judging by the socket, had not fully erupted. He did not doubt that the skull, jaw, and teeth all came from the same kind of creature, *Eoanthropus*, but he thought more than one specimen of that creature might be present. However, others disputed his idea about the wisdom tooth and pointed out that the two remaining molars were heavily worn, like the canine. Keith seems to have accepted this. There was agreement that X rays showed the molar tooth roots to be short, as in man, not long as in an ape.

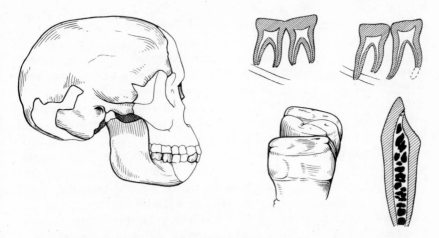

The Piltdown Man. Left, the skull and jaw, as restored to form *"Eoanthropus."* Right, above, the molar tooth roots, showing the human appearance in old X rays, and the true, ape-like appearance in later X rays. Below, left, a close view of the molars, showing that the "wear" is unnatural, being in a different plane in the two teeth. Below, right, an X-ray section of the canine, showing the pulp cavity (packed with sand grains) extending to the worn surface of the tooth, without secondary dentine. After Le Gros Clark, Oakley and Weiner.

Eoanthropus Reinforced

Nothing more of interest turned up at Piltdown. Dawson died in 1916. In 1917, Woodward reported a last find. "One large field, about 2 miles from the Piltdown pit, had especially attracted Mr. Dawson's attention, and he and I examined it several times without success during the spring and autumn of 1914. When, however, in the course of farming, the stones had been raked off the ground and brought together into heaps, Mr. Dawson was able to search the material more satisfactorily: and early in 1915 he was so fortunate as to find here two well-fossilized pieces of human skull and a molar tooth, which he immediately recognized as belonging to at least one more individual of *Eoanthropus dawsoni.*" Later, it proved impossible to identify this field for further search. And Hrdlička always thought it strange that these particularly small fragments should have been caught up by a rake. But there was no mistaking the striking similarity of the small bit of forehead to the parts of the first skull, nor of the new molar tooth to the teeth in the first jaw, and so this clear evidence of a new *Eoanthropus,* found at some distance from the first, settled many doubts as to the combination of man-like skull and ape-like jaw. Nature, said Elliot Smith, would hardly play such a trick twice.

One other thing, I think, strengthened *Eoanthropus'* scientific pedestal. Smith Woodward had provisionally put the skull together, getting a smallish brain case with a capacity of 1070 cubic centimeters, about what Pekin Man had in his much more brutish cranium. When Keith got a copy of this reconstruction, he disapproved of certain details: it was not symmetrical, and too small for the size indicated by the temporal bone in the ear region. He worked over the parts, opening out the top for various anatomical reasons, and arrived at a rather positive preliminary estimate of "about 1500" cubic centimeters, or at least the size of modern man in this respect. Smith Woodward rejected Keith's figure, supported by Elliot Smith.

Keith continued to disagree. At length Professor Parsons of St. Thomas's Hospital suggested that Keith test his procedure (which involved locating the mid-line of the top of the skull accurately) by making a restoration of a modern skull of known size, after it had been cut up into pieces corresponding to those from the pit at Piltdown. Keith was delighted with the idea and decided to make it the subject of a talk he had already promised to give at the Royal Anthropological Institute early in 1914. He was given the test pieces, from the skull of an Egyptian woman. He fell to work and produced an estimate of 1415 cubic centimeters, against an original measurement of 1395, an excellent approximation and nearly within the limits of precise measurement on a complete skull. This triumphantly accurate result carried the field for Keith, and Smith Woodward came eventually to accept Keith's figure for the Piltdown skull (which the latter, as a result of all this study, finally brought down to 1400 cubic centimeters). I think it is likely that Keith's tour de force, because it showed that Piltdown Man's brain size could be estimated with reasonable accuracy, indirectly and fallaciously invested everything about Piltdown Man with greater scientific sanctity.

Clear Followed by Cloudy

At any rate, harmony reigned among the British anthropologists, a few years after *Eoanthropus* was brought to London. A new kind of man stood recognized on the stage of our history, to become so well known in the popular mind as to star in a comic strip as well. With his high forehead and his entirely ape-like jaw, he was in shocking contrast with the Java or Neanderthal men. But, half a century after Darwin, and soon after the Java and Heidelberg discoveries, a feeling of bright expectancy suffused museums and universities. The time was ripe, the stars were in conjunction, to welcome *Eoanthropus* and to be instructed by him: if he could combine so modern a head with so antique a mandible, then that was part of the story of evolution. After all, a truly great anatomist, Elliot Smith, could hold the opinion that the brain had outstripped the skeleton as man was rising from the apes.

And how old was Piltdown Man taken to be? Both flint tools and animal bones had been discovered in the pit, along with a large tool or pick of sorts, made from a slab of bone from an elephant's leg, sharpened to a point. The flints were crudely shaped flakes, still sharp, but brown in color, like the rest of the lowest gravel. The animals (fragments and teeth) were a faintly bizarre group. It contained mastodon, rhino, and hippo, all good early Pleistocene. It also included a distinctly early elephant, *Elephas planifrons,* heretofore a stranger to England, as well as a beaver of the modern and late Pleistocene genus, *Castor.* Mr. Dawson himself, however, suggested that the oldest animals were probably late Pliocene, and had been washed out of an old fossil bed and into a new one together with the Piltdown skull and the beaver in Pleistocene times. Years later, in 1935, Dr. Hopwood (namer of *Proconsul*) went over all the bones again without being able to resolve the difficulties, but concluding that the skull actually belonged with the earlier animals, not the later. At any rate, the date was never settled on exactly, but was supposed to be in the first half of the Pleistocene, perhaps First Interglacial, perhaps Second.

Nor did the clouds ever wholly leave the skies of the Dawn Man himself. In spite of the satisfaction and delight over his discovery, doubts remained. He was among friends in England, but even Keith was never quite comfortable. Abroad he had fewer adherents. Boule in France, Mollison in Germany, Giuffrida-Ruggeri in Italy, all said his jaw was not his own, but a fossil ape's. Gregory in New York felt so at first, but later took an intermediate position more benevolent to *Eoanthropus.* In Washington, Gerrit Miller would use the name *Eoanthropus* only for the skull; he separated the jaw and named it *Pan vetus,* as a new species of chimpanzee, while Friederichs in Germany gave the jaw a whole new ape genus, *Boreopithecus* (Ape of the North). Hrdlička kept finding small inconsistencies and always remained a doubter. He noted that the molar tooth of the second specimen, reportedly found in 1915, was so exactly like those of the first that he suggested an error in the records: perhaps it had actually come from the original pit. Sir Ray Lankester had already remarked that both tooth and frontal fragment might conceivably be parts of the first specimen, except that the 1915 specimen also had a piece of the occiput, which duplicated that in the original lot and so must have come from a separate head. And Mr. Marston, finder of the Swanscombe skull, kept pointing to the incongruities in the maturity of the Piltdown person: the skull was definitely middle-aged; the jaw, in spite of the wear of the teeth, seemed young and recently adult; while the canine was frankly immature, with an uncompleted root, still open at the end.

Against all these prickly points, and a host of others, were arrayed the powerful, simple arguments of the nature of the find itself, arguments which, as the years went by, tended once more to make even the doubters doubt their doubts. Here, in gravels of seemingly early Pleistocene times, had lain fossil animal remains, mostly taken out under the careful eye of Smith Woodward of the Natural History Museum. Among these fossils were bones of ape-human nature, the only relics of any such highest primates of the early Pleistocene from anywhere in the British Isles. And there were remnants enough only for one individual. If the jaw was a chimp's, why no chimp head parts? If the skull was a modern man's, why no human teeth? And the combination had been repeated again, a mile or so away. Who could arbitrarily throw down the plain evidence from the soil, and turn his back on it?

Weidenreich could. As early as 1932, before going to China, he had decided flatly that the combination was too incongruous, and never mind the geology; he noted that, in human fossils, the jaw tended to shrink, and become more human, as the brain grew, and that Piltdown Man was the lone exception to this rule. (I think it is fair to say that Weidenreich was an acute and deeply experienced student of physical form, and not much inclined to let geological scruples interfere with anatomical conclusions.) At last in 1943 he wrote:

"I am only wondering why, if a human vault, a simian mandible and an anonymous 'canine' were combined into a new form, the other animal bones and teeth found in the same spot were not added to the 'Eoanthropus' combination; I do not believe in those miracles whether offered by anti-Darwinian [sic] or Darwinians. The sooner the chimaera 'Eoanthropus' is erased from the list of human fossils, the better for science."

But the redoubtable Weidenreich was by this time virtually alone in taking so positive a stand. Others continued to feel a sympathy for the geological evidence. And the discovery in 1935 of the modern-looking Swanscombe skull, of Second Interglacial date, renewed attention to Piltdown Man and to the possibility of putting him into the family tree somehow. But there was no real Restoration. In fact, mere bewilderment over the meaning of Eoanthropus, after prevailing for a generation, gave way finally to mounting distress, distress which became acute by 1950.

This was not due to anything new about Piltdown Man himself. In all these years he had gone on as an object of prime anthropological interest, though only through reconsideration, re-examination, rehashing of the same original evidence. None of the old arguments or objections settled the matter; instead, the tree of knowledge put out a lot of new foliage. Rhodesian and Pekin Man were found, and then more jaws of Java Man, and *Meganthropus;* finally, from 1947 on, copious remains of the australopithecines (still no apes in England). And all of these things were entirely consistent, in their general story of development, as well as on one particular point: early man *never* had a jaw like a chimpanzee. (I have already noted that a simian shelf was probably a late pongid acquisition rather than an ancient primitive trait.) Piltdown Man became at last quite incomprehensible. Remember that the gentlemen who gathered at the Geological Society in December 1912 had been imagining an early kind of humanity which had, roughly speaking, the skull of a man and the jaw of an ape. But the fossils have since taught us that early hominids had, again roughly speaking, the skull of an ape and the jaw and teeth of a man. The man-apes of South Africa finally outdid even Weidenreich in the harshness of the questions they asked of *Eoanthropus.*

Beginning of the End

And so a new conjunction of the stars had come about for Piltdown Man, a new stage of knowledge and of inquiry. Now, in 1950, Kenneth Oakley asked him another point-blank question. Oakley had begun to apply the fluorine test to various important fossils: Swanscombe Man passed; Galley Hill Man failed it and resigned from the club. Oakley tested the Piltdown skull, jaw and teeth, using infinitesimal amounts of the precious fossil. The result was astonishing: only a low degree of fluorine was present in any of the remains, much less than in the other animals of the pit. Judging from the not too reliable figures, this meant a) that the skull and jaw *did* belong together, since they gave similar results, and b) that they would have to be moved up in date, making Piltdown Man not earlier than the Third Interglacial! Did he go with the beaver after all? (One more little point: drilling showed the inside of the canine tooth to be unexpectedly white, considering the dark, fossilized color of the surface.)

It would be hard to invent an outcome more aggravating to the whole Piltdown problem, whatever view you might take. So vexed was Oakley, in London, mulling over his results, that he exclaimed to a colleague, "This thing's bogus!" But the appalling spark did not take light: Oakley was aware that the tooth of a fossil hippo from Piltdown, an animal which could well have been there in the Last Interglacial, likewise showed almost no fluorine. Quite independently, it was J. S. Weiner, who had never discussed Piltdown Man with Oakley, who thought things out a little more thoroughly.

Weiner, ex-student of Dart's and Reader in Physical Anthropology in the Department of Anatomy with Le Gros Clark at Oxford, did his thinking while driving back from London to Oxford, late one evening in the summer of 1953. He was wondering about *Eoanthropus,* and the impossible situation which now existed, a ridiculous mixture and a ridiculous date. He looked at the two old explanations. A real creature, ape in the jaw, human in the skull, in the Last Interglacial in England? A real ape in England, at the same time—a million to one chance— mixed naturally in the same little pit with a man's skull—another million to one chance? Both actually impossible. What else could conceivably have happened? Could this have been a dump—could someone have tossed a modern ape's jaw behind the hedge by accident? No, the ground-down molars and the odd canine were too striking. Well then, could it have been made and put there deliberately? Certainly a wild and extravagant idea.

Once come, however, the idea would not go away. And in fact, seen beside this one, it was the other two hypotheses which looked wilder and more extravagant. Weiner turned it over in his mind for a while and then mentioned it to Le Gros Clark. It struck the latter, naturally, as wild and extravagant; furthermore, Le Gros Clark recalled that other evidence in the jaw was against faking. In the first place, X rays had shown that the molar tooth roots were short and human in form. Secondly, although the canine might give the appearance of having been radically ground down and reduced in size, X rays had also indicated that secondary dentine had formed inside the tooth, in the pulp cavity at the center. This is the natural reaction which reinforces a tooth when the outer surface enamel wears away slowly from use. Therefore, the wear of the tooth seemed natural, not artificial.

Still, they had to think about it, and they began going over the Piltdown evidence once again. Then, just to see, Weiner took a chimpanzee jaw from the collections and filed the molar surfaces a little. He was surprised to find how easy this was, how readily any chimpanzee details were removed, leaving only the common hominoid pattern of the worn cusps, and the appearance of flat human wear. He dipped the teeth briefly in permanganate, which gave them a fine fossil appearance.

He was delighted. He took the "fossil" into Le Gros Clark's office, put it on the desk, and said with a great air of innocence: "I got this out of the collections. What do you suppose it is?" Sir Wilfrid, not an unperceptive man, perceived exactly what it was, and exclaimed: "You can't mean it!" Clearly, it was time to go to London and to visit Oakley and *Eoanthropus*. That moment, when these two men could persuade themselves that the hypothesis of deliberate forgery was really worth looking into, was the precise moment of the fall of Piltdown Man.

Such a hypothesis, of course, meant that there would have to be real signs in the jaw and teeth of the work of a forger, signs which had never been noticed, or which had been wrongly read. All this was, as they started out, well within the realm of possibility, for several reasons. In the first place, the jaw had never been fully studied: Oakley's test for fluorine had been admittedly inadequate, and meant only to compare the F content of the mandible roughly with other bones from the site. So the men began to make a little list of things they must find if, in fact, the jaw was no part of a primitive Pleistocene man, but only the stained-up, filed-off hand-me-down of a thoroughly recent ape. They found them; the little list soon became a big one.

The Walls of Jericho

Let us look at the canine, that tooth found in 1913 which so neatly fitted what Smith Woodward had said in 1912 it should be like. X-rayed once more by modern methods, it appeared clearly a young tooth which had been heavily ground down, since the pulp cavity was that of a much larger tooth. There was *no* secondary dentine under the ground areas, and in fact that grinding had carried right into the pulp chamber itself, near the tip, something which would never happen through wear on a living tooth. On the surface, under a magnifying glass, there could be seen the fine scratches left by the abrasive, whatever it was. And this tooth was actually painted!

The molar teeth in the jaw also showed fine scratches from artificial grinding. And that "flat human wear" could now be seen as entirely too flat, so that the edges of the crown were sharp, not smoothly beveled as they would be in any naturally worn tooth. Another thing: though very flat, the flat surfaces of the two teeth were not in the same plane but slightly out of kilter with one another. Now the whole meaning of primitive human chewing is the rotary motion which wears all the teeth in the jaw to a smooth, common plane. This could not have taken place with the Piltdown molars; on the contrary, they show just what could happen if a forger had filed one tooth, and then shifted his grip a little before filing the other. These things, the different planes and the sharp edges, are easily visible to the naked eye, once they have been pointed out, and yet they had escaped forty years of inspection when nobody was looking for them. Finally, of course, the new and better X rays showed that the molar roots were long, as in apes, not short as in man after all.

Oakley attacked the chemical nature of the fragments resolutely, not tenderly as before. At once new evidence appeared. On really biting into the bone, the drill drew powder and dust from the skull parts, but the jaw gave microscopic shavings, like fresh bone, together with a burning smell. When adequate amounts of bone were tested for fluorine, the skull showed the presence of a low degree of this element, but the jaw and teeth (including the 1915 tooth) showed almost none, or only what is present in new bone. Contrariwise, a test for nitrogen, which is present in the amount of about 4% in living bone but is lost over a few thousand years, showed the jaw to have 3.9% of nitrogen and the skull to have 1.4% or less.

The color of the bones also betrayed the hand of man. They all make fine fossils on the surface. The dark color comes largely from iron oxides, which are present both in the ground and in the chemist's laboratory. This oxide color runs deep into the skull bones, but lies only close to the surface of the bone of the jaw. Another substance gives some color to the bones: bichromate of potash. In the last century, fossil bones were sometimes soaked in a solution of this, in the erroneous belief that they would be hardened; Galley Hill Man was so treated. Mr. Dawson had dipped his first pieces of Piltdown Man in chromate, before Smith Woodward told him it was pointless. Therefore, as you might suppose, chromate can be detected in the parts found in 1911 or before. It is not present in the skull parts found in 1912, when Smith Woodward was on the scene. But it is present in the jaw, also found in 1912, and in the 1915 remains. The chromate could hardly have got into the jaw after it was found. It could not have entered while the bone was in the ground. So it must have got there before the bone was in the ground, and for purposes of pigmentation, not of preservation.

With all this and more in hand, the three men announced to the press in November 1953 that the Piltdown jaw was a hoax. A grateful sigh of happiness and relief must have left the throat of every anthropologist on the globe. *Punch* printed a most *Punch*-like cartoon, complete with Du Maurier overtones: a dentist, saying to Mr. Piltdown seated in the chair, "This may hurt, but I'm afraid I'll have to remove the whole jaw." (Collapse of 600,000-year-old party.) The exasperating dilemma had been resolved; *Eoanthropus* was no more.

All this, of course, revolved around the mandible. The skull was clearly not as recent, being slightly fossilized or mineralized. Momentarily the possibility remained that some crank had adulterated a perfectly good discovery of fossil man by inserting a bogus jaw (though how could he be sure that the real mandible might not also come to light?). But as Le Gros Clark, Oakley, and Weiner continued their several and joint investigations, Piltdown Man continued to unravel. The skull itself could not be trusted, with so many oddities about the staining; the frontal fragment found in 1915 is too likely to have been part of the original skull, and the occipital portion found with it does not match it, in nature or in fluorine content. The puzzling fact of finding the delicate nasal bones and the still more delicate turbinal, in 1913, in gravel which should by rights have pulverized them, ceases to be a puzzle in the new light, as does the missing joint of the jawbone, which a forger *had* to knock off. On top of all this, Le Gros Clark examined the "turbinal" fragments minutely and found that they were no turbinal bone at all, but merely some bone splinters of uncertain origin.

Turning to the tools, the hunters found things which really should have been noticed long before. The strange elephant-bone pick had cut marks, where it had been fashioned to a point, which could never have been made on a tough fresh bone with a stone tool but only, as a little experimenting showed, with a steel knife or hatchet on a bone already fossilized. Another fraud. And the stone "tools," seemingly having the dark patina which comes from lying in the soil for hundreds of thousands of years, were found instead to be superficially colored with the same iron salts as the bone. Except one: this was colored with bichromate of potash! Now there was a time, as I said, when it was thought that chromate would harden bone. But nobody has ever imagined a reason for applying it to flint. Nobody, that is, except a forger.

The animal bones, at last, turned out to be the craziest aspect of the whole fossil pudding. They had always been a strange-looking lot —mixing early mastodon and late beaver, and featuring *Elephas planifrons,* much more at home around the Mediterranean—but at least they had a general Pleistocene flavor. Oakley reanalyzed the fossils. He found many of them liberally dosed with the same pigments, chromate included, as the skull and the tools. And, getting the cooperation of atomic-energy scientists, he tried another new chemical test, one for the accumulation of radioactive uranium salts, something like the fluorine test. Here he found every grade, from very slight up to one fragment so radioactive that he made it take its own picture by setting it on a photographic film. The radioactivity was especially high in the teeth of *E. planifrons,* higher by far than anything he could find for any fossils from the British Isles, or even Europe. At last he found some fossils which would rattle a Geiger counter at the same rate. They were from a site in Tunisia. Here the uranium salts are particularly abundant. And here *Elephas planifrons* is particularly abundant as well.

Evidently, the *planifrons* fragments originally came from this very place, probably through a dealer or dealers. And evidently the pit at Piltdown was nothing but a salted mine from top to bottom. The man who salted it could have bought all the materials from dealers of one sort or another: animal fossils, the jaw of what almost certainly was a female orang utan, and the skull from an ancient tomb, perhaps even Neolithic, of a sufferer from Paget's disease, which causes a thickening of the bones of the cranial vault. What kind of man did all this? Obviously, someone who knew a good deal about geology, paleontology, and anatomy. He knew very well what to use and what not to use. The jaw was a perfect job, since he had to remove the joint, and all the teeth except the molars: and he could only dare to introduce a canine tooth after Smith Woodward had stated publicly, in so many words, what it should be like.

Why did he do it? Out of plain deviltry? This is a lot of trouble for a silent laugh. Was he an "anti-Darwinist?" Hardly: anyone who knew as much as he did does not sound like an anti-evolutionist. Did he do it simply to attract attention to himself? Quite possibly. Even the saintly Darwin says that as a little boy he was given to inventing deliberate falsehoods for the sake of causing excitement. But this Darwin was a little boy. Conceivably Piltdown Man was meant originally as a joke to be confessed to, but a joke which ran so far ahead of the joker that he could not bring himself to confess. Indeed, the discovery of the "turbinal" bone in 1913, so outlandish on the face of it, almost looks as though the forger were trying to wake everyone to the absurdity of it all, without standing forth himself. But no: he followed this up at once with the canine tooth, the most labored item in the whole scheme.

Who did it? Nobody knows. Keith and Father Teilhard, both now dead, were in 1953 the last surviving actors of the drama, and they could only express blank astonishment at the news. Weiner went down to Sussex in the spring of 1954, to see what he could turn up, and recounted his findings, and the whole story, in a delightful book, *The Piltdown Forgery.*

Never mind the name. The real moral of the story has nothing to do with the ethics of a man. Rather, it points to the progress of a science. Some of my colleagues feel that the whole affair was a tragic waste of time. I do not agree, although it was indeed an injury to Smith Woodward, who spent many of his later years in fruitless further search. Under totally false colors, Piltdown Man created great interest in ancient man and problems related to him. He was largely responsible for Keith's important work, *The Antiquity of Man,* and he was a constant spur to thinking, which is not wasted time even if a lot of the answers are wrong.

More than that. The Piltdown business was carried out as a fraud. But if it had been done as a test, to measure the reality of the advances in knowledge of fossil man, it could not have been better devised. The anthropologists were fooled by *Eoanthropus* for a long time, since they accepted the apparent evidence of nature, and were playing according to the rules. Because of this, it eventually became clear that *Eoanthropus* himself was not playing the rules.

And because of the outcome, we can see the soundness of most of the rest of our knowledge, and the importance of certain principles. The falsity of Piltdown Man does not cast a shadow on Swanscombe Man, for example; quite the reverse. And we can see how significant is our understanding of the australopithecines, since this was such a factor in forcing the exposure of Piltdown. At the same time, we are reminded of the supreme importance of having exact information about dates, whether from careful geology, or from tests like the F test, or from reliable animal associations.

18. RACES OF MAN

THE EARLY MEN go back into the cupboards now, for we are done with them. The rest of human history is that of *Homo sapiens* alone. No other kind seems to have lived long beyond that same point, about 37,000 years ago or less, at which modern men were making their appearance in Europe. Our concern now is with another kind of difference, the differences among races; and with another kind of history, the arrival of these races where we find them in historic times.

So we have passed through a doorway. But we have not shaken off the problem that bothered us in that other room; it is still with us in the new one. When, how, and where did *Homo sapiens* originate? The First Man, as he is painted on the ceiling of the Sistine Chapel, is unquestionably a handsome White man. But what did the first man of our own species actually look like, back in the long Pleistocene? Our knowledge of race and of racial history is obviously all tied up with this, and one side of the problem asks questions of the other.

We can be sure of this: races have become different from one another since the time when the species *sapiens* took shape and came to occupy different regions. We do not know just why, whether through gradual divergence or through mixture with other kinds of men. We do not know how different they were at any one time, say ten thousand years back, or thirty-five thousand years back, or more. We do not know which of the important racial forms may be more recently developed and which may be quite old in their present guises, though I would be willing to guess. We do know, for example, that the Upper Paleolithic people of Europe already had the character of Whites, or Caucasoids, simply from their skulls. And this is one of the strong arguments for the considerable age of *Homo sapiens*. We must conclude either that the Whites are the oldest and most primitive—the first—sapient men, brand-new then, and that they have not changed materially since then; or else that the first of sapiens were older, and gave rise to the White stock as one of several of their branches.

Weidenreich believed the first racial division in man was very ancient, as you have seen. Hooton also seems to have felt that races were at one time more distinct and well defined, since he believed most racial types of the present were due to mixtures among such more ancient races. "We are not presently in the primary race-making phase of man's evolution, nor have we been at that stage of the evolution of *Homo sapiens* for the past ten thousand years or more."[1] This of course does not hold a candle to Weidenreich's estimate of the whole Pleistocene since races first diverged. But both views strongly suggest a day when races were pristine and pure. It is an idea which needs re-examination. We cannot examine it in the light of history, since the evidence from the skulls is too fragmentary, one of the worst gaps in human history. We must look at it through what we know of living people, and of evolution.

Various Views of Race

The whole subject of race in modern man has been surrounded by ignorance and perverse judgment. This is another case where common sense and everyday observation have been inadequate, lacking a well-developed body of real biological knowledge, so that ill-founded theories, ill-advised references to the classics, and a lot of plain poppycock were all mixed up together. You will remember the confusion of ideas which attended the findings of the Neanderthal and the Java men. The same confusions rallied around the subject of race, and they did not stay within the relatively polite fencing salons of scientific societies, but got out into the vulgar brawls of politics, and have caused decade on decade of race-generated misery.

Races were recognized in antiquity, but roused no great interest and were shrugged off with some fabulous explanation. Any foreign land was thought to be peopled with ogres or cannibals (the Anthropophagi), and a man who differed from yourself merely in having a black skin and fuzzy hair was by comparison nothing to look at twice. Little of the world was yet known. Race was really discovered from the fifteenth century on, in the great age of exploration. "Indians" were found who did not live in India. Hairy aborigines came to light in the antipodes. This was, of course, before anything like an evolution for man had been suggested, and the stunned voyagers from Europe ascribed the many new kinds and colors of men to a series of separate creations, in other Edens which the Scriptures did not mention.

[1] E. A. Hooton, *Up From the Ape* (New York: Macmillan, revised edition, 1946), p. 634.

There was, in fact, a seesaw battle on this point, when some writers began to think that man might somehow have changed in different places, given a fairly long time and a not too strict obedience to the Old Testament. The great Blumenbach, jack-of-all-sciences, in 1775 made one of the very first reasonable classifications of man, and he suggested that the Whites (whom he dubbed the Caucasians, because of admiration of the appearance of natives of the Caucasus) were the original type of man, from which had drifted away, largely under the influence of climate, the Yellows (Asiatics) and Reds (American Indians) on one side and the Browns (Malays) and Blacks (Africans) on the other.

After about 1860, when evolutionary theory broke out of its egg with Darwin, and the Neanderthal Man broke out of his cave, serious attempts by scientists to relate human origins to Adam and Eve quickly stopped. Classification, however, continued apace. Anthropology was born, giving itself the job of seeking out and describing the varieties of mankind, until virtually every last Pygmy had known the stare of the camera lens and the feel of the calipers. However, while succeeding in its field objective of learning about all the earth's peoples, racial study was gradually bogging down because of some theoretical defects.

One was soon apparent: nobody could agree how many "races" there were, estimates of the number ranging from two (the "Handsome" and the "Ugly") to over sixty. Another defect was more subtle: after abandoning the idea that the different types of man had been created separately, just as they are, and the other Biblical idea, that they were the descendants of the several sons of Noah (whence the use of the terms Semitic, Hamitic, and Japhitic) or of the Lost Tribes of Israel, the students of the subject neglected to supply themselves with any other plausible explanation. (One other suggestion was made: races descended from the different kinds of apes!) For a long time there seems to have prevailed simply a hazy understanding that somewhere in the past there had been ancient races which once were pure. This mythical atmosphere made it possible for certain German and French writers to develop their groundless philosophy (long before the Nazis) of ancient Aryan purity as the secret of civilization.

And so a great deal of good and careful descriptive work was done, with no very clear problem in the mind of the doer—no questions as to the basic nature of races or as to how they had come into existence. It is obvious that anthropologists were mostly trying to separate races and types, to make them as distinct and clear-cut as possible, so that the "hybrids" and "mixtures" of the present day might better be understood. Only late in the game was it realized that all the overlapping and intergrading, and the difficulty of deciding just how many races one should count, might in themselves be significant. Eventually a "scientific" view began to grow up, by which I mean the awareness that racial differences and racial theory must be made to jibe with what is known about evolutionary processes, genetics, and biology generally. But this was not the happy ending. We have a scientific view, but not a complete scientific understanding. Anthropologists began to attempt definitions of race. But these turned out to be refractory. For race is not just a thing. It is a whole situation in a biological process, and to understand it demands a pretty full explanation of a lot of evolutionary principles, only partly stated in the early chapters of this book.

Therefore, defining race is like "defining" human history. I would say that definitions drawn up to be understood by a newspaper reader are long, rambling, and inadequate, and that short, accurate, and meaningful definitions can be understood only if you know the background. For example, this one, by Dobzhansky, is highly acceptable: "Races are populations differing in the incidence of certain genes." To an educated person this probably means that races differ in some of their hereditary traits. But, in its suggestions and limitations, it means a great deal more than that, if you understand the full sense of "population" and the theoretical processes by which gene incidences are maintained or changed.

This difficulty of defining is no false bugaboo. To discredit racial doctrines in modern politics, UNESCO in 1950 assembled in Paris a panel of anthropologists and others, to draw up a general statement on the nature of race, as it is understood today. This was to be a long and full definition and explanation, a scientific reference for laymen of any sort. The panel did its work and made public its statement with hopeful satisfaction. But the other anthropologists fell upon this document with such vigor that the English journal, *Man*, was for some months running what amounted to a department of criticism, correction, and amplification, in the form of letters from Great Britain, France, and the United States. So UNESCO quickly got together another panel in 1951 to do the Statement over again. This time the draft was circulated widely, so that the rest of the profession could get its comments and abuse in early. By compressing the results UNESCO was able to publish the statement and the gist of the exceptions to it—a sort of minimum anthropological description of race—in a relatively small volume. When, a few years later, I submitted the statement to a seminar of educated but non-anthropological European graduate students, presumably a worthy sample of ultimate consumers, it was still good for a barrage of further criticism from this quarter, which was impressively well informed. So perhaps, in defining race, the policy of containment is not too successful.

Human and Animal Variety

Perhaps in fact the whole endeavor to define, in descriptive terms, is a futile one. Supposing we were to forget old arguments and definitions, and begin afresh, looking at humankind as though we were setting out to collect beetles or seashells. We notice different-appearing men in different parts of the planet's geography. We examine them for their fundamental characteristics. Are any of them as different as orang and chimpanzee, who belong to two different genera, *Pongo* and *Pan?* No, evidently not. Are any of them as different as two species? That is to say, have they significant distinctions in physique—more than you could find in cattle or in dogs? Can you see boundaries of some kind between them, so that overlapping is slight, and so that, even if mingled in the same territory, they tend to breed separately, not together? No. Human racial distinctions, however marked they may seem at the extremes, shade into one another and tend to be lost, both in geographic overlapping and in ready interbreeding. This last applies to all contact, whether it is local and special, like Danes and Eskimos in Greenland, or is a vast zone of intergrading, like Africa just south of the Sahara, or a great melting pot, like Latin America.

We see only a big, world-wide species which, like other animal species, is both polymorphic and polytypic. That is, its individuals are highly variable in any place, and the average of individuals also differs from place to place. Both of these things are natural to any species, and the place-to-place variation, the existence of races, is the more likely, the more widespread is the species.

To the ordinary observer, all this variation is not so obvious in other kinds of animals, but it is there, and zoologists know it; ordinary observers do not look very hard at any species but *Homo sapiens*. In fact, after several generations of anthropologists had believed that man, in his skeleton and skin, was an extraordinarily variable animal, Professor A. H. Schultz demonstrated that chimpanzees are at least as variable, if not more so. And chimpanzee "species" have been fallaciously named and described, literally by the dozen, because of the finding of a specimen or so with an unusual combination of coat, size, and features. These species do not exist; they are known to be merely variant individuals of the general population. Possibly other chimpanzees stare at them, as we notice a man who is very tall or very red-haired.

So these two kinds of variety, in-group and between-group, are not peculiar to man. Rather, they are usual to all animals, and in fact needful. Without this variety, you may recall, evolution could not take place at all. Furthermore, the keeping-up of such differences is an aid to the health of the individuals and the strength of the species.

Consider the in-group heterogeneity, which has often been construed as lack of "purity," as departure from the ideal type of a race as it supposedly once existed. Such a purity never did and never does exist. For the variety rests on the possession of different kinds of genes in a group, which is important to it, both to meet new situations or to form protective combinations. "Purity" in fact means nothing, unless it means homozygosity, the eliminating of all but one kind of gene. This is interesting in the laboratory, but if you want to apply it to man it means brother-sister mating. And this is viewed as dimly by the geneticist as by the layman, since it tends to uncover detrimental genes in homozygous form. Heterozygosity, the pairing of different genes, protects against this, and broadens the resources of the whole group.

And different groups also diverge in the whole pattern of their genes, that is to say, in the proportions and combinations they possess. I will be specific in a minute. This comes from a variety of causes. It may come simply from the group being isolated, and also from natural selection working to favor one combination in one place, a second combination in another. And so we have races, in animals or man. Some such races eventually become so distinct from each other as to change into new separate species. But that is not the necessary fate of races. They are present in the nature of things when a species is widespread. Human races are really a kind of local limitation in the total variety of mankind.

Now these two kinds of variation occur together, an important point. Groups may differ from one another, but the individuals in each also differ so much that the overlap is wide. So we can speak only of average differences in groups, in racial traits. In some things (such as skin color) the average differs so greatly between European Whites and African Negroes that the individuals do not overlap, and there is no question as to which race a man belongs. In other things, the overlap is so broad that we cannot tell if the averages actually differ at all. But the features of race we study generally lie in between.

Blood and Genes

We come at last to these features, the way in which different races differ, more or less. Let us begin with the engines of life, the internal organs and their behavior. Here, even the anthropoid apes are strikingly similar to man. Individual human beings differ considerably in size and shape of viscera, but it is not known whether there is any average difference between races. In blood chemistry there is a little more difference from apes: it is possible, by introducing human blood serum into a chimpanzee's blood stream, to develop antibodies in his blood serum which will then show a reaction in the presence of human serum. But no such thing can be done with the races of man: human blood is all the same in this respect.

However, our blood has different sets of individual antigens and antibodies, like A, B, and O, or the Rh system. This illustrates nicely what we have been talking about. Individuals in a population differ in their blood types, according to the two genes they have inherited, so that you are type O, or A, or B, or AB. Most racial groups, however, have all these kinds of individual (some populations have no B, and a few have O only). So they do not differ in an absolute way, as though there were an "A race" and a "B race," but only on the average; or better, in their proportions of the same things. They differ, as Dobzhansky says, in the "incidence of the genes," not in having totally different genes. The blood types are the same, wherever you find them, so that a member of your own family might very well be a greater menace to you, if you were having a blood transfusion, than a Hottentot.

One of the fascinating discoveries of recent years is another blood oddity, the "sickling gene," or the sickle-cell trait, also called Hemoglobin S. Somewhere, in a pair of genes having to do with the development of hemoglobin in the red blood cells, there took place a mutation, or change to a new gene. If, instead of having two of the usual, or normal, genes, you inherit from your father or from your mother a sickling gene, your red blood cells will have a peculiar property. If their oxygen is reduced (as will take place if you let a drop of blood stand on a glass slide), they will lose their round form and take on abnormal shapes, especially crescents or sickles. And you will have another peculiar property as well: you will have a high childhood resistance to the most severe type of malaria.

Clearly this will be to your advantage, if you live in a malarial region, and beyond the range of the best medical treatment. And you would expect that this gene, this trait, would become very common, through Darwin's principle of natural selection. So it has. You might expect, in fact, that it would become universal and supplant the "normal" gene.

But wait. Suppose it is fairly common and that both your mother and your father are the proud possessors of it; suppose that through the laws of chance you inherit the sickling gene from *both* your parents, and so are homozygous for it—have two sickling genes and no normal gene. This is too much. You will have no normal hemoglobin. You will have a severe anemia, sickle-cell anemia, and you will almost certainly die from it before you grow up. And so you will hardly pass the gene on to your children.

That is why the sickling gene does not become universal: it kills itself off. Where malaria exists, it builds itself up, by natural selection, because people who have it in the single dose are healthier, with larger families, than people who do not have the gene at all, suffering malaria severely or dying from it. But then, as this happens, the smaller proportion of homozygotes will also rise. That is, more infants with the double dose are born, only to die; and so some of the sickling genes are picked out of the population and thrown away. The gene cannot rise up beyond a certain level before it drops out faster than it increases; obviously, if it could somehow get near the point where everyone had two sickling genes, then everyone would die, and that would be the end of gene and population alike. A balance is struck: one part of the population is more healthy and vigorous for having the gene against malaria, which helps the whole population to survive; but at the same time the population cannot survive unless the other part acts as custodian of the "normal" gene.

Why do you not see these things all around you? Because you are probably not an African or a South Asian, and so you will not have played in this lottery of life and death. The sickling phenomenon is at home largely in Negro Africa, here being in a broad way commonest where malaria is worst and less common elsewhere. It occurs virtually throughout Negro territory, and on the fringes; it is found in the ordinary Negroes, in Pygmies, and in the tall Watussi and their ilk. It is not found in the Bushmen of South Africa. But it came to the New World with the American Negroes, among most groups of whom it seems to have been declining, since their new environment is not sufficiently malarial to encourage it, and so to offset its lethal effects. With control of mosquitoes through DDT, the gene may be expected eventually to fall sharply in Africa as well.

Does all this mean we have hit on something which distinguishes the Negroes as a race? Not really. The same gene turns up widely in India, notably among some of the backward peoples. It is not uncommon in Greece and has been found in malarial regions of Italy, Turkey, and Arabia; one suspects it came to these places with an importation of Negroes, however small. This makes it look like a Negro tracer. But it should be looked on rather as a trait which spread (and was still spreading lately) among the Negro populations of Africa, simply because it appeared there, in some region exposed to malaria. It did not expand in certain other parts of the world where malaria exists, because it was not there to expand, not because the inhabitants were not Negroes. It could have spread. It probably did so in Greece and Italy quite independently of other Negro traits, once it arrived somehow from Negro Africa to start with.

Oddly enough there is another such gene, though a different one, in Italy and other Mediterranean countries, causing Cooley's anemia. But we cannot be on this all day. The sickling trait is sufficiently instructive, teaching a variety of lessons. Aside from being as beautiful an example of natural selection as is known, it shows how genes are not the special property of only one race, but can be passed to any, without limits. Rather, genes may accumulate in one direction or another, as genes for lighter skin accumulate in one region or population and genes for darker skin in another. That is the actual nature of race, the way in which populations begin to become distinct.

Function and Adaptation

When we come to matters of function, there may be some general differences from race to race and place to place. Little is known. Research on basal metabolism, or rates of growth, has found considerable average differences among different peoples. But these differences seem to be very much a matter of climate and diet, and individuals of the same group will change in metabolism if you move them around. Therefore such differences cannot be called "racial." The same thing is apparently true of most diseases, like tuberculosis or hypertension.

But Negroes do seem positively more resistant to infection from a variety of skin afflictions, including some skin-related or skin-implanted diseases like scarlet fever or diphtheria. This is resistance to infection, not to the disease itself, since they will be as sick as the next man once they catch it. Nobody knows the exact source of the resistance, but it would appear to lie in the skin itself and to be a real racial distinction. Eskimos appear to withstand cold in the tissues of the hand better, by a better regulation of the blood supply than in Whites; but it is not known whether this is an acquired hereditary—a racial—trait or results from long personal acclimatizing, during the life of each Eskimo.

The human figure is also "functional" in a related way, as I have said before, because it seems to help out with the regulation of body heat by changing its shape to the best form under the circumstances. You do not get long, lanky Eskimos in the frigid north: a short and roly-poly seal hunter keeps his heat better, and in the awful cold he can get emaciated fast enough without starting that way. Contrariwise you do not find chubby and stumpy camel drivers in the Sahara. Instead, the tall and slender people of broiling deserts are much more

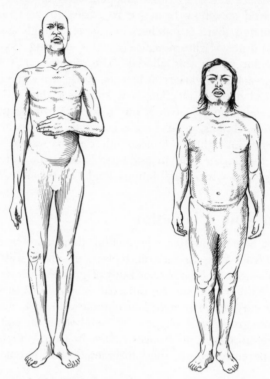

Contrasts in body form between a Nilotic Negro (Shilluk) and an Eskimo. From photographs.

likely to avoid heatstroke by being stretched out, and presenting as much skin as possible, per pound of flesh, for body heat to escape through. So we may reasonably assume these body forms to be real effects of natural selection. And they are real "racial" traits, having come to be the hereditary equipment of certain peoples. But they are not exclusive, for the desert lankiness belongs to Arabs and Tuaregs, of the White stock, to the Nilotic Negroes along the White Nile in the Sudan, and to the desert-living aborigines of Australia, three quite different kinds of men. We have, rather, a racial trait which is a climatic adaptation.

Skeleton and Skull in Race

There are probably other shape differences like this, whose significance does not suggest itself so easily. Indeed, the Negroes in general tend to be longer in the leg and in the forearm than the

Whites, judging by comparisons made in the United States, so that this could be looked on as a vague but persistent difference between the two stocks. But one needs to get the averages of large numbers to find such a distinction, and the fact is that the bones have no really characteristic differences from race to race. Mankind is very uniform in this regard, as you might suspect from knowing that even Pekin Man did not differ discernibly from us below the neck. And the anthropologist who looks at a headless skeleton and ventures a guess as to the race it represents is making a stab in the dark, nothing more.

He will do better with the skull, and particularly its facial parts, if he has some experience. Mongoloid peoples generally have a flattish face region with wide and angulated cheekbones and little canine fossa, but with some projection just at the bony gum. Negroes have more such projection and larger teeth, as well as a receding chin, rather delicate cheekbones, broad nose apertures and low but vertical foreheads. Whites have the most vertical faces and prominent chins, as well as good brow ridges. And an especially primitive combination, of projecting face, smaller brain, heavy brows, and receding foreheads, appears in the natives of Australia and of some other parts of the western Pacific, like New Britain and New Caledonia. So the several main races of man tend to differ a little in the things which have made *Homo sapiens* what he is: in the degree, that is to say, of the lightening up of the brows, of the diminution of the teeth, or of the pulling in of the face.

Even these descriptions are a little too pat. I said before that sapient man is really much alike everywhere in skull and skeleton.

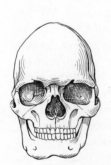 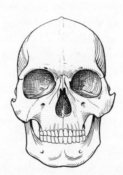 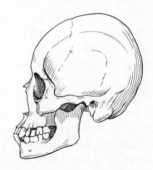

Skulls of modern races. Left: an Australian, with narrow skull, heavy brows, low face, eyes and nasal opening. Center: Eskimo, with flaring cheekbones, wide jaw, narrow forehead and nasal cavity. Right: African Negro, with prognathism of the lower face, and small brows.

It might be instructive to you to leave the book open at this page and try to identify the next cranium you see. The anthropological eye can generally spot the narrow, poorly filled skull of the native Australian or the very wide face and peculiar high pitched cranium of the Eskimo without difficulty. But he, or anyone, will begin to have trouble with Europeans and Negroes, and more still with the generally nondescript varieties of Asiatics. If a strange skeleton is dug up in your vicinity (North America), look first at the front teeth in the upper jaw. If they are just a little projecting, not vertical, the person is more likely to be an Indian.

Skin and Color

It is only when we come to view the human exterior that we see the features we have always called "racial," the things which give races their distinctive appearances. Foremost is skin, so prominent in our hairless species and so varied in pigmentation that it has been the popular handle for race since the beginning. Now skin is a most useful material, and does not exist merely to keep your insides inside and the bath water outside. It is an envelope, a bacteria-killing agent, a sense organ, a heat regulator, and, probably most important here, a light filter. It admits limited amounts of ultraviolet light, which is needed to form vitamin D, but presumably diminishes or diffuses dangerous doses by a screen of pigment granules.

This pigment, melanin, is present in everyone excepting pure albinos, and everyone has both a fixed amount as well as some ability to form more temporarily—in other words, to tan. It is the basic amount in which racial groups differ so noticeably (and in which individuals within a racial group also differ among themselves). We are used to talking about Whites and Blacks, but Sallows and Dark Browns would be more like it. The White stock as a whole has a considerable range, although it is generally so light that tanning is more prominent than any basic light brown tinting of the skin, and the blood can show through to give varying degrees of ruddiness. In northern Europe the whole pigmentation can be very pale indeed, since so little melanin is present. At the opposite end of the scale the Negroes also have a considerable range of color, in the dense brown shades. Skin which actually looks black, or nearly so, is rare in the somewhat diluted American Negroes, but is occasional in Africa and Melanesia.

This variety in outer color has all the earmarks of an adaptation, of a trait responding to the force of sunlight by natural selection. The dark-skinned racial types are distributed in the tropics of the Old World. And the bleached-out Europeans are swarthier in the south and reach their extra degree of depigmentation, true blondness, in the cloudy north where sunlight is not only not a danger to body tissues but is actually at a premium. It looks as though here the skin has stripped itself of its usual defenses in the hope of gulping up the little supply of ultraviolet light.

But at the same time, there is not as good a correspondence with climate as exists in body form, as I described it a few pages back. White and Black have approached the same body form in the Afro-Arabian desert belt, but they have not approached the same color. And the American Indians in their vast range from the Arctic to Tierra del Fuego also reflect climate in body size and form, to a discernible degree, but not in color. There are other reservations: are the tropical forests really so sunny as to encourage their inhabitants to be dark-skinned? Therefore, some of the racial differences in skin color may be more deep-seated, and possibly more ancient, than a direct tie to sunlight might suggest. It may well be that other things, not yet detected, bear on pigment; and I have already mentioned the superior resistance to infection of Negro skin. If so, then skin color probably answers to a complex balance of forces, a little like the sickling gene, and not simply to the persuasion of the sun.

In fact, it is just in skin color and the other most obvious trappings of race that we find the greatest difficulty in finding explanations. In hair and eye color mankind is more uniform, with dark brown eyes and dark brown or black hair the mode; only certain sections of the depigmented Europeans have lighter shades of these. By excluding more light, a dark iris may make a more efficient camera out of the eye than a light one; and so blue eyes and blond hair, with no apparent advantage to them, probably tag along after fair skin as accidental side effects. Hair varies in shape as well as color. Among Mongoloid peoples generally it is perfectly straight. In Europeans it may also be straight, but the hairs are more apt to twist in unison at intervals along their length, giving rise to waves or curls. In Negroes there is a continuous curl to the hairs, which do not lie parallel; thus they do not form curls but intertwine vigorously and make a woolly mat. Possibly this acts as a natural pith helmet.

Other Familiar Features

Some differences in form are incomprehensible. Why are Negro lips rolled out and thick? Why do Whites and native Australians retain full beards and a certain amount of body hair? Why is the head itself differently shaped: long, round, high, or low, in different localities? Why does the face vary in the same way? One cannot escape the feeling that there has been some accidental evolution in these things, although invisible causes are always to be assumed.

Here, however, is a difference which does seem to make sense: the narrow nasal cavities of the north Europeans and the Eskimos seem to warm and moisten air for the lungs in dry and cold climates, as a protection. At any rate, there has been shown a strong statistical relation between nose shape and the average temperature and water vapor in the air, when studying peoples who have been a long time in their present climates.

Racial differences, then, taken altogether, seem to result from a mixture of things. Part of them are surely mementos of evolutionary journeying: differences in shucking off brow ridges (and perhaps body hair). Part are almost certainly adaptive, reflecting the demands of different climates and habitats. Part of them could be, and probably are, due to chance. A "race," or better, a local racial form, is a population with its own combination of average physical characteristics. Such a thing is a sort of corporation of genes, a breeding stock. You might convey its appearance through an individual, but a race is not an individual, a single set of genes. Nor is it an ideal type, a photograph of its average member. At the same time, it is not the people of a whole continent. It is a population which actually exchanges its genes in breeding, and thus changes or evolves as a unit. Still it is never, in mankind, cut off from others, and so it keeps exchanging its heredity somewhat with other populations, be they tribes, or villages, or islands.

All over the world this has been going on. Such segments of humanity, real but ill-defined and borderless, have been undergoing slight changes, allowing their neighbors to partake in them, and producing local racial differences. And by virtue of distance, of contrasting environment, and probably of a good many thousand years, this process gave rise to four main population groups or racial stocks, at the four corners of the Old World: the Whites in the northwest, the Negroes in Africa, the Mongoloids in northeastern Asia, and the dark, hairy, primitive-looking Australians in the southeast.

19. THE EUROPEANS

CLASSIFYING the Europeans into types or subraces is an old sport. One of its roots goes all the way back into the eighteenth century, when it was first realized that every language from Ireland to India (excepting those of the Finns, the Turks, the Hungarians, and the ever baffling Basques) belonged to a single family. Scholars eagerly began studying one of its earliest recorded forms, Sanskrit, which had been handed down from the Aryans, ancient invaders of the Indian peninsula. Thus the family came to be called the "Aryan" languages (the name has since been changed to "Indo-European").

This discovery, by the rules of the game as played in the nineteenth century, allowed everyone as many guesses as he liked as to who were the first Aryan-speakers of Europe and where they came from. Writers took the map of Asia and dotted it all over with imaginary homes. The legend grew. The Aryans became the inventors of civilization, coming out of the Hindu Kush, or the Urals, or wherever, shouting Aryan encouragement to Aryan oxen pulling Aryan carts full of Aryan household goods. By the middle of that century Count de Gobineau was giving the Aryans credit for every civilization on record—Egypt, China, the American Indians—through their ennobling influence and their ennobling blood. On and on jounced this fairy tale, until National Socialism in Germany fashioned its most recent edition. Early in the Nazi regime Arthur Guiterman, in the following poem, made the whole matter about as clear as can be done:[1]

ETHNOLOGICAL

The valiant pre-historic Aryans
Suppressed all neighboring barbarians.

Their progeny, the Indo-Germans,
Preached culture, using swords as sermons.

From them derived the warlike Teutons
Who cut the Romans up in croutons,

[1] From "The Conning Tower," New York *Herald Tribune*, June 8, 1933.

And they begat the Goths and Vandals
Whose raids are celebrated scandals.

From all these strains and many others,
Diverse, yet close as sons and brothers,

Arose our modern Nordic heroes,
To whom all other breeds are zeroes.

The Nazis contented themselves with defining Aryans as those who were not Jewish. It was older writers who tried to discover what Aryans might actually look like. At first, as in de Gobineau's book, the Aryans were simply misty demigods from a vague Valhalla, locality unspecified. But racial classification was going on, and the obvious and valid variations among the Europeans were being noted, especially that tendency to extreme blondness which centers on the Baltic. In fact, by the end of the century there were recognized the three races everyone has heard about: Nordics, Alpines, and Mediterraneans. The Nordics (or Teutons) were tall, longheaded, longfaced, and fair; the Alpines were stocky, roundheaded, of medium complexion; the Mediterraneans longheaded, but slight and dark. And while perfectly honest anthropologists were trying to analyze the population of the European continent in terms of these races, some of the Aryanists ran off with the scheme and subverted it for their own ends.

Two early writers, Pösche, a German, and Penka, an Austrian, had felt that there was no need to bring the godlike Aryans out of backward Asia when more godlike countries were available (Germany, for example). This in turn suggested that the Aryans might be a specific racial type of Europe, rather than the faceless wanderers of de Gobineau's book. And the obvious candidates were the Nordics, whose singular blondness suggested the notion that they were most likely to have been the "original" Europeans. And so the Nordics, wearing a surprised look, became the heroic builders of civilization.

This kind of "history" was perpetrated in several countries. H. S. Chamberlain, an Englishman who went to live in Germany, wrote the fattest book, and perhaps the most famous, *Foundations of the Nineteenth Century*. In America, Madison Grant published *The Passing of the Great Race*, in which the supposed unseating of the Nordic founders of this country by later immigrants from southern and eastern Europe was good for a pail of tears on every page. Much more interesting and sophisticated was *L'Aryen; son rôle social*, by the French political scientist Georges Vacher de Lapouge. In this scientific-sounding version, which had a good deal of general, probably unconscious, acceptance, at least among the Anglo-Saxons, the three races have their biological differences in ability. The Aryans (read "Nordics") are the natural leaders and creators, rising to the top like cream, unless their society or nation is so unfortunate as to have diluted them too far. The Alpines are stodgy, but sound; the perfect subjects for any ruler. The less said about the Mediterraneans the better; they belong at the bottom of the scale, with Mongolians and other invertebrates. Lapouge took several volumes to say all this. Hilaire Belloc got it into three verses,[1] viz.:

> Behold, my child, the Nordic Man,
> And be as like him as you can.
> His legs are long; his mind is slow.
> His hair is lank and made of tow.

> And here we have the Alpine Race.
> Oh! What a broad and foolish face!
> His skin is of a dirty yellow,
> He is a most unpleasant fellow.

> The most degraded of them all
> Mediterranean we call.
> His hair is crisp, and even curls,
> And he is saucy with the girls.

This ended with the First World War, except in the Nazi camp. Between the wars the anthropologists, with growing information about living peoples and a far better knowledge of the past, were examining the European population from a more educated and expert position, culminating with Coon's fine study, *The Races of Europe*, in 1939. It is no longer possible to accept the time-honored scheme of three races. The objection is not simply one of new complications. Rather, the scheme suggests an old frame of mind. It puts the em-

[1] Dr. Gottfried Kurth of Braunschweig did me the honor of translating the original version of this book for the German edition. I cannot resist citing his deft rendering of Belloc's poem:

> Sieh da, mein Kind, nordische Eichen!
> Versuche ihnen stets zu gleichen.
> Die Beine lang, der Geist so so.
> Die Haare schlicht aus schierem Stroh.

> Hier haben wir nun die Alpinen.
> Wie breit und töricht doch die Mienen.
> Die Haut, gemischt aus gelb und braun,
> Es lohnt sich nicht, sie anzuschau'n.

> Am tiefsten aber, kaum zu ahnen,
> Steh'n stets nur die Mediterranen.
> Ihr Haar is kraus, fast negerkratzig,
> Und zu den Mädchen sind sie patzig.

phasis on the differences among the Whites, not on their likenesses and relationships. And it clearly assumes, once more, that Nordic, Alpine, and Mediterranean were originally "pure," having mingled since then in different ways in different places to form the stream of European history. This is almost as bad as falling back on the sons of Noah; there can hardly have been such a day of purity. The root of all the trouble lies in starting at the end of history—with the living people—and trying to work backward. That is the wrong end. Let us start at the beginning.

Rounder Mesolithic Heads

Back we go to the break in the Würm glaciation, and the advance guard of the invasion of western Europe by *Homo sapiens*. In the time just before, we must suppose, there was a broad area of varying Neanderthals, in Europe, North Africa, the Near East, and an unknown portion of Central Asia. If it is a correct view, it suggests the Central Asiatic plain, or perhaps India, as the possible sources for the newcomers. Conceivably they might have arrived from Africa, through the Near East or even Gibraltar. But there are considerations, principally archaeological, weighing against these alternatives.

At any rate, the invaders were not home-grown. We have seen them immigrating at the opening of the Upper Paleolithic, and this was evidently the pattern for later times as well. The Upper Paleolithic men, tall or short, all had large, long skulls. Men of the same kind appeared in North Africa; and from the beginning to the end this southern shore of the Mediterranean has been White, racially, continuing its bond with Europe from Neanderthal times. For thousands of years the new Europeans hunted big game and painted caves, until the glacier eventually withdrew from the continent, lingering on the Scandinavian peninsula before giving up its last grip.

Now the forests grew up in Europe, and the herds of mammoths, horses, bison, and reindeer were gone or going. In spite of chilblains, life in the old cold days had been easier hunting. About 8000 B.C. the culture took on a different look. New tricks in hunting and new kinds of food were discovered. Bows and arrows, canoes, nets, fishing lines appeared. People settled on shores where shellfish abounded. Stone tools show there were new contacts with Africa. This phase of history is called the Mesolithic, and in Europe it carried on until after 4000 B.C.

As to the people themselves, there were no striking changes and no signs of further immigrants of importance. However, two new notes were struck. Although still rugged by modern standards, Mesolithic heads from Portugal and Brittany were diminished in size from those of their Paleolithic ancestors somewhat, and were in fact about what you would expect to find gracing a well-built Scot or Swede today. Secondly, the first rounder heads appeared. This is another grisly archaeological drama: in a cave at Ofnet, Bavaria, were found thirty-three skulls—nineteen children, ten women, and four men—all cut off from their skeletons, and all packed together in a circle like a clutch of eggs. Holes in the skulls, just the shape of a stone axe of the time, show that these people did not die of the measles.

Every skull was broken, many badly so. Such as could be put together agree with the impression given above: they hark back to the older Paleolithic people but are smaller, and in size and ruggedness are like recent North Europeans (such as Irish or Anglo-Saxons). On the average, however, they were rounder, or shorter, in shape than the skulls of their predecessors.

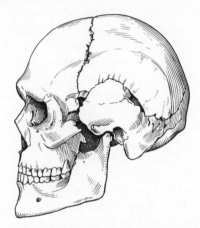

Teviec skull No. 11, a Mesolithic skull from Brittany. A particularly rugged male, in a small-statured group, he represents a group of Mesolithic descendants of the Paleolithic people. From a photograph, courtesy of Dr. Henri Vallois. ¼ natural size.

Since some are quite long, some quite round, the curious Ofnet skull nest used to be looked on as a mingling of different tribes, and as signaling the entry of roundheads into Europe. But the variety, I think, has been exaggerated; statistically it is not unusual, and some of the heads were accidentally slightly flattened in back when the owners were infants. In addition, there is a broad likeness is appearance among them all. Also, there is no good archaeological evidence of immigrants. Finally, a constant tendency to change from longer to rounder heads has appeared in many of the world's populations in

Europe and out, during post-glacial times. So, even if we actually have a mixture of trophy heads from different tribes (which I doubt), we have no dependable sign of new people arriving in this quarter.

Smaller Neolithic Heads

At this same time great changes had been taking place in the Middle East, of which the backwoods Europeans were unaware. The European Mesolithic was primarily the extension of the ancient hunting life of the Paleolithic, striving to meet new conditions and to find new food resources and ways of using them. But in the Fertile Crescent, from Palestine around the northern flank of the Tigris-Euphrates plain in Iraq, the Neolithic had been dawning, with the invention of farming, undoubtedly the most important thing ever to happen to man.

"Neolithic," the name invented by the early students of prehistory, means New Stone Age, and indeed some stone tools came to be polished, which allowed the making of efficient axes or adzes for woodworking. And before long, also, the arts of pottery and weaving were discovered. But these are nothing—mere conveniences—beside the domestication of animals and plants, which is the foundation of modern life and of all recorded history. Because of agriculture we can live together in large numbers, and manage a civilization based on writing, mathematics, science, and trade. Without it we might still be bending every thought upon the next meal, still living a Mesolithic life such as was led by our own European forefathers barely six thousand years ago, a life which would be pitied by the New England Indians or the natives of the Congo. To return today to hunting, and to a dependence on natural food alone, would call for the extinction of all but a handful out of every thousand persons now alive. So the Neolithic saw the beginning of a gradual great increase in human numbers.

This was happening more than ten thousand years ago. By about 7000 B.C. there was already a sort of town at Jericho, with a wall around it. Dr. Gottfried Kurth, who studied the skeletal remains, found a gradual change from a coarser to a lighter type, and a decline in body height. The known remains of the Natufian people of the same area, wandering Mesolithic gatherers on the verge of agriculture, had long, fairly large skulls and were of medium size. So it appears that, in this part of the Near East, the Mesolithic people were already somewhat less in size and ruggedness than their contemporaries in Europe, continuing to diminish to a sort of standard Mediterranean form of more recent times.

This tendency to reduce the average size and heaviness of the skull from the rugged type of the Upper Paleolithic has no explanation.

Coon suggests that the Paleolithic people owed a strongly built physique, in some cases quite tall, to a combination of things, including a plentiful meat diet and the fact that a large body (with or without the short limbs of the Eskimos) is more efficient at retaining heat in a cool climate than is a small one. If so, the large skull may be an expression of the general body size, as in large northern Europeans of today. We simply find that skull size went down, and by Neolithic times had reached modern standards.

In the Near East the new way of life took hold and became productive. Here was a basis for civilization: city dwellers and traders, who could live emancipated from all direct work in the raising of food. The first city states, in fact, grew up in the centuries after 4000 B.C. in Sumer, at the head of the Persian Gulf. Civilization soon followed the Neolithic into Egypt as well, being fully established there by 3000 B.C.

In the northern lands the Neolithic, like the coming of day, was slow. A first blush, without pottery, appeared early in Greece and in places along the Mediterranean. The people of the Near East were already writing and building temples when agricultural life really took root in the west. Impulses now arrived by different routes. One came up from the region of Spain and southern France into Britain, giving rise to the famous pile-dwelling villages along the shores of the Swiss Lakes as well. Another rose in Hungary and moved up the Danube, clearing the oak forests on the easily worked loess soil of eastern Europe and planting settlements which might have made you think of the Iroquois long houses. A third seems to have sprung up in South Russia, from Mesolithic people there who were touched by Neolithic influences from further away; these came west about 2000 B.C. into the region of Denmark, apparently with warlike intentions and stone battle-axes. All this early farming was simple and crude, unable to cope with much of the deciduous forest of Europe, and banned entirely from the northernmost coniferous zone.

It is not now possible to say how far these streams of influence were actual migrations, bringing new people, and how far they were merely the transmission of new ideas, like Paris fashions. They did result in a larger population. And the population was physically less like its predecessors and more like that of the Near East, a modern longheaded skull form, especially along the Mediterranean shores and on the Danube. Perhaps these were not the skulls of invaders, but only the result of a similar diminution in size taking place in Europe. In the west slightly larger heads prevailed, or persisted, in a form called the Atlanto-Mediterranean. The Battle-Axe people from the east were also large in the head, and large in the face, and these were probably real newcomers: battle-axes are all too apt to travel gripped firmly in aggressive right hands, not in peaceful trade. And here and there, in the north and on the Swiss Lakes, round heads carried on from Mesolithic times.

The Bronze Age

During the Bronze Age, Europe continued to trail its barbarous way behind the Near East. The full civilizations of 3000 B.C. only began to be reflected in the west about 1800 B.C., with a knowledge of bronze casting brought by traders, and some renewed movements of peoples. From the Mediterranean and up the Atlantic shore there came a cult of building tomb structures—dolmens or megaliths—of large rough stones, at the close of the Neolithic. Another such religious structure, Stonehenge, was started at the beginning of Bronze times in Britain, and carvings of daggers and axes on the stones, of a particular kind, betray a contact a few centuries later with Mycenaean Greece and Minoan Crete, about 1500 B.C.

More important for racial history was the coming to the British Isles of the Bell Beaker people. They were bronze makers and traders from Germany, and their presence there, in England and elsewhere, can be read from the sort of earthenware tumbler they made, known as a bell beaker. The people were tall and well built, and they had round skulls. Or rather, their skulls were short, not long; they had too much modeling or angularity to be called "round" in the sense of globular. They seem to show that there was a new florescence, in Central Europe, of the tendency of heads to change in shape from long to round. They had a considerable effect in Britain, which had been purely longheaded before, judging by the crania from the old megaliths, or "long barrows." The Bronze Age people buried their dead under round mounds, and the archaeologists used to be able to say, "Long barrows, long skulls; round barrows, round skulls." This is a little too neat, but it is one sign of the fact that the early Bronze Age was a time, in western Europe, of rounder heads.

The chances are that the Bell Beaker people were the first bringers of an Indo-European language, early Keltic, or Q-Keltic, to Great Britain. For this was the time when languages of the family were being established in many places, stemming from a home which was probably the Balkans, perhaps South Russia, possibly both. Greek is now known to have come to Greece in the Bronze Age, perhaps as early as 1900 B.C., and the language of the Hittites, in Turkey, was already being written. Probably Germanic, parent of English, had already arrived in the Baltic region with the Battle-Axe people; at any rate, this is the most obvious incursion of new people who might have brought that speech.

In the latter half of the Bronze Age a new culture took shape in southeastern Europe, the Urnfields culture. It moved into the west, eventually into France and Spain, probably bringing the Keltic language of the Gauls which prevailed until it was erased by the daughter tongues of Latin, after the Romans. The Urnfields culture and its spread were important in other ways and were probably related to similar excursions elsewhere, like the Dorian Greek's coming down into Greece from the north, or the Villanovan people entering Italy. For this culture seems to have represented a renewal, a stepping up of agriculture, capable of supporting larger settlements, and so it was perhaps the last major development in barbarian culture history before the Roman conquest.

The Iron Age

But we can hardly tell what the Urnfield people looked like. For during late Bronze and early Iron times the thoughtless Europeans were cremating their dead, and burying only the ashes in urns in large cemeteries. That is the frustrating meaning of "Urnfield." In the Iron Age weapons of the new metal were added to European arsenals, without other essential changes in the life of the people. Burial of the ordinary kind was resumed in the Hallstatt phase of the Iron Age, about 700 B.C., named from a large cemetery in Austria. The remains of these warrior folk show them to have been of somewhat more than average skull size, and longheaded—a rather old kind of European, which Coon calls "Nordic," meaning, in the skeletal sense, a longheaded resultant of mixture in North and Central Europe of various Neolithic longheads, including the strong-faced Battle-Axe people. Over in the west, however, the Kelts, or Gauls, coming down to Roman times, were evidently more influenced by the roundhead tendency, their skulls being of medium shape, and rather low.

The alarums of the Iron Age carried on, in spite of Roman legions. The "Nordic" longheads of Europe had something of a reinforcement, with the eruption and spread of the Goths and Vandals, and the crossing of the Anglo-Saxons into England. But now, in historic times, roundheadedness, or brachycephaly, began to assert itself powerfully. This cannot possibly be ascribed to the entrance of a "brachycephalic race," because the change to rounder heads took place in other parts of the world, in other racial stocks as well. Nor did the new roundheads have bigger brains. The explanation is, perhaps, that a rounder shape gives a more economical way to contain the already large brain in the smaller skull of modern man, with his decadent brow ridges and lighter neck muscles. And natural selection yearns for economy in structure. All over central Europe the same peoples got rounder in the head. The great Slav tribes, originally settled in Poland and the Ukraine, are known to have done so. Invaders of the Balkans and Turkey—Huns, Avars, Mongols—might have brought roundheads, but if so, they themselves must have come by the roundness in the same fashion. In any case, it is evident that the process was going on everywhere, unconnected with movements out of Asia. By modern times the whole central zone—France, Switzerland, South Germany, and out into the eastern Mediterranean and Central Asia—had become brachycephalic, or "Alpine" in classic terms. Three main regions resisted the trend: the north; the shores of the Mediterranean; the further Middle East.

As to blonds, we do not know their real age. They are not new, and are probably very old. Blondness pops up in many groups of the White stock, in a sort of incipient way, as in lighter-eyed or fairer-haired men in North Africa, indicating that the variation, and the genes for it, are present widely. But blonds became pronounced, and common, in a great sphere of Scandinavia and Russia, most probably (says Coon) under the cloudy skies of late glacial and post-glacial times. It is found particularly in some of the old northern longheads (of the large medium size) but also in the "squareheads" of the Prussian-Finnish zone, recognized as the "East Baltic" type by race classifiers. So blondness is imposed over and above other variations: not all "Nordics" are blond, and not all blonds are "Nordic," by any means.

There, I think, you have the real best explanation for the "races" of Europe, the visible combinations of form and color. They are not three ancient, pure races, ideal molds. Rather, says prehistory, we have these things: preservation of a basic White type, a light-skulled, brunet Mediterranean, in the south and east; a strong prevalence of roundheadedness (with some lightening of complexion) in the broad middle zone running out into Asia; and the building-up of blondness in the north, especially among old larger-bodied and larger-headed longheads of Neolithic and Mesolithic derivation. These things all cause an impression of *types*, where in fact they are tendencies and combinations of tendencies. And the seeming variation and untidiness (dark-haired Danish "Nordics," blond French "Alpines") are not the result of mixture alone; rather, they are the only possible result of all these trends, like size reduction, roundheadedness, or blondness, none of them absolute and all of them working independently of one another. Gregor Mendel found out, in his original plant-breeding experiments, that wrinkling of the pea skin, or the color of the pod, or size of the pea plant, were inherited separately, in total independence. Why, then, need fair hair be accompanied by a long skull? It need not. So much for Aryans.

The Asiatic Whites

And so much for Europe. For this, of course, has not been the only home of the Whites. They have occupied Egypt and North Africa from the first appearance there of *Homo sapiens*. The Middle East, we have seen, has always been White in post-Neanderthal times. But the Whites have reached much further into Asia.

We know that the cattle-driving Aryans entered India from the northwest, singing Vedic hymns in an early Indo-European language, and, by their own stories, bringing castes and Hindu gods. This was about 1400 B.C. Since "Aryan" and "Iran" derive from the same word root, we have more than a hint as to where they came from. Their culture and traditions were something like those of the barbarous west and even, it has been suggested, like the very early Greeks. So their own view of themselves, bequeathed to posterity, is as the civilizers of India: a very "Aryan" view. But they were actually rude herders and warriors, who on coming into the Indus valley found a civilization with large brick cities, already a thousand years old. This had Middle Eastern connections, and a people of Middle Eastern type. The Aryans evidently overthrew it, and doubtless appropriated some of its gods and traditions. All this shows how far the Aryans were from being either the civilizers of India or the first western Whites to come in. Who the latter might have been we cannot even guess, because Indian prehistory is almost unknown, and without ancient skeletons.

India today is basically "White," meaning that head and face have the general Mediterranean form, though there is an increasing darkness of skin from the northwest out to the south and east. This darker skin may be partly an adaptive increase of pigment, due to the climate, which has not affected other physical traits; we do not know. But it is certainly traceable in some degree to mixture with old, dark-skinned peoples, if only enough to provide a leaven of genes for darker color. For there are still wild tribes, primitive natives speaking non-Indo-European languages, dark in skin, and certainly the true aboriginals.

It is probable that the Whites, coming in from the northwest, largely erased the primitive hunters whom they found, while absorbing enough of them to cause a perceptible darkening of their own skins and, in some places, other physical effects. It is as if the European colonists of America, on arriving on the east coast with Anglo-Saxon language and culture, had also mixed with the American Indians as they displaced them, more and more as they came to California, until there was some American Indian blood in all of us; yet leaving, as we have actually done, islands of the aborigines with their original languages and ways of life in the remoter parts, like the Arizona desert or the Everglades of Florida. I do not mean that, in India, Whites brought in modern Indian civilization already formed, but only that this civilization, the property of the mixed Whites who are India's population, is a single culture, and that in going among the wild tribes one leaves this and steps into an aboriginal world. Who these aborigines are, or were, we can leave until later. They were assuredly not Whites.

Russia and Central Asia are old White territory. According to Russian anthropologists, the Cro Magnon variety of the Upper Paleolithic men—large of skull and broad of face—persisted through the Neolithic out about as far as Lake Baikal in Central Siberia, and, if Thoma's reading of the skulls is right, all the way to the Far East still earlier. In the Ukraine this continuity was breached briefly, in the Mesolithic, by the kind of narrow-headed and narrow-faced Mediterranean of moderately large size which later characterized the fringes of Europe and parts of the Near East. Eventually, the Upper Paleolithic type reduced, or gave way, to the smaller, still rugged form of the "Nordic" variety of northern Europe, with which it was probably actually continuous in Iron Age times. At any rate, Indo-European languages were spoken in Chinese Turkestan until about a thousand years ago, and the Chinese annals speak of blonds.

Up to the founding of Chinese civilization, then, and later, the Whites may have reached right into China in the region of the Yellow River, serving as a transmission belt for the idea of agriculture from the Middle East, the idea on which civilization in China was founded. But then these Central Asiatic Whites underwent some marked changes. For one thing, the same kind of brachycephalization as in Europe seems to have translated the population into a roundheaded one. For another, Mongoloid peoples, who were present beyond Lake Baikal in Neolithic times, began pushing west, sometimes in waves of invasion like the Huns and the Mongols, crowding and partly mongolizing the older Whites, until nowadays there are people of Mongoloid appearance all the way to the lower Volga River.

There is at least one more reason for thinking the Whites once extended far to the east: the Ainus of Japan. A submerging remnant now, they recently lived a simple Neolithic kind of life in the northern islands, Hokkaido and Sakhalin, enjoying certain trade privileges with the peoples of the mainland coast. Their appearance classes them as White. Today almost all of them exhibit signs of mixture with Japanese, partly from their custom over recent generations of adopting Japanese babies. But many individuals show no trace of this, and could pass for Europeans without question. Their principal characteristic is, in fact, their great hairiness—a non-Mongoloid feature of the White stock which the Ainus carry to almost indecent extremes. But they themselves admire this. The older men, wearing a long coiffure and beard, manage to look a good deal like Tolstoy, and the women, who do not grow real mustaches, used to tattoo themselves with false ones in a tasty shade of blue.

The Ainus are stockily built brunets, with a medium head form. They have no outstanding characteristics except for the hair, and, again except for the hair, they are not "primitive" in any obvious way. Their skulls are also rather nondescript, without the beaky noses usually associated with Whites, and with some of the flatness of face so characteristic of Mongoloids. The Ainus evidently go back to the Jomon period, a sort of pottery-using "Mesolithic" which may have begun as early as 7000 B.C. Mathematical comparison of a number of the skulls from this period shows that they were not Japanese, who apparently began arriving only about 300 B.C. These early people were not all Ainu, however, although they have resemblances. There were probably varied primitive tribes in the region, some of whom at least had connection with the Whites further west.

20. ASIANS AND AMERICANS

BLUMENBACH called it the Mongolian variety and Linneaus, the first classifier, called it *Homo sapiens asiaticus*. Even more than the Whites, it runs off into vague or mixed forms on its fringes, but it is probably the most numerous kind of man today. We know the Mongoloids have been expanding, but where and when they first took shape is harder to say. Very little has been found in eastern Asia by way of human remains. There is Pekin Man, of course, and Weidenreich thought him a parental Mongoloid; but in fact he is so very pre-sapiens that there is no real basis for such an idea. An Upper Pleistocene woman's skull comes from Tzeyang, Szechwan. She was certainly sapiens; her large brows seem non-Mongoloid, but her face is missing and so her racial connections are difficult to tell. What is probably a still earlier skull comes from Liukiang, Kwangsi Province. It is somewhat Ainu-like in its appearance and characteristics; Thoma, as I have said, detected this and also found it close to the Cro Magnons. At the same time it has a wide nose, and is probably associated with a skeleton of small size, facts which even suggest connections with Negritos, or possibly the Niah Cave boy. Its finders call it a proto-Mongoloid, but the description does not seem to fit it well. The final important find is three good skulls from one of the Choukoutien deposits near Pekin. This is the Upper Cave, just above Locality 1, the cave of Pekin Man, but much later. The skulls are believed to date from the end of the Pleistocene, or roughly the last of the Upper Paleolithic. They are slightly Mongoloid in nature, but on the whole rather indefinite. Let us leave them for the moment.

The Mongoloid Face

How would you describe a Mongoloid? Yellow skin. Slant eyes. Oh yes, and "high cheekbones." These common ideas are not a precise or informative description, nor do they convey the variation which exists. Take the skin and eyes. Mongoloids vary from an actual brown

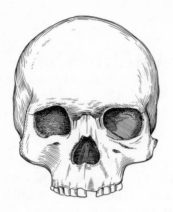
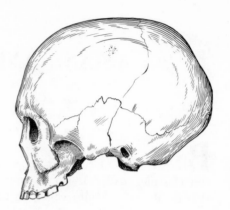

The Liukiang skull, Kwangsi, China. ¼ natural size.

to something quite as light as the average European, as a small amount of observation will show you. However, there is more opaqueness, less ruddiness from blood showing through, than in Europeans, and this, more than anything else, gives the impression of yellow. As to the eye, there is a tendency for the inner corner to be partly or wholly covered by a continuation of the fold of skin, in the socket just above the eyelid, or even by a continuation of the lid itself (in American Indians); and since the lower border of the fold slants up toward the side, the opening looks oblique.

Such a fold may be marked, or slight, or absent, in the bulk of Chinese or Japanese. But it is evidently commoner to the north of these countries, where in fact the whole face takes on a character which is exaggeratedly "Mongoloid," a specialized face which my colleagues Coon, Garn, and Birdsell ably argue to be a mask against cold. It is, they say, a remodeling of skeleton and soft parts into a combination providing the greatest possible protection, in very cold dry air, for the nasal passages, for the eyes, and for the sinuses in the brow and cheeks. Everything has been done to flatten the face, to decrease its area of exposure to frostbite, and to pad it. The nose is low. And the cheekbones have been brought forward, and widened (become "high"), so that the nose is recessed that much further into the face, and the eyeball is recessed similarly, at least relative to the flesh. Fat pads cover the sinuses in the cheeks and help fill the eye socket below. The sinuses above the eyes in the frontal bone are reduced and the brow ridges flattened out. And the upper part of the eye socket is sheathed by a well-developed Mongoloid fold, which also narrows the eye opening to a slit.

Given such an analysis, and the known insulating properties of fat, the argument that the extreme Mongoloid visage is a climatic adaptation looks very strong. It is not proved, but it is good. And this is a face which is at home in the coldest part of the world, northeastern Siberia (and also among the Eskimos of the American Arctic). It is common in Korea, and it crops up less often in Japan and China. But it is very obvious among the rather primitive hunters and fishers of the northeast forest and shore: Chuckchis, Koryaks, Goldis, Gilyaks, Kamchadals, and others. Coon and associates think it is likely to have developed, by natural selection, at a time during the last glacial phase, in Siberia, when some populations were caught, ringed in by glaciers in mountains to the south, though still able to live in the open lowland tundra between. Here they would have been subjected to intense, inescapable cold, with pneumonia and infected sinuses acting as the selective agents.

After the ice ring melted, these specialized Mongoloids could escape and spread, carrying their new flat faces with them. We have seen that they reached the borders of Europe in historic times. Earlier, they had also moved west through the forest zone along the shore toward Scandinavia. All through three thousand years of Chinese history, there are known to have been movements of peoples southward in the Far East, and the living natives indicate that the frost-adapted face influenced not only China and Japan, but also Tibet and tropical Southeast Asia and Indonesia, including the Philippines and Formosa. Waves of contact and culture are known from archaeology, and certainly the best explanation of the strong Mongoloid stamp of the whole Far East lies in the expansion of a segment of the northern population, beginning in the Mesolithic and Neolithic, particularly with their probable incorporation into the founders of China.

Mongoloids and American Indians

But this is almost too tidy a story, this hypothetical tale of exposure, escape, and expansion. Does it suggest that the very emergence of "Mongoloid" peoples awaited the late glacial alchemy of cold selection? I think not. I think it likely that the specialized Mongoloids—what writers have been inclined to call the typical, or classic, Mongoloids—were probably built on a less specialized form but one already Mongoloid in nature. Take away the Mongoloid mask, and what have you? You have a medium-skinned, dark-haired man with slight prognathism in the tooth-bearing part of the upper jaw, and more positive brow ridges. If he is already a sort of incipient

Mongoloid of the recognizable sort, he may have some lesser variation of an eye fold, and he may have a broadish face (as did the Cro Magnons of Europe as well). Now give him skin clothing and some wampum, and what have you got? As far as the above description goes, you have an American Indian.

Hooton, great student of the Indians, concluded that they resulted from an ancient mixture of several other varieties of man: Mediterranean Whites, the type of the native Australians, a Negroid or perhaps a pygmy Negrito element, all topped off by a final Mongoloid strain of the classic type, which determined the superficial appearance with its straight dark hair and moderately Mongoloid look. He emphasized that it was in such surface traits that the American Indians had their greatest unity, while they varied in size, proportions, head shape, nose form, and so on: a very useful point.

Hooton did not necessarily mean that entirely different kinds of men had come into the Americas, there to fuse, but rather that such fusions had taken place over a period of time in Asia, the product or products finding their way into the New World over the Bering Strait as time and ice allowed. As I have said before, he found the notion of ill-defined races repugnant and considered much of present humanity to come from the mixing of more definite types, developed in an older period of primary race-making. But I cannot escape the opposite view. Just as the Ainus look White externally but have a very nondescript character cranially, so do the American Indians look somewhat Mongoloid externally but nondescript cranially, and I doubt if they have looked otherwise in most of their past. I think that, most probably, they, the Indians, are the primary race, and the Siberian Mongoloids and Eskimos are a specialized form of it. Human races are surely not obliged to have a strongly special, easily classified character.

But this does not mean the Indians are "pure." I believe they could be called "mixed," in a sense remotely like Hooton's idea. That is, they were probably a sort of mixed bag to begin with: small populations drawn from Asiatic tribes which ranged from something frankly Mongoloid toward something suggesting the Whites. Certain of the recent Indian tribes, on the Northwest Pacific Coast, in California, and in New England, had a more European look than the majority. I think it is most probable that the parent Indians, in Asia, were in contact with Ainu-like Whites, from whom they were not profoundly different in the first place. Accordingly, to state it very broadly, I would say that the Indians were somewhere in the middle, between the Whites and the specialized Mongoloids, both in origin and in the effect of any later mingling of such strains.

Indian Varieties

The American Indians of historic times, like the Europeans, refuse to fall into a neat scheme of types. Those of the eastern United States, who looked a little "White," were generally tall and long of head. Also tall were the Sioux, and other Plains Indians, of striking appearance, with a high and narrow nose set in a face extremely broad across the cheekbones. Elsewhere Indian noses usually lacked a high bridge or a high root of the nose, and in the west of North America and Mexico people were typically short-statured and round-headed. The Mayas of Central America portrayed themselves accurately on their stone monuments, for their peculiar physiognomy is the same today. Their faces are large and long, their noses high and convex, and their upper lips prominent; the eyes are large and heavy-lidded; the whole face, though large, has a soft and feminine look. In South America the Indians of the Andean highland, who were largely included in the Inca Empire at one time, are again rather nondescript. But in the Amazon Basin, to the east, there is more variety. Here, short people with a Mongoloid flatness of countenance and more frequent suggestion of an eyefold, whose faces might almost be matched in Borneo or the Philippines where many natives are frankly Mongoloid, contrast with other tribes or people having unusually wavy hair, and features something like those of a dark European.

Certainly a large part of all this variety should be looked on as the result of local settlement, development, and mixture in the last few thousand years—the same things that went on in Europe. Marshall Newman has shown, for example, that body form has undergone regional responses to climate and temperature in the Americas, being slighter near the equator, bulkier in colder regions. Of course, some of the variety must be imported variety. But I think it would be dangerous to use these "types" of American Indians in trying to find ancient ancestors in the Old World, except in the general way I have suggested above, or to base history on the present. Too many changes have taken place, over and over, in the American continents.

If you would know about prehistory, consult prehistory. Dr. Georg Neumann has studied the skulls of Indians, early and late, devotedly and minutely, and he has been able to set a few landmarks for North America, wherever enough crania from one place and time have been found to show what the population was like. The Plains Indians, with their very broad faces, he believes to be a minor racial type recently and locally developed from other strains, a probable enough explanation. The Eskimos, also with very broad faces, but having the browless foreheads and the long low noses of the other specialized Mongoloids, are known to have taken up their home along the arctic rim of America only about two or three thousand years ago, so that they are actually recent. Other types of this time span in North America do not seem to diverge significantly from historical inhabitants, with tall long heads in the north and east, and smaller, medium heads in the southeast and southwest.

But in some of the earlier people, faces were less broad and rugged than recently. In the eastern United States the inhabitants of about 3000 B.C., living a late "Mesolithic" existence before the arrival there of pottery or agriculture, are known from a huge cemetery at Indian Knoll, Tennessee. They were small-skulled, medium to long in the head, and without heavy brows or faces. A still older population in North America was widespread and long enduring—nobody at the moment knows how long. Neumann calls this type the "Otamid"; it had a large, long skull, and a long face with a high nose, in his typical group from the Texas coast. But all the above types are variations on a theme. None of them look like anything but Indians, from first to last (always making a partial exception for the Eskimos).

Here the evidence peters out, before we have come to grips with the actual antiquity of the Indians. But there are gathering signs from archaeology that this antiquity is considerable, and we are not without a few ancient skeletons. Time was when the evidence seemed to be diminishing, and leading to a conclusion that the Indians had come from Asia only day before yesterday. It is a lengthy and often funny story, with a plot a little like the search for ancient *Homo sapiens* in the other hemisphere. By this I mean that, in the old gullible days, a long line of skeletal claimants to great age came to court, all sooner or later exposed as imposters, and so casting doubt on the whole idea of such claims. However, just as the corridors were finally cleared of this rabble, a very few more came forward with the stamp of real authority on their credentials. There are also certain cases which have never been settled either way.

Calaveras Calvarium

The most notorious of the buffoons was surely the cranium from Calaveras County, California, which, in view of the Jumping Frog, is probably the most implausible place in the Americas to furnish an Indian of honest geological age. This particular skull came back from glory in 1866, in circumstances which will never be quite clear. The following account, the best I can furnish, is certainly part fable. A Mr. Mattison, by trade a blacksmith, sank a shaft for a gold mine in Bald Mountain, near Angel's Camp. At 128 feet he came on some old wood and vegetable matter, and a human skull, barely recognizable as such, broken and with a lump of gravel cemented to it, which he took back to his house out of curiosity. His wife endured the gravelly head for a space and then told him to get rid of it. He foisted it onto a pair of shopkeepers he knew, who accepted it with little more grace than Mrs. Mattison. One of them, however, a Mr. Mathews, thought of a use for it. His own digestion had lately got into a bad state, apparently from drink, and Dr. William Jones, physician at the nearby town of Murphy's, had given him some powerful medicine which made him feel worse yet. Now Dr. Jones was a keen collector of antiquities, and Mathews decided to avenge his digestion by deluding the doctor into thinking the skull was a scientific treasure.

He did not actually try very hard; he simply sent the skull over to Murphy's in a potato sack. Dr. Jones took a look at it, saw cobwebs on it, and forthwith flung it out into his yard, where it lay by itself in the weather for weeks. At last Mr. Mattison, passing through Murphy's, recognized the forlorn cranium, asked the doctor how he got it, and told him where it had been found. Now the shoe was on the other foot. Dr. Jones gathered the skull up, and sent it to the state geological office in San Francisco. This was directed by Professor James Whitney, also newly appointed to a chair at Harvard. Whitney investigated, accepted the skull at face value, and introduced it to polite society as "Auriferous Gravel Man"—a Tertiary human being! The ensuing commotion inspired a satirical ode by Bret Harte, of which the following is an abbreviated version:

TO THE PLIOCENE SKULL

Speak, O man, less recent! Fragmentary fossil!
Primal pioneer of pliocene formation,
Hid in lowest drifts below the earliest stratum
    Of volcanic tufa!

"Eo-Mio-Plio-whatsoe'er the 'cene' was
That those vacant sockets filled with awe and wonder,—
Whether shores Devonian or Silurian beaches,—
    Tell us thy strange story!

"Speak, thou awful vestige of the Earth's creation,—
Solitary fragment of remains organic!
Tell the wondrous secret of thy past existence,—
    Speak! thou oldest primate!"

Even as I gazed, a thrill of the maxilla,
And a lateral movement of the condyloid process,

With post-pliocene sounds of healthy mastication,
Ground the teeth together.

And, from that imperfect dental exhibition,
Stained with expressed juices of the weed Nicotian,
Came these hollow accents, blent with softer murmurs
Of expectoration;

"Which my name is Bowers, and my crust was busted
Falling down a shaft in Calaveras County,
But I'd take it kindly if you'd send the pieces
Home to old Missouri!"

The confusion went on for years. By the end of the century many claimed to know that the skull had been planted in Mattison's mine by other miners for a joke, or that it had been mixed up with another skull while it was in Mathews' store. But these storytellers have been denounced by still others as attention-seekers who could not have known the true facts. With this wild background, the skull cannot be taken seriously. It is physically unremarkable, resembling other Indians of California. The natives are known to have placed their dead, during recent centuries, in caves or tunnels, where the bones become mineralized or gravel-coated, and whence they also turned up occasionally in mine diggings, leading to suppositions of great antiquity. The Calaveras skull long ago lost the respect of everybody, and now it sits in abashed obscurity in a cabinet in the Peabody Museum at Harvard.

There were plenty of other cases. Some were as bad as this one, or worse, like the fragments which a South American savant wished to derive from the Pliocene or the Miocene. Others were much less gaudy and more reasonable, and were usually at fault only through some misreading of the nature of the deposits in which they were found. The famous Dr. Hrdlička, of the U. S. National Museum, did a great service to all of us by examining such cases, good, bad and indifferent, and pitilessly fracturing their claims, one by one. Semi-officially, he became Bouncer of First Americans at the Court of Antiquity, developing an ease and polish in his art from the very fact that his victims always had a fatal flaw somewhere.

Signs of Indian Antiquity

Practice eventually made too perfect, however, because Hrdlička convinced himself, and many others, not only that no old Indians had been found but also that none ever would be, or could be, found. There was good reason for this impression. Not a single "old"

Indian remained upright; all lay in the alley where Hrdlička had thrown them. Furthermore, the developing archaeology of the first quarter of this century had discovered nothing but older remains of the existing kinds of Indian culture, so that the earliest knowledge still dealt largely with peoples of a "Neolithic" stage of existence, and the only "Mesolithic" remains were those of people who are hunters still—there was no sign of a real Paleolithic hunting stage underneath it all. Therefore students were disposed to great caution, and tended to think of a relatively few thousand years as the term of the occupation of America.

At the same time, they could not help being a little suspicious. Ancient-looking javelin points had been picked up in many places. And although the Indians of most regions were in a "Neolithic" culture stage, this was not a Neolithic imported from Asia. It was based on native plants and gave clear signs of having grown up, on a simpler base, in Central and South America, spreading from there. Logically, this suggested a fairly long time during which early Indian hunters spread from the port of entry at Bering Strait, in Alaska, down through North and South America, becoming acquainted with American foods and eventually learning to breed them, so that they finally developed Indian corn out of the stubby little seed ears of a wild plant, the size of a child's finger.

Such things, culminating in the rise of cities from Mexico to Peru, could not have happened in three thousand years. They did not, as we now well know. Ancient early corn has been found. And hunters are known to have reached the Straits of Magellan, two continents away from Bering Strait, before 8000 B.C. The real break came in 1927, when a projectile point with a special shape called "fluted," because of flutings or channels running up each side, was found near Folsom, New Mexico, among the bones of *Bison antiquus*, an extinct bison with wide-spreading horns. Such Folsom points had been found on the surface of the ground already, in many places, but this was the first real establishment of the Folsom culture, now known to have been that of big game hunters in the Great Plains, and to have begun about 8000 B.C. In fact, we are aware that it was only one such culture in a series, and by no means the oldest. Many well-dated finds of such things, in camp sites or caves, have since come to light, among the bones of American horses, camels, mammoths, and other extinct animals of Pleistocene appearance. It is strange now to remember that the first announcement from Folsom was greeted with the habitual disbelief of the time.

Dr. Hrdlička firmly and coldly rejected the Folsom discovery as an "illusion," and only at the very end of his life, sixteen years later, did he admit that a crack had appeared in his defenses. When the

Minnesota Man turned up in 1931, our Inquisitor bore down upon it with his accustomed hostility. This skeleton, actually the earthly remnant of a fifteen-year-old girl, was uncovered in the gravel bed of a vanished glacial lake by a road scraper, which was engaged in relaying a frost-disturbed road by cutting a trench ten feet below ground surface. The circumstances of the find were well noted by the foreman on the job, an experienced and intelligent man, and the bones were turned over to Professor Jenks of the University of Minnesota. The body had lain too deep for any ordinary grave; and its position did not suggest burial, but rather drowning and subsequent covering by lake silt. So if it means what it seems to mean, then an Indian girl jumped or fell into the icy waters of a lake which was fed from the edge of the last glacier, standing at the time only half a mile from the spot.

The great difficulty has been that the road-scraping machine innocently removed all the overlying gravels, making it impossible to say whether the body was buried as deep as it seemed, and whether the levels of gravel directly above it were truly undisturbed, showing their natural lines of deposition in the ancient lake bed. Drs. Hrdlička and Jenks argued for ten years, on other grounds. Hrdlička claimed the skull belonged to the type of the Sioux, not a really accurate description of it. Therefore, he said, it must be a Sioux burial of recent times, since a body lying on a lake bottom would have disintegrated before being covered up naturally. To this Dr. Jenks retorted that being like a Sioux did not make it a Sioux, and he cited from police records the case of an identified sailor who had fallen overboard in chilly Lake Superior in 1930 and floated ashore again in 1936 without having lost so much as a toe bone.

Six years would have been ample for the Minnesota girl to have been covered by the rapid silting of a glacier-fed lake, and such a lake was still colder than modern Superior. The gravel close to the skeleton clearly showed the banded nature ("varves") of such silt, resulting from successive summer meltings of glacial ice. If the body had been buried in the last few thousand years, traces of pollen from local vegetation, such as is always present in the air, could have been detected by a microscope in the soil around it. Yet the silt enclosing the bones and within the skull was sterile, bespeaking the almost plantless, arctic climate of the glacial fringe.

Still, doubts must remain. Perhaps the best evidence of recency is the fact that, along with the skeleton, there was found an ornament made of a shell occurring today in the Gulf of Mexico—a not unlikely trade object of later Indians—and also a group of random bones of small animals also living today in Minnesota, seeming like the con-

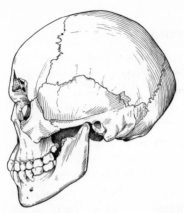
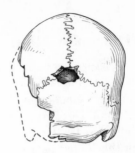

Ancient American Indians. Left, the Minnesota Woman, after Jenks. Right, rear view of the Midland skull, from Stewart's restoration. ¼ actual size.

tents of a medicine bag such as was well known in the region in historic times. Some way will be found eventually of dating the skeleton. In the meanwhile it hangs in suspense, and reminds us strangely of the Galley Hill find. In that case also, the argument revolved around a burial versus a natural coverage by glacial gravel. In that case also, Keith argued that the skeleton showed a group of primitive traits, which Jenks did for Minnesota Man, an argument not really justified in either specimen. The skull does, however, resemble Neumann's "Otamid" variety, the longheaded, not especially Mongoloid type which seems early. And a late Pleistocene age for the Minnesota girl is by no means as unlikely as the supposed middle Pleistocene age of Galley Hill. But time will tell.

The Punin skull, found in 1923, is another vexer. Certainly not a burial, it was discovered all by itself in the side of a ravine in Ecuador, in a layer of volcanic ash. Elsewhere roundabout, the same ash contained various extinct animals: American horse, mastodon, camel, sabertooth cat, and others. Anyone would call this fauna "Pleistocene," except that in our hemisphere some of the animals involved do not seem to have recognized their exit cues in time to get off stage with the ice, as they did in the better disciplined European company. Witness the mastodon, who vanished from the Old World even before the Upper Pleistocene but lingered on until very near our own day here. At any rate, this leaves the Punin individual's age uncertain. In addition, none of the animal bones were found very close to the skull. But the chances are that the skull is respectably old, and belongs with the animals.

Tepexpan Man, Midland Woman

These cases, and certain others, are interesting and perhaps important, but we do not have to depend on them. We have two stronger champions. The Tepexpan Man was found in 1947 by Dr. Helmut De Terra, not by luck this time but by strict attention to business. De Terra was looking for stonework of early Indian hunters in the Valley of Mexico, when he got involved in a mammoth hunt. Skeletons of these beasts have been coming regularly to light from the old bed of the Lake of Mexico. Only shriveled fragments of the lake remain now, even from Montezuma's time, but at the end of the last glacial phase the mountains around the valley had ice on them, and the lake was large. It has bequeathed us a dusty plain whose northern rim meets the foothills near the railway station of Tepexpan, on the road from Mexico City to the pyramid city of Teotihuacán. Led here by mammoth skeletons, De Terra went to work, with the help of a Swedish geophysicist and a sort of mine detector. They were able to detect, by differences in electrical conductivity below the surface, some of the features of the shore where, in the old days, lake and swamp had met. They marked three points where particular irregularities seemed to lie. De Terra hoped he might find more mammoths, with spear points in their bones. He dug under two of the "X's," and found water. He dug under the third, and found his long-dead Indian.

The Indian lay on his face. De Terra thinks he was engaged in hunting mammoths and got hopelessly mired himself. Apparently vultures picked at his back as he sank into the water and muck, because the bones of his shoulder blades, pelvis, and back were fragmentary and largely missing. But his skull is in fine shape. There is really nothing to say about it: he was an Indian of Indians with, in fact, a rather round head, not a long one. His only distinction is his age. The soil levels in the old lake floor reflect several stages of relative dry and wet, especially at a hard layer of caliche left by a very dry interval which here followed the end of the Pleistocene. The skeletons of the man, and of two mammoths found nearby, lay lower down, in the sands of the actual lake of the late glacial or pluvial stage. Therefore we have strong evidence of a real Pleistocene man. His age, by geological estimate and by radiocarbon, is set at about 10,000 B.C.

Here he is outranked by a lady from near Midland, Texas. Her badly smashed skull, and a few fragments of arm bones, were spotted as they were being exposed by wind, blowing the sand away from around them (like the Saldanha skull in South Africa). The spotter was Mr. Keith Glasscock, an expert amateur, and the time of spotting was June 1953. Excavation by him and other archaeologists showed that the site had several layers of sand, deposited both by wind and by lake water. The skull parts came from a series of gray sands which also contained horse teeth and stone tools; above these lay red sands, and above the red lay signs of the Folsom hunters and the bones of their great quarry, the long-horned bison. So, clearly, the Midland Woman lived and died well before the time of the Folsom people, which was about 8000 B.C. Several attempts have been made to date her more exactly, by radiocarbon and related means. All of them show that she is old, and one of them gives her a *floruit* of 18,500 B.C.!

If anyone could put Humpty Dumpty together again, it would be Dr. T. D. Stewart of the National Museum (Hrdlička's successor). He put the Midland matron (she was not particularly young) together again, from sixty of her pieces, and when he was done he had seventy pieces left over, too tiny to make sense out of, or too distant from the next part. The face is missing, for example, so the upper jaw fragments are isolated. But the result is very satisfactory. She was delicately made, with an extremely long, high skull, rather peaked in the mid-line and rather projecting in the back. Her brow ridges were light, and her teeth and jaws were small. So there are several interesting things about her. In the first place, she agrees very well with the "Otamid" type of Dr. Neumann, agreeing with a previous impression that the type is both important and really old. Second, for all her antiquity there is nothing non-Indian about her. Third, for all her antiquity she does not exhibit any of the ruggedness or specially large size of the Upper Paleolithic people of Europe and elsewhere; if there is anything "primitive" about her, and about the "Otamid" population generally, it is the kind of thing which can be called primitive in the Swanscombe skull—the fact that the high ridging and flattish contours of the skull seem to be archaic features in *Homo sapiens*, although they do not constitute signs of relationship with other human types. But this is only an impression, not something known to be a fact.

It will be of enormous importance when we finally know when the first Indians came, and what they were like. The last word is not in. The Midland skull is certainly old, but the highest figures for its age are unreliable. All that can be said with complete confidence is that the Indians had made their move by about 12,000 B.C. In fact, many archaeologists believe this is the whole story. Certainly no older radiocarbon dates have so far withstood all scrutiny.

But it is probably not the whole story. The firm dates relate to the well-defined and specialized culture of the big-game hunters, with their fluted projectile points, an American invention though probably built on much older traditions from the Paleolithic of western Russia. But there are also dim signs of other cultures, existing at the same time as the hunters and apparently earlier, the signs being groups of cruder stone tools not of the fluted point tradition. One such tool was recently found in Fulton County, Illinois, apparently safely embedded in silts of the last glacial (Wisconsin-Würm). These particular silts are known from several localities in Illinois and their place in the geological sequence is clear; and a number of $C14$ dates from this and higher levels seem to give the tool an age of 35,000 to 40,000 years.

Also important is this point: ice barriers would have kept immigrants from getting south into the Americas, from Bering Strait, from about 21,000 B.C. to about 11,000 B.C. And yet, just at this later date, there begins to flourish in North America the specialized native tradition of projectile points, which could not be a recent import because there was nothing like it in Alaska or Siberia. Thus the argument is that the Indian population actually arrived quite early, at the most favorable time of 24,000 B.C. or just before (perhaps earlier still), being isolated from the Old World for a long period thereafter. The failure of the strongly "Mongoloid" face to penetrate the Americas—excepting for the Eskimos—seems to me a forceful argument for just such an interpretation.

Indian Beginnings

At the least we have reached well back into the Pleistocene, to a time when the Upper Paleolithic people in Europe still had several thousands of years of hunting before them. So the American Indians are no longer, as in the nineteen twenties, to be looked on as latecomers, interesting only for certain cultural developments in this hemisphere. On the contrary, if they care to tell us anything about the rest of the world in the late Pleistocene, we had better let them speak. We have already seen that, as far into the past as we know them, they are all Indian, and all sapiens, with no suggestion of anything Neanderthal-like, no suggestion of large brows, and not even, as Dr. Stewart has stressed, the cranial heaviness of the Old Worlders of their time. The same for stonework: finely made projectile points give way in earlier remains to cruder flake tools of no special character, which however do not suggest a Lower Paleolithic nature.

How should we imagine the immigration of early Indians? As hunting bands who came long before Mesolithic inventions such as bows and arrows, but with equipment like their European contemporaries of the Upper Paleolithic: lances and spear throwers, and a knowledge of skinworking. The date was certainly Pleistocene, and possibly middle Fourth Glacial. Crossing would actually have been easier in glacial times, when the sea, lowered by glacier building, would have exposed a land bridge, and when Alaska and the Bering Strait region were in fact not ice-covered, northerly though they are. Crossing, and fanning out in the new country, would have been difficult, and the first migrants were probably small isolated bands, few in number.

Now at last, if we run the film backward, we bring the Indians back to Asia. What can we relate them to there? In the first place, we find rather Indian-looking people in various parts of Asia, especially the south, like Burma, or Tibet. Here there are unspecialized Mongoloids who, though recognizably Mongoloid in a general way, with brownish skins and broad faces, have a nondescript character and lack the facial traits of the Siberians. There may be other reasons to explain the racial nature of these people, but I think it likely that they, and the Indians, represent the basic Mongoloid from which the cold-adapted specializers sprang.

In the second place, there are those skulls from the Upper Cave at Choukoutien. Thought to be late Pleistocene, they are not likely to be much older than the Midland Woman, if as old. Of several individuals found here, all of whom died unnatural deaths, as fractures in the skulls show, three are excellently preserved (and, fortunately, did not take tickets on the train to Chinwangtao). They are an odd group. The male skull strongly suggests the Upper Paleolithic men of Europe. One of the women looks faintly Negroid ("Melanesian," Dr. Weidenreich called her). The other woman looks Eskimo-like. Weidenreich made much of these distinctions, as bearing on race formation. But in fact, the "Eskimo" does not really look like an Eskimo on careful examination, the "Melanesian" is less "Negroid" than the Punin skull from Ecuador, and the very White-looking man has rather prominent cheekbones, and a definite prognathism of the upper jaw.

Now it is characteristic of Indian populations, with their nondescript cranial form, to give such pale imitations of other racial types, as Dr. Hooton proved with his famous study of the skulls of Pecos Pueblo. Actually, this apparently strange assortment in the Upper Cave really looks like a group of American Indians. More, Dr. Neumann has examined them minutely, and he finds that in a series of small details they have a specific, particular resemblance to his "Otamid" variety of Indians. Certainly the "Eskimo" woman looks like this group. Neumann being one of the least excitable people I have ever known, I am sure this is a reliable and informative conclusion, and not a wishful effort to make a nice fit between early Chinese and early Americans. Even without this, the Upper Cave people, in any calm view, look like unmigrated American Indians.

As to the appearance of the specialized Mongoloids of Siberia, these Upper Cave people seem to say the same thing as do the Indians. Dating from some time not long before the emergence of Mesolithic culture in the Far East, they are not "specialized," but only

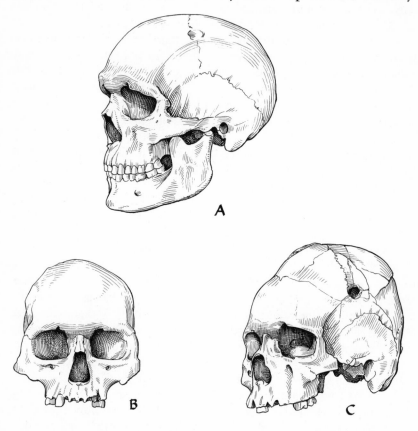

The Upper Cave Skulls from Choukoutien. A, the "Old Male." B, the "Eskimo" woman. C, the "Melanesian" woman. From casts. ¼ natural size.

moderately "Mongoloid." The Indians, arriving in America about this time or somewhat earlier, are also not specialized. The Eskimos are specialized; they are late, not before about 1000 B.C. in America. Thus, whenever the specialized Mongoloids became established, they were not general in eastern Asia until late times, as we saw earlier in this chapter. This raises the unspecialized, basic Mongoloids to a still higher plane of importance: it is hard not to see them as an old Asian population of considerable importance, later overrun and affected by the specialized type. I think one might say the older Mongoloids were probably more like the Whites in early days, and the Whites more like them; that is to say, like the American Indians.

But this is rank speculation. The Far East, an enormous region, has been less than generous with human skeletons of the late Pleistocene. We can imagine almost anything we like. We could even imagine an Asiatic population, possibly late Third Interglacial, something like the Indians, not too different from the Whites. It was probably continuous with Whites, on the west and south, and perhaps on the east. (Physically, it might have had the characters of a long, narrow head, projecting occiput, with a face of moderate breadth; characters found in the earliest Upper Paleolithic people of Europe—Lautsch, Combe Capelle—and in the earliest American Indians.) We might imagine that the ice, forming in the early Würm, split this population, pushing part of it over a land bridge into open Alaska, trapping the other part to produce the flat-faced Mongoloids, who later came to rule so much of Asia. Fortunately, imagination is cheap.

21. DARK CONTINENT, DARK PAST

SOUTH of the Sahara, Africa holds out a promise of simpler kinds of racial history. The promise is not fulfilled. In a relatively isolated part of the world we find two well-defined kinds of men: the Negroes and the South African Bushmen. But in South Africa we find a picture of early men too broad and complicated to explain. And in the territory of the Negroes—a major stock of mankind, fully distinguished from Whites or Mongoloids—we find virtually no history at all.

The living people are not hard to describe. The great populations of Negroes, beginning at the Atlantic bulge of Africa, run from the savannahs and woods of West Africa through the Congo forest up to the highlands of the east and south. Like the American Indians, they vary somewhat in size and features. But they have the classic Negro features: woolly hair; thickened lips; heavy pigment; a broad, short nose; and prognathism, or projection of the middle and lower face. The head is rather flat-sided, and the forehead is also narrow and tends to be vertical, if not high, and to be lacking in brow ridges. They are of medium build and rather well muscled, not lanky, though the arms are relatively long. In all this central territory, it would be hard to make even the kind of tribal distinctions which can be loosely stated for the American Indians.

Negroid Contrasts in Size

Along with these medium-sized gardening Negroes of forest and savannah, the Negroid stock as a whole also contains the tallest and shortest of men. Among the very tallest tribes in the whole world are the so-called Nilotic Negroes. Including the Dinka and Shilluk, they raise grain and keep cattle, inhabiting mud villages in the open plains along the White Nile, in the southern Sudan. They are long of head, long of face, and perhaps relatively longer in the nose than the ordinary Negroes, whose features they otherwise share. Herding their cows, they lean on spears or staffs under the flaming sun, clad only in their dense pigmentation. Thus they are one of the people used as evidence for the hypothesis that, in such sunny, hot environments, the body's system can function best in a slender physique which can lose heat rapidly, avoiding heatstroke. Supposedly the giant Nilotics have adapted their bodies to their hot plains by becoming generally skinny. Their great height is, I judge, not the result of good food and exercise, but simply a necessary part of their becoming lanky and attenuated.

Actually, the lankiness, with a fairly tall stature, is characteristic of all the peoples of this eastern section, radiating in a semicircle around the Horn of Africa. It is true of Ethiopians and Somalis. But these people are only partly Negroid, judging from their appearance, and they have traditional connections with the north and speak languages of the Hamito-Semitic family, like the Egyptians and the Berbers. While they may be dark in skin color, and curly or woolly-haired, their features vary from Negroid to Mediterranean White, and their skulls are more White in type. So, without knowledge to the contrary, they appear to be an extension along the Nile and Red Sea of the White zone of Africa, paralleling the Arabian shore, but a White contingent which has been affected by Negro admixture.

Conversely, there are tall Negroid tribes which seem to have been affected by White admixture, to accept this interpretation for the time being. The Nilotics have their own relatives extending southward into Kenya and Uganda, into the general region of such more typical Negroes as the Kikuyus. But there are other people, also cattle keepers, who are tall but who look different from the Negroes. In particular, these are certain tribes which have set themselves up as a ruling aristocracy among farming Negroes, notably the Bahima in Uganda, and the spectacular Watussi in Ruanda and Urundi, southwest of all the others, on the line of lakes which makes the border of the Belgian Congo. The Watussi (who has not seen pictures of them?) are tall and skinny like the Nilotics, but their long faces are clearly less Negroid, especially in their prominent and narrower noses.

The Watussi (their name is more properly Batutsi) live as ruling clans among the much more numerous Bahutu, crop raisers of typical Negro form and appearance. And, in forested parts of the same territory, live Pygmy hunters, the Batwa. To the west, as the land slopes from the open uplands down into the shade forest of the Belgian Congo, there are many other groups of Pygmies, living in small bands, wandering in search of game of every kind from birds to elephants. They are proficient little huntsmen, and they trade their meat to the Negroes of the Congo, who are settled farmers and who hunt only occasionally themselves. The Negroes sometimes take Pygmy wives, because they are cheap, but there is not general mixture; the Pygmies do not take Bantu wives, and the two peoples live essentially different kinds of life.

The Pygmies, obviously, are short, though they cannot be looked on as dwarfs of the circus variety. In some groups the males average four feet eight inches. They differ from the Negroes in certain other ways, sometimes having more beard and body hair than the Negroes. Their heads are apt to be round and their foreheads bulbous; their faces may or may not have a rather infantile look, but the nose is relatively big, and especially broad relative to its length. All these last features are probably reflections of small size, and thus not to be counted on as important racial differences from the Negroes.

The Pygmies seem simply to be a branch of the Negro stock, typical in all ways except that they have become reduced in height. Nobody knows why. It has been suggested from time to time that ancient mankind was once of pygmy size and that modern races grew up from smaller prototypes, but a look back at chapters you have read already will show you how worthless this suggestion is. It has also been conjectured that the Pygmies are the victims of dietary deficiencies, perhaps due to something in the soil, so that a sort of stunting has become a racial property. But the fact is that their diet is good and well rounded, with plenty of meats and wild food plus trade vegetables, while that of the Negroes is more starchy and restricted, deficient in fats and meats. There is probably some good cause for Pygmy minuteness. They are definitely a forest-living people, and Carleton Coon suggests that small size is a real and important advantage in moving quickly through the thick growth when hunting. Certainly, men of standard size cannot match them at this.

It is not an unlikely explanation. Indeed, there are good signs that simple body size can change fairly quickly in short-term evolution. Many animals have produced giant or dwarf strains having all the other particular traits of their "normal" forms, and there are, in fact, pygmy chimpanzees in the bend of the Congo, as well as pygmy men, though little is known about them. So it is perhaps not surprising that human strains should become very tall or very short under pressure of the appropriate environment, by natural selection. But we are still in ignorance of precise causes or of the length of time needed for Pygmies to become Pygmies.

Bushmen and Hottentots

In southernmost Africa we leave the Negro stock and come to quite a different kind of man, the South African Bushmen, and their relatives the Hottentots. The Bushmen, though still numerous, are remote from the general view because, except for remnants of tribes in other parts of South Africa, they are now confined to the Kalahari Desert. Here some of them still live by nomadic hunting. Their stage of life is truly Mesolithic, if you note the exception that they get a little metal by trade and work it into arrow points with stone tools. The Hottentots on the other hand are, or were, keepers of cattle, a kind of existence which they can have acquired only from regions to the north. It made them natural enemies of the Bushmen, who were just as happy to use their poisoned arrows on a cow as on an eland.

Taken together, however, Bushmen and Hottentots should be looked on as another major racial variety of man. They have traits which are Negro-like, such as broad noses, full lips, and tightly curled hair. But even these traits differ in detail. The nose is very low. Lips are everted, but this is not marked or typical, and the lips are flattened against the face. And the hair out-Negroes the Negroes, being so tightly curled as to form little individual spirals (called "peppercorns"), rather than a mop, leaving much scalp exposed. I would say, as a manner of speaking, that the Bushmen resemble the Negroes no more than American Indians resemble Europeans.

In skin, Bushmen vary around a warm tan, some darker brown and some yellow, but in the average much lighter than Negroes. They have a most characteristic head and face form. The skull is full and five-cornered, with marked angles at either side of the narrow forehead, at the sides above the ears, and at the pointed back. The whole gives the impression of an "infantile" skull, accentuated by the vertical, rather smooth brow. The face is also "infantile," being flat, small, and markedly pulled in under the skull; the jaw, like the forehead, is small, but the cheekbones are typically wide and prominent, so that the front edges of the temples slant outward in a pronounced fashion, giving the lower face a triangular form which is a racial hallmark. Ears are very short, and square in shape. Finally, the skin over the upper eyelid tends to cover the lid itself, sometimes by a fold over the middle, sometimes by a "Mongolian" fold over the inner corner.

The light skin, the flat face and brows, and the eyefolds have led some writers to think that a true Mongoloid strain has entered Bushman lineage. Aside from the problem of bringing Mongoloid parents from northeastern Siberia to South Africa, over staggering distances showing no sign of them present or past, I cannot see any real resemblance between this group of traits and the specialized Mongoloid complex, and I think the correspondence is fortuitous and illusory. The Bush face is thin, not fat; the eyefolds do not suggest the Mongoloids as much as all that; and it is hard to be impressed by the skin color.

Certainly the Bushmen have a problematical ancestry, but I am sure we can leave the Siberians out of it.

Two other Bushman traits are important. Steatopygia is one. If this is Greek to you, it means "fat on the buttocks." Bush and Hottentot women, when eating well, store fat on the backside until they stick out very decidedly in that direction. Hottentot house servants looked splendid in the days of the bustle, but they look odd when dressed otherwise or not at all. Other human beings pack their surplus calories all over, and especially on the torso. But the Bush or Hottentot female can be thin and fat at the same time. Once more we may be viewing an adaptive advantage for human beings in a special climate, in this case hunters in sunny plains or desert. Like camels, and some other animals, they can keep a reserve of energy, stored as fat, without suffering the consequences of having the fat act as a heating blanket on the body. Instead, the fat is tucked into one lump, and stuck where its effect on the heat economy of the body is at its very least, whatever may be the effect on the fore-and-aft trim. Unfortunately, we do not know if the Bushmen have long been exposed to desert heat. In addition, it is only the women who develop marked steatopygia, leading to the suggestion that it may be primarily a fortification for pregnancy, among these people whose food supply is so precarious.

Such careful disposition of extra fat might be especially valuable in a small-bodied people, in whom a little fat goes a long way. And the Bushmen are small, another of their significant traits. They are not pygmies: they are quite different from the Pygmies of the Congo, and there is no reason to see any close connection, and many reasons to doubt one. But they are short, with light bodies and delicate skeletons. Male averages for Bush tribes run around five feet two inches, the Hottentots being very slightly taller. Their small size may contain the answer to some of their other peculiarities, especially the counterfeit Mongoloid look. At the same time, it is one of the question marks in the problem of their origins.

South Africa's Past

We have been observing the natives of modern Africa, seeing the Negroes dominant everywhere, the Hottentots as shattered survivors, and the Bushmen as refugees in the Kalahari. Let us begin turning the clock back from what we know and can surmise of recent history. Rouse Cecil Rhodes from his grave in the Matopo Hills and send him back to England, and the English after him. Pull the Boers out of the Transvaal, out of the Cape, and send them back to Holland. This is only a few centuries. But it also takes the Bantu Negro nations back from the south, for they were just moving into the last great Bush-Hottentot territory as the Europeans were landing on the Cape. In the centuries before that, they had been taking various routes down through the Rhodesias, where they must have been established over a thousand years ago. For the spectacular granite brick "city" of Zimbabwe was built by the Bantus, in Southern Rhodesia, perhaps as early as the sixth century A.D., if the radiocarbon dates are to be trusted. Beyond these dates the signs become dim. Such as they are, they carry the Negro peoples back in the direction of West Africa. Negroes were known, of course, in ancient Egypt, but they were evidently not established in very early times in East Africa, judging from Stone Age skulls.

With this evident contraction of older Negro territory, there was certainly a considerably expanded former territory of the Bushmen. In the Later Stone Age there was a wide area of stone cultures using small flakes or microliths, and beads, throughout South and East Africa. This is highly suggestive of Bushmen, but it is neither extremely ancient, nor was it necessarily the property of Bushmen alone, wherever found. Nevertheless, there are other signs of a once broad distribution of the Bush race. For example, the Hottentots must have got their cattle via East Africa, though of that we know nothing. Further, there are definite Bushmen remains, and Bushmen cave paintings, over a wider range of country than the recent Bush habitat. Also, remnants of peoples exist in East Africa who speak languages resembling those of the Bushmen and Hottentots. The resemblance lies in the use of "clicks," or consonants made by sucking the breath in, rather than pushing it out.

The question now becomes, not How widespread were the Bushmen? but rather How long have they been Bushmen? All over the same region, East and South Africa, the Late Stone Age was preceded by cultures of the Middle Stone Age, largely of the Still Bay tradition. This tradition goes right back to the Proto-Still Bay found in the cave at Broken Hill, some time toward the middle of the last glacial phase of Europe. That is not very old, of course: we might guess 40,000 years or less, though unfortunately we do not know much about dates in this part of the world. But in South Africa, within the same period, a good number of skulls and skeletons have come to light, and they run a gamut between two extremes, the delicate browless Bushmen on one hand, and the Rhodesian Man with his big face and truly enormous brows, on the other. Except for these extremes, however, and the Florisbad skull, all the crania are ordinary *Homo sapiens*, of medium to large size, varying in brow-ridge heaviness. A few of them, notably the Boskop skull, have the typical Bush shape, but on a giant scale, and one of this type was found far to the north, at Singa on the Blue Nile, in the Sudan!

Because of this, and certain other skulls of the north and east in which he sees Bush traits, Coon thinks that Bushmen origins are actually to be found in North Africa, among the Neanderthals of Morocco and their successors. Caucasoid expansion, he believes, eventually drove the Bush stock to the other end of the continent via East Africa, passing by the territory of the forerunners of the Negroes proper, so that they have now reversed positions. For Coon, Rhodesian Man is a Negro, not a Bushman ancestor.

The complicated state of affairs has led to other interpretations by Dart, Broom, Drennan, Wells, Tobias, and others in South Africa (land of wonderful anthropologists), of some complexity. They involve two main hypotheses. One is that the essential Bushman derived his small size and his shrunken face, bulbous forehead, and little jaw, by a process of infantilizing, or the retention of infantile traits, called "pedomorphism." The other views the Bushmen as the final result of the mixture of several—as many as six or seven—different racial types arriving or developing in South Africa. This hypothesis notes not only the different Stone Age skull types but also slight differences within the whole Bush stem, which includes the following forms: typical Kalahari Bushmen; an almost extinct western variant, the Strandloopers; the Hottentots, of larger size; and the Koranas, a Hottentot nation with slightly heavier faces and stronger brows.

This mixture theory, of the mingling of once purer strains, is exactly like Dr. Hooton's explanation of the American Indians. I feel the same way about it, for the same reasons. I do not doubt it altogether, but I believe it is greatly overdone: it imagines types so potently fixed and defined as to crop out in mixed descendants, even while its proponents can accept the idea of easy and drastic change in type, through "pedomorphism."

This last, the diminution in size, seems much more important in interpretation. Such a change must have taken place somewhere, for the Bushmen are smaller than average human beings. It is only reasonable to suppose their larger ancestors were the men, known to have lived in the same place in the Middle and Later Stone Age, who in fact resembled them in form of skull. As I suggested for the Pygmies, the key seems to be general diminution in body size, with particular lightening of the skull and of the face, since such diminution, it is known, will affect the brain less than its envelope, the skull. The result is to produce a swollen forehead jutting over a small face, and a head the shape of a Bushman's.

Since these are the proportions seen in infants, the Bushmen look infantile.[1] Now it is one thing to call the Bushmen "pedomorphic," meaning that they look infantile. But I object to calling all this "pedomorphism," suggesting an actual infantilizing process, or the retention by some special biological process of a more infantile stage of development (a kind of larvalizing which has indeed taken place in some animals). I believe that reduction may occur, both in general size of the skeleton and skull, and in particular features, like the brows, or the face, by small-scale evolution or natural selection of some kind, without any special process of infantilizing. Probably the infantile appearance is coincidence, flowing from the proportions. As we have seen, the Australopithecinae appear ape-like in skull form because of their brain-jaw proportions. However, we would hardly refer to this as resulting from a process of "chimpomorphism," since it simply follows from small brain size.

Actually, I have oversimplified the views of my South African friends. Some of them, particularly Drs. Wells and Galloway, do not stress the type differences very strongly, and Galloway finds that practically all the prehistoric skulls have a general kinship. The crania vary considerably, which is natural in any major group of mankind, like the American Indians. But if any of them are not ancestral Bushmen, it cannot be said what else they may actually be. Varying degrees of the tendency to reduce size are perhaps the most important cause of difference, as I think is the case in the living. That is to say, just as some of the Whites are more extreme—perhaps more pinch-nosed, or lighter in pigment—or some of the Mongoloids more Mongolized, so we might view the Kalahari Bushmen as more "Bushmanized" than the Hottentots or Koranas.

Of course, the above are suggestions, and Bushman origins and history still remain obscure. Some students begin the line of descent with Rhodesian Man himself (unlike Coon, who makes him a "Congoid," or Negro) since he certainly occupied the right territory. I think this is rash, since enormous doses of "pedomorphism" or any other kind of reduction would be called for to diminish his brows and face to the size prevailing in the Middle Stone Age not long after, to say nothing of getting down to Bushman delicacy. Although Rhodesian Man clearly survived into the Middle Stone Age, it looks as though there had been a break here, rather like the one which saw the disappearance of the late Neanderthals at about the same time, with

---

[1] If one wonders how the large "ancestral" Boskop skull comes to have the typical Bush shape, if diminution is suggested as the main cause of the Bush shape, the answer is that the Boskop (and the similar Fish Hoek) skull had an extraordinarily large brain, so that the infantile proportions prevailed.

sapiens men presiding in the rest of the Middle Stone Age and Late Stone Age. These last do not show signs of continuing and rapid evolution such as recent descent from Broken Hill man would require, but constitute only a varying sapiens group in which Bushman traits of form begin to be exhibited. (This excepts the early Florisbad skull, a very heavy-browed sapiens. If he was not partly descended from the Rhodesian type it is difficult to explain him.) We do not know where or when the main size reduction of the Bush stock took place. Nor, though this reduction looks like the kind of adaptive evolution the Mongoloids supposedly went through, can we say clearly what kind of selection caused it. But we may regard the Bushman, early or late, large or small, as a racial form of some antiquity, wherever it came from.

East African Queries

If we go now to East Africa, we are in another province with its own great importance, and its own great problems. By East Africa I mean the modern Sudan, plus all the eastern uplands: the Horn (Ethiopia and the Somalilands), East Africa (Uganda, Kenya, Tanzania), and Ruanda and Burundi. It is a sort of crossroads, open to access from all points, but especially from the Nile to the north, from the forest to the west, and from the grasslands to the south. Arabia to the east, though close by, appears to have been less in contact in prehistoric times. Note also that East Africa is an area where cattle can exist, free of tsetse fly.

This is all a province of people partly White, partly Negroid, though generally dark-skinned. And the traditional assumption has been that aboriginal Negroid peoples were affected by the arrival from the north of "Hamites," that is to say, people speaking languages of this branch of the Hamito-Semitic family who were believed to be Mediterranean Whites. The appearance of things justified the assumption. Certainly cattle must have come into Africa here from the Near East. I have pointed out that the Hottentots could have got them ultimately from no other source, and the same applies to the Bantu and other cattle breeders. And certainly such Hamitic-speaking peoples as the Gallas and Somalis, dark of skin but "White" of skull, came down in the not very ancient past. So there grew up the notion of the "Hamites" as an important culture stimulus and racial element, absorbing something from older East African Negroes to produce the tall cattle-driving aristocracy, such as the Bahima or the Watussi. In other words, a Neolithic importation of tall, longheaded African Whites, and a "Hamitizing" of a part of Negro Africa.

This is all wrong, as has been known now for some time. To put it simply, if skulls mean anything it is the Whites who have been solidly entrenched in East Africa since the later Pleistocene, and anyone else is an interloper. A long series of skulls, early and late, has been recovered in the region as a whole, largely through the indefatigable work of Dr. and Mrs. Leakey in Nairobi. There are plenty of puzzles and complications in the known prehistory, such as the indication that cultures of Upper Paleolithic type run back, not simply to the middle of the last pluvial period, but to its beginning and perhaps to the preceding one, which supposedly corresponded with the Third Glacial. But in the main the complications make sense. They are what would result from quite different peoples coming from quite different parts of Africa.

The ever-problematical Kanjera skulls, of course, should be viewed as the oldest. If they are to be labeled at all, they should be called "White," though they are hardly in good enough shape to be called anything but sapiens. However, from the last pluvial period comes a small group of longheaded, long-faced, high-nosed skulls which cannot be placed anywhere but with the Whites. They were mostly found in caves, along with an Upper Paleolithic blade culture whose only connections are also with North Africa, and possibly with the Near East and Europe. It is not like the Still Bay culture of the south, which does however reach into East Africa. The same general kind of skull carries on into a period of "Mesolithic" cultures, about 10,000 B.C., and into a subsequent "Neolithic." These cultures appear to be a single line of descent, like the men involved. They are local, but vigorous, and it is interesting that archaeologists think the Neolithic in the eastern Sudan was early, about 4000 B.C., so that the region was anything but isolated and stagnant. At any rate, there is reason to suspect northern connections along the Nile, early and late.

But these were not the only contacts. East Africa was probably the edge of Bush territory at some time. If we follow the rules, the Singa skull shows the presence of a Bushman, or something like one, right up in the Sudan. And at a few places in Kenya, skulls suggesting Bushman traits have come from graves or caves of general Neolithic date, associated with a stone culture of South African affiliations, the Wilton. As to Negroes, there is no sign of them before the Mesolithic, and nothing positive then. Only with Neolithic remains does there appear a skull (Nyarindi shelter) which really looks Negro. This, with a somewhat less Negroid-looking companion, came from western Kenya, and the culture accompanying it, Dr. Desmond Clark suggests, was derived from the Congo. So this, too, seems to work out nicely. Later, in the last thousand years B.C., there had come a much heavier

Negroid visitation, in the form of a large settlement at Jebel Moya, in the Sudan between the White and Blue Niles. From their skulls, the dwellers here were clearly Negroids and like some of the tribes of West Africa, but in appearance they lacked something of being pronounced Negroes, not having a marked prognathism. Nowadays, of course, Negroid peoples live all across the Sudan grasslands to the west, as well as in much of East Africa.

The net result, the important conclusion, is that peoples of a basically White stock have been the holders of this strategic area, at a sort of communications hub for South Africa, for Egypt, and also for southern Arabia, if this route had any meaning. They need not have been White in the sense of being pink and blond. Indeed, they may have been strongly brunet to begin with, and probably got darker and more curly-haired in later times as Negroids, or Bushman ancestors, came to call, until they might in this way have produced just what we now see in the Watussi. But originally they must have belonged to an Upper Paleolithic, large-skulled White stock of a longheaded variety, somewhat different from the Cro Magnons, and perhaps more like the Combe-Capelle longhead. Men like them were in South Russia in the Mesolithic, and perhaps in the Near East. But the train of connections with the other Whites, and the problem of the Neanderthal territory, remains to be worked out.

The Home of the Negroes

This also bears on the history of the other peoples. These East Africans must have been on the scene immediately following the Rhodesian Man in South Africa, especially if the Eyasi skull was of the Rhodesian type. Also, they would, by their presence, have isolated the Bushman stock from the rest of the world from that time on. The same for the Negroes. If recognizable Negroes are only rare and late visitors, bearing cultures which seem to look back to the Congo, this suggests a long history for the Negro peoples in West Africa, bounded on the east, as on the north, by Paleolithic and Mesolithic Whites, and bounded on the south by Bushmen.

Going at last to Negro territory, and trying to view Negro origins from there, leads to similar conclusions. We are hampered by the fact that human remains from the past hardly exist. One thing we do know: the Negroes have had a marked expansion east and south in recent times, and indeed the whole picture of the Negro populations of Africa may be deceptively new.

In the first place, the tribes speaking Bantu languages are the result of a broad increase and spread. I have talked about Bantus coming through the Rhodesias and into South Africa in the middle of the Christian era. This was surely one of their latest moves, following their penetration of the Congo earlier, and of parts of the east as well. Careful study of the whole large language group indicates that its spread started, not before 2000 B.C. (and probably rather later), in West Africa, in the eastern part of Nigeria.

In the second place, the face of things in East Africa may not be very old. The Kikuyu of Central Kenya are farmers speaking a Bantu language, and thus hardly ancient settlers. The tall Sudanese Nilotics speak languages quite different from Bantu or any of its western relatives of the Niger-Congo family. However, some of their own relatives, like the Luo of Kenya, are less tall than the Nilotics, and, if blood-group types may be taken as a sure guide—an uncertain proposition for any long range purposes—they, like the Kikuyu, resemble the Negroes of the west. I think it quite possible that the tallest of the Nilotics may have become so tall and lanky in a relatively short time— something like two thousand years, more or less—since the Berber Tuareg of the Sahara must have undergone a similar change during the Christian era. On the other hand, some of the earliest Negroes may have been rather tall and slender, as we shall see.

At any rate, it seems logical to connect the tribes I speak of to a Negro stock placed further west. Other East Africans, like the Masai, are different, in form and blood, and are probably of mixed parentage. Still others, like the stringy, horse-faced Watussi, though Bantu-speaking, may be basically traceable to the ancient "White" strain of East Africa, having become strongly negrified, and adopting a Bantu speech from contacts in Uganda, where they lived before moving down into Ruanda-Urundi, some centuries back. Dr. Jean Hiernaux has been able to demonstrate that they have since then become mixed still further, to a slight degree, with the Bahutu—a typical Negro tribe—among whom they settled.

Constantly we are led back to West Africa, south of the Sahara, for a Negro homeland. In fact, the Sahara itself, and the open country and grasslands on its southern edge, may have been as important, or more so, in Negro history than the forests which are the characteristic Negro habitat today. That is what gathering evidence points to. The Sahara was a far more hospitable place in much of the Pleistocene, supporting the typical large game animals; and this state of affairs lasted until quite recently, allowing elephants to survive in North Africa into classical times. And there is much evidence of human occupation in the Sahara. So the Negro territory probably suffered a contraction here before, or while, it expanded to the east and south. Thus many of the seemingly mixed Negroid peoples living on the southern edge of the

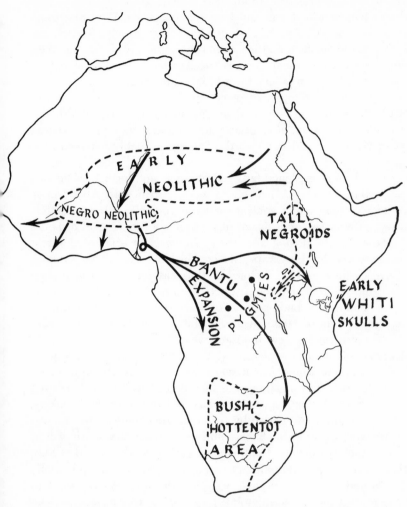

A map of some probable prehistoric events in Africa.

Sahara today, or even within it, like the Teda of the Tibesti plateau, may be old inhabitants there. Thus it is that the tall and slender body form of many Sudanese peoples, contrasting with the more heavily built, muscular forest Negroes, may after all be an ancient property of the Negro stock, or of part of it.

At any rate, this was the shape of the oldest Negro known. He is not very old—possibly Mesolithic in culture—but he is almost unique. He got drowned in a stream in what is now the open Sahara, near the military post of Asselar, about two hundred and fifty miles northeast of

Timbuktu. He was definitely a tall, rather slenderly built Negro, with long lower legs and forearms, and long slender hands. West and south of this an incomplete "Neolithic" skull comes from Tamaya Mellet; this has a Negroid lower face and is apparently more typical for the West Africans, as we know them, than is the Asselar Man. The skull was associated with harpoon points, for fishing (in the Sahara!), which have also been found in a number of places in the southern desert, and as far as Khartoum on the Nile, and in Fayum basin in Egypt. All this forms another suggestion of Negroes partaking in a widespread African variety of Neolithic, and living in the Sahara, probably between 4000 and 3000 B.C.

Here the skeletal evidence fails us. There is nothing more, beyond dim suggestions of Negroids such as I mentioned in East Africa, or in the Sudan. Nothing really ancient, or even very clear. Unfortunately the forest, with its acid soils, is not likely to allow the survival of bones of ancient men, even if they were there. However, in spite of the poor evidence, we can hardly escape the conclusion that the Negro stock must have existed far back before anything as recent as the Asselar Man. It is too well-defined, too distinctive, to have emerged in a short time span. Changes in body size or form are one thing; the characteristic hair, lips, form of face and ear, all bespeak a racial lineage running back more than a few thousand years.

But about this we can say nothing. We can only imagine a scheme of events for recent times, which seems reasonable in the light of all we know. In the following there are included ideas I have borrowed from Dr. Frank Livingstone,[2] who has put together archaeology, malaria, languages, and geography to reconstruct some of the events.

Negroes were living in the Sahara and in open country south of it at the end of the Pleistocene, hunting and gathering their food. (Note that this might be the kind of area to which their dark skin and woolly hair is adapted.) They may have occupied the forest in the west to some extent. But the great equatorial forest of the Congo was successfully peopled only by a special branch of the Negro stock, the Pygmies, who were, or became, better adapted to forest life and hunting through small size. (Whites in East Africa, Bushmen in the southeast and south.)

Then agriculture and the Neolithic arrived in Africa, through Egypt. The Negroes of the Sahara and Sudan soon took it up (before 3000 B.C.), but they domesticated millet and sorghum and grew them in place of the wheat and barley of Egypt and the Near East. So farm-

[2] Frank B. Livingstone, "Anthropological implications of sickle cell gene distribution in West Africa," *American Anthropologist*, vol. 60, pp. 533–62. Menasha, Wis., 1958.

ing moved over to West Africa. But it stayed out of the tropical forest, to which millet and sorghum are not suited; the only Negroes present on the forested Guinea coast, to the south, were still hunters.

The Sahara became too dry at last for much farming, but events made it up to the Negro tribes in other ways. In the first place, the Negroes in the west domesticated new crops which were well suited to the forest, especially yams. And then, before the beginning of the Christian era, knowledge of iron arrived there, and with iron the forest could be efficiently cleared for planting. At last, and only now, could the Negroes move into the forests with a way of life which would sustain them there in force. (And only now, Dr. Livingstone suggests, did malaria become a plague, since only now did clearing of the forest create pools of unshaded water which the malarial parasite's host, the mosquito *Anopheles gambiae*, needs for breeding. Thus Livingstone finds evidence of the recency of all these events in the fact that the sickling gene, a human reaction to endemic malaria, has just lately been reaching and becoming common in some of the more isolated tribes of West Africa.)

So yams and iron are the explanation of the explosion of the Bantu-speakers into Central Africa and beyond. (They have adopted various other crops since then, of course.) And thus we have the probable key, not only to the striking spread of this one language group, but also to the great shift of the Negro populations. We understand how, starting from the Sudan, they have in the course of only about two thousand years thrust themselves into the complexities of East Africa, surrounded the Pygmies in the Congo, and overrun the Hottentots and the Bushmen in South Africa until they finally collided head-on with the Boers moving up from their settlement in the Cape.

22. THE EASTERN TROPICS

WE HAVE one piece of earth still left to look at: a belt of the tropics running off to the east, through India and Southeast Asia and right across the Pacific. It is not big, compared with the ground we have covered, but it is important. The main question is one of getting more light on the dark-skinned kinds of man.

Let us go about this by trying to peel off some of the later peoples so as to look at the older layers where the dark-skinned races lie. By the later peoples I mean the lighter skinned Whites and Mongoloids, who have evidently penetrated the natural defenses of this whole area at a few likely spots: the Whites at the northwest of India, the Mongoloids down the coast in the Far East, and the two together by water in the Pacific. And the Pacific is the best place to begin, because it is an island world.

On a continent where the country is open, one kind of people may be swept away by another, if the latter is more numerous and stronger, with a higher culture. Or else the two may mingle to form a well-stirred daughter racial group. If the country is broken up, the sweeping or the stirring may be uneven, so that pockets showing ancient differences remain. Islands are better still for such survivals, and so the South Seas have become a museum of human races.

More than that, the Pacific has been something like a coal grader, for the further out you go from Asia, the smaller and farther apart the islands become, and therefore the more difficult of approach by really primitive peoples. If you stand at Singapore, the logical point of entry from Asia today, and look off east by south into the ocean, the Indonesian islands at your feet will appear huge and close together, readily accessible to any kind of an Asiatic who has a small boat or even a raft. Further away, however, the distances call for greater skill and better boats, and the islands themselves become so poor in natural food that any invaders must bring their own sources of food with them.

The Polynesians

We may start at Easter Island, nearest to South America, and work slowly back around the world to the strait of Bab el Mandeb in Arabia, just over the way from the Horn of Africa, where we spent some puzzled moments in the last chapter. Reaching Easter Island was one of the crowning achievements of the Polynesians, who sailed out in big oceangoing canoes to populate the whole eastern half of the Pacific Ocean, or everything beyond Fiji and the international date line. Not far from Fiji are the island groups of Samoa and Tonga. Further off is Tahiti in the Society group, and beyond that stretch out the corally dots of the Tuamotus, the Low Archipelago, pointing toward Pitcairn Island. Far out on the edges lie the points of a great triangle: Easter Island, beyond Pitcairn; Hawaii on the north; and New Zealand, the only sizeable Polynesian territory, at the southwest.

The Polynesians came to their islands fairly late in human history. A highly developed skill in navigation, and the plants they brought with them, allowed them to settle and to produce the large population and the lusty culture which so attracted the imagination of eighteenth-century Europe. The plants were, principally, breadfruit trees, taro, yams, and bananas. All are native to Southeast Asia, where they were domesticated by the Neolithic peoples. And the Polynesians themselves were "Neolithic," for their islands held little, other than fish, on which non-agricultural people could have lived.

Now Polynesian history is by no means unknown. It was not written down, of course. But it was remembered, in a somewhat glorified form. Genealogies were kept, and lists of ancestors were recited on ceremonial occasions (the oldest ancestors having become gods, by a gradual canonization). And myths and traditions told of explorations and of visits between distant islands. The anthropologists have collected all this and added it up. They have also made estimates of the length of time needed for the different dialects of Polynesia to drift apart. On top of this, there is a growing number of radio-carbon dates of great importance. There is a good deal of uncertainty, but everything points to the outlines of the story. Perhaps before 1000 B.C., Polynesians arrived in Samoa and Tonga, going on later to Tahiti in the center, and then to the Marquesas, still several centuries B.C. The islands at the corners of the great triangle—Hawaii, Easter, and New Zealand—were all reached from 500 to 1000 A.D. There was some internal migration, and in places such as Samoa heads changed from longer to rounder; however, it does not seem likely that later waves of Polynesians ever entered the area from somewhere else.

There have been plenty of interesting and fanciful books trying to show that the Polynesians are the Children of Mu, or the last remnants of Alexander the Great's fleet; and also that the Polynesians were American Indians, or vice versa. Let us snub the more riotous of these ideas and consider only the Polynesian-American Indian connection. It is of course possible that Polynesians, exploring to the east and missing Easter Island (which I should think would have been the fate of more than ninety-nine per cent of the explorers) might have survived the extra two thousand miles, and all the adverse winds and currents, and have brought up on the South American coast. They would have found Indian civilization in an advanced state: peoples who, by the Christian era, already towered over them culturally, and to whom they could have brought nothing of consequence, though they were admittedly superior in boatcraft. Contrariwise, it is conceivable that some of the Peruvian Indians might have set off on a raft into the setting sun, involuntarily or voluntarily, even though lacking a radio and the knowledge that there were islands to the west. If they did this, and washed ashore at last, they have had no visible effect on Polynesia. For Polynesian traditions and culture are all of a piece, and point back to Southeast Asia. Even the supposedly mysterious statues of Easter Island are in the Polynesian tradition, though of giant size because light volcanic rock allowed them to be made thus. The Polynesian plants are from the west. And so is the language; it is a member of the large Austronesian stock, including most of the languages of the whole Pacific and Indonesia.

The Polynesians are tall and rather like the Whites in body form, though a little more solid. In this, but mainly in the head and face, they strongly suggest a mixture of Mongoloid and White, with possibly a little Negroid causing occasional frizzy hair. This is going by appearances; we do not know what actually went into the recipe, but it is hard to mistake the force of the White elements. The Polynesians have large, deep faces, with noses both long and broad and eyes without Mongoloid folds. Skin is light brown to brown, but hair is wavy, and beards are usual. If anything, the "White" appearance is strongest in the Maoris of New Zealand, who are well bearded and look like nothing so much as a brunet European. (Polynesians do not at all resemble American Indians, which is a reason I doubt that the Indians are in fact a mixture of White and Mongoloid, with a little Negroid, as often claimed. I am using a strange kind of reasoning here: judging Indians by something assumed to be known about Polynesians, which is not really known at all. I can only say that much of racial anthropology still consists of educated hunches.)

The traditional theory of Polynesian origins involves a migration from the west, beginning on the mainland of Asia, anywhere from China to India, or from Indonesia. Their languages are closely related, as with the Eskimos; their physical type is different from that of their Melanesian neighbors; their cultural and religious ideas are at various points striking and distinctive. This might argue that, once they had mastered the art of blue-water voyaging, they set out on a great eastward migration from an undiscovered home, passing through island groups already taken up by earlier settlers, reaching the area of Samoa and Tonga and fanning out from there.

But if this is so, the evidence for it has never been discovered. There is nobody of a real Polynesian appearance in all the regions of Asia; only a few areas where physique recalls them a little. Of course, their homeland might since have been occupied by other peoples; any remaining "Polynesians" might thus have become mixed beyond recognition, perhaps by being mongolized. Or else the Polynesians themselves changed somewhat (growing larger in size) due to their new environment. It is quite likely that eventual affinities with ancient peoples of Japan or the China coast may be found. Japan evidently has some kind of a White element, in the present Japanese population, aside from the Ainu. Formosan aborigines have certain likenesses, physical and cultural, with Polynesians, though this is not strong. In Southeast Asia also, we may find, cropping up in certain individuals, suggestions of a White type, lacking Mongoloid fold and features entirely, looking both White and Polynesian in a very general way.

But all this yields nothing very specific. Polynesian gardening derives from the old Neolithic garden culture based on the pre-rice plants of Southeast Asia, which is shared by Melanesians and the most primitive Indonesians. Other Polynesian traits, like tattooing and bark cloth, seem to belong to this same culture layer. In fact, there is nothing positive to demonstrate that the Polynesians, as we see them now, did not originate in the Central Pacific itself. That is what language students now suggest: Polynesian seems to be related to a particular subgroup of Melanesian languages of the general Fiji region, recalling the fact that the widespread Bantu languages of Central Africa similarly appear to belong to a small subgroup within the much more varied Niger-Congo stock in Africa. Now, Melanesia was certainly occupied, even in the east, before 1000 B.C., possibly much before. And it must be remembered that language and physical type are not reliable guides to one another, certainly not in the Pacific. Therefore, it is the physical type of the Polynesians which remains unexplained. If this could be placed, a thousand years B.C., somewhere in the region of Fiji or the New

Hebrides, then the phenomenon of the later Polynesians, spreading their uniform physique, language, and culture over their wide domain, following on the achievement of expert navigation and big canoes, is easy to comprehend. We remain baffled largely by Polynesian physique. Is it really based on a White ancestry? Is it possible that this is an illusion, produced by a parentage which is partly Mongoloid, coming down from the Northwest, and partly Melanesian or Australian, since this latter element is today present in the region, in New Caledonia?

Little Negroes in the East

We have peeled off the top layer of people in Polynesia and found nothing below. Peeling in the large region of Southeast Asia and Indonesia is more rewarding. Possibly the Polynesians represent something from the middle of the pile in Indonesia. It is a region, running northward to Formosa, where new arrivals have been stacking up for perhaps a million years. Recent times have seen the coming of Americans, Portuguese, Spanish, British, and Dutch. Earlier, while the Polynesians were spreading through Polynesia, Southeast Asia was getting invaders from India, and waves of the Chinese who form such a powerful part of the population today. Removing all these historic layers of two thousand years, we find ourselves at the top of a series of descending steps of culture going down to a simple "Neolithic" base, preceding the use of paddy rice and woven cloth, and constituting the kind of thing the Polynesians carried with them on their voyages. The Malays and proto-Malays associated with these steps are a hodgepodge of Mongoloids, unspecialized Mongoloids, and near-Whites who make up the older people from North Burma to Celebes and the Philippines.

Then, under the whole thing, we find the Negritos. They are pygmy Negroids, with all the typical traits of the Negro stock: dark skin, broad noses, woolly hair, full lips, and so on. They differ in appearance somewhat from the African Pygmies; or rather I should prefer to say the Pygmies differ from the Negritos, because to my eye the Negritos are more faithful mimics of full-sized Negroes. I see no good reason to consider them as anything but eastern representatives of the same group. But there is strong disagreement on the point. Their proportions of several blood-group systems are quite different from those of African Negroes or Pygmies, and much more like the proportions of other peoples in the areas they occupy in the east. There are therefore two diametrically opposed explanations. If you believe that blood-group proportions stay the same over many generations, while skin, hair, and body size change more readily, then the Negritos have become what they are through natural selection working in a forest environment upon full-sized Mongoloid or Negroid inhabitants of this or that region. If on the other hand you think size, hair, and skin change more slowly, and that blood groups are more readily acted upon by selection (for disease or other causes), then the Negritos are members of one population, differing in different places (including Africa) in blood groups because different blood-group combinations may have special advantages in different areas.

There is no reason, certainly, to doubt their importance in this part of the world. They are found in the mountains of the Malay Peninsula, where they are called the Semangs. They are widespread in the Philippines, under the name of Aeta. And they were, until our own times, the only inhabitants of the Andaman Islands in the Bay of Bengal, because the natives here had the good sense to destroy anyone who landed or got shipwrecked on their shores.

These are the places with living populations of real Negritos. Elsewhere they suggest their presence in mixture only, through small size, curly hair, and suggestions in the face; indeed, they may have combined with lighter-skinned people coming in after them, in greater amounts and more localities than we think. And one other racial element can be detected, though faintly. Individuals suggesting the Australian natives may be seen in the Timor Archipelago, on Indonesia's southeast border. Otherwise, the only sign of the Australian type is found in the Wadjak skulls, brought back from Java by Dubois and thought possibly to date from the late Pleistocene. Unfortunately, the past of this whole vital territory is still only slightly known for the important period since the end of the Ice Age, and human bones are almost lacking. We know only that both Negritos and Australians must have been early inhabitants of the region, from the evidence above, which is good enough, and from the fact that they had to go through Indonesia to get to Melanesia and Australia.

Melanesia: Islands of the Black

You can almost jump the various straits between islands in Indonesia. At times during the Pleistocene, when the sea fell, they were largely joined to one another and to Asia, in any case. But getting to Melanesia and Australia means crossing open water. For they lie on the other side of "Wallace's line," with a very different animal life, including marsupials, which shows they have long been totally separate. Once in Melanesia, water distances begin to open up still more, as one goes from the very large island of New Guinea (the interior natives know nothing about seas) out toward the Solomons, the New Hebrides, and finally New Caledonia to the south and Fiji to the east. This makes a central track out into the Pacific. To follow it demands considerable navigating ability, though not that which is needed to overcome the distances in Polynesia. And the people have a gardening economy which, like that of the Polynesians, goes back to an older stratum of life in Southeast Asia.

Melanesia ("Black Islands") is inhabited by peoples, dark-skinned and superficially Negroid, who are nevertheless so varied physically, and so graded by the arrangement of islands, as to make a wonderful racial layer cake. It would tell us volumes about the racial history of man altogether, if we could analyze it to our satisfaction and get the layers straight. But this is almost as hard as getting the eggs, flour, and sugar out of it again. The people run a gamut in size from the tall and handsome Fijians to some very small people (Negritos?) of the mountains of New Guinea. In Fiji the people are outwardly Negroid, in color, frizzliness of hair, and so on, including a considerable breadth of nose; however, in the bone below, as in many aspects of their features, they are Polynesian in size and form, and specifically close to their neighbors the Samoans and Tongans, with whom they have evidently long intermingled.

In the Solomons group, and the New Hebrides and the Bismarck Archipelago (New Ireland and New Britain), the appearance of people seems basically Negroid, though the hair is bushy rather than woolly. People are of medium size. In much of New Guinea, coastal and interior, it is clear that the population is a mixture of the Australian and Negrito strains: many men are small-bodied, with coarse faces, frequent beards, heavy brows, receding foreheads, and narrow, long heads. Finally, in northern New Britain especially, and in New Caledonia, there is another type. It is larger-bodied, and of Negroid appearance, but here the skull below the skin is much more Australian than African in appearance.

This is only an outline, and Melanesia, though it has had much attention, deserves more still. We can pick off the top layers easily: some regions have been strongly affected by settlements or contacts from Micronesia on the north and Polynesia on the east, so that a number of small and isolated islands are hardly Melanesian at all. And the last settlers on the New Guinea coast have a considerable dose of Indonesian blood, showing in light skin and straighter hair. Also, there is a group of Melanesian languages, spoken largely by coastal peoples, which belongs to the Austronesian family. But in many inland areas the languages are non-Austronesian, a totally different lot of unrelated or loosely related tongues possibly having affinities with those of native Australia. All this makes it plain that anything having to do with the Polynesians, or the Mongoloid Indonesians, or their languages, is late. The Melanesians stem from a definitely older dark-skinned population. Possibly they partook in the original "Neolithic" of Southeast Asia, but they settled in Melanesia before the arrival, or the formation, of the Austronesian language family, and before the coming to Indonesia of the first Mongoloids, specialized or unspecialized. Archaeology in New Guinea is only just beginning, but already it is known to have been occupied about 10,000 B.C. at the latest, and in fact it must have been reached at least as early as Australia.

The lowest layers, then, are evidently the types of the Negrito and the native Australian. Were there also true Negroes? There are tribes who seem to be such in Melanesia, but there are no traces whatever of Negroes (in contrast to the Negritos) in Indonesia, nor indeed anywhere westward until you get to Africa. This undeniable fact has convinced some of my colleagues that the Oceanic "Negroes" are synthetic—that they are not Negroes at all, but either a mixture of Negritos and Australoids (which the eastern Melanesians do not actually look like), or else more or less pure Negritos who have become enlarged again. In other words, they are the world's largest pygmies.

Aborigines of Australia

Certainly there are no Negroes in Australia. There are apparently Negritos in the rain forest of Queensland, near New Guinea, discovered long ago but only brought to general attention recently by Norman Tindale and Joseph Birdsell. The rest of the continent was occupied by the Australian aboriginals proper, primitive men with a primitive hunting culture, lacking even the bows and arrows of the Negritos of other parts. They are dark-skinned but hairy, with thick, ridged, poorly filled skulls and heavy, though fully sapiens, brow ridges; and with broad noses, short projecting faces, large teeth, and receding chins. In every way they conform to a picture of *Homo sapiens* at his most backward, before recent racial specializations and before a final lightening of brows, reduction of teeth, and expansion of brain.

Dr. Birdsell, who knows these people thoroughly, believes they are actually composed of two strains, equally primitive. One is predominant in the north, and he calls it "Carpentarian," from the Gulf of Carpentaria: this is the essential Australian, tall, dark, less hairy, and very lanky. The other, concentrated in the south, is fleshier and stockier, very hairy, and not so very dark; and Birdsell believes it is an antique White strain, related to the Ainu, and derived from North

China or Manchuria. Here, once again, we have a theory of origin by a mixture of diverse strains, though in this case with more justification, since one man was able to examine a whole continent personally, and make a real distinction between populations.

I think the theory remains to be demonstrated conclusively. The distinctions Birdsell finds are not reflected in the skull, nor in the blood types; and there remains the possibility that the Australian population has been on that continent long enough to become physically adapted to different climates, a possibility to which Dr. Birdsell himself is very much alive. That is to say, the stockiness, hairiness, and lighter color of the south might be related to the chilly temperate climate of that part, while the extreme lankiness of the Carpentarians might, as Coon and Birdsell have suggested, be another case where such a body form, as in the Sahara and the Sudan, has been emphasized by natural selection, in the hot, sunny, plains and deserts of the north. So the question is open, and the open part of it, as we shall see, is whether Australia, and the whole region, was invaded by an ancient and primitive White stock, via the China coast, or not.

At any rate, the general Australian form is the one element which can be traced back into the past. Several skulls expressing it have been found in Australia, which clearly or probably are of Pleistocene age. The most important is the Keilor skull, found embedded in the Keilor terrace of the Maribyrnong River near Melbourne. There have been arguments about this terrace; it was once claimed to be of Third Interglacial date. It is, however, clearly one which was built up in the late Pleistocene when the sea was lower. At the river's mouth it dips under the present flood plain, whereas the later terrace flattens out at water level. Also, in the region of the skull there have been found hearths at various levels, with charcoal and charred meat bones, and C14 dates the earliest of these back to 16,000 B.C., with the skull level being approximately 13,000 B.C.

The skull itself is entirely Australian in appearance, though of large size. There have also been arguments as to whether it actually belongs in the terrace or was intrusive, but the detailed evidence entirely supports its position, and another skeleton was found in 1965 in the same terrace, though higher up. Dr. Edmund Gill of Melbourne, who has studied this case in detail, has also reviewed a few other signs of equivalent antiquity for Australian aborigines. In addition, a recent excavation in the Koonalda Cave in South Australia has revealed a deep series of human implements; the oldest radiocarbon dates are over 16,000 B.C. but the tools continue down beyond this to a point which suggests a total age of 30,000 years.

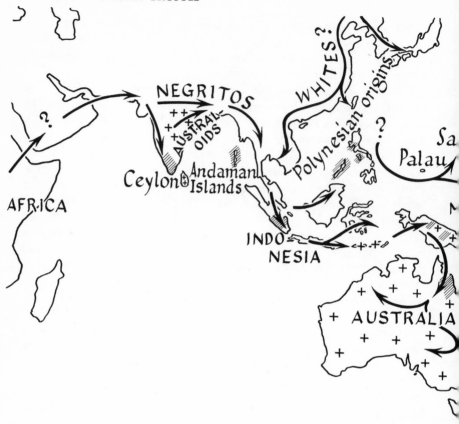

A map of some probable prehistoric migrations in Asia and Oceania. Areas showing signs of an Australian-like element are shown by crosses; those with Negritos by shading.

Another supposedly Pleistocene skull is a frontal bone from Aitape on the north coast of New Guinea, which does not appear to differ from present-day natives of the region in general, or possibly from the Australian aboriginals. In any case its finder, after revisiting the site, recently reported a C14 date of only about 3000 B.C. Then there are the well-known Wadjak skulls of Java. Thus we have heady footprints leading back to Asia's doorstep, and demonstrating an age for Australia's native population which is greater, from what we know today, than that of the first American Indians, and may even compare with *Homo sapiens* in Europe.

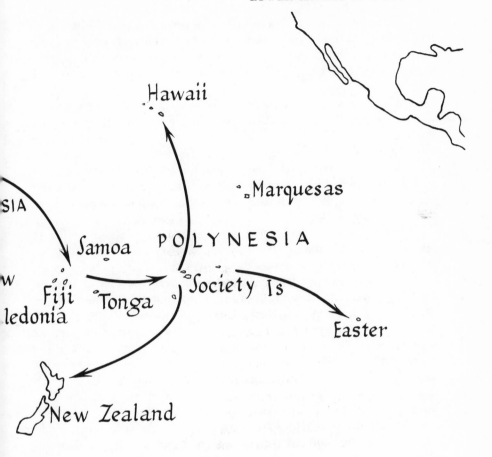

Lower Layers in India

Pursuing the dark-skinned peoples westward, we come to India. Here, we have seen, the great bulk of India's people are dark-skinned Whites of the western, Mediterranean variety. But far down, in the lowest castes and in the still-wild tribes, familiar faces appear: Negritos and Australians. The latter type is evident, much refined, among various of the Dravidians, who speak languages of this non-Indo-European family. It occurs again, also in delicate form, in the vanishing primitive Veddas of Ceylon.

Elsewhere, among other backward hill tribes, there are many groups marked by very short stature, dark skin, bushy hair, and broad noses who, though not recognizable as pure Negritos, are clearly their mixed descendants. These descendants even look something like other adulterated Negritos, in Malaya or the Philippines. So in India, as in Southeast Asia, Indonesia, Melanesia, and Australia, we have insistent signs of former populations both of the Australian and of the Negrito varieties, without, possibly excepting Melanesia, any vestige of true Negro.

Evidently, then, both of these racial forms, Negrito and Australian, were once established in southern Asia, and went from there out into the Southeast Pacific. Dr. Birdsell, from his studies, has reconstructed this history on a hypothetical basis, as follows. One can raise objections along the line, of course, but anyone undertaking such a hypothesis is obliged to go in for such sweeping guesswork in the first place that we might as well pass over most of the objections, sit back, and enjoy ourselves.

Birdsell thinks that the Negritos are particularly adapted for life in thick rain forests, and have always been associated with them, as they are today. He believes they were the main population of Southeast Asia in the late Pleistocene, and were the first of modern men to go out into the Pacific itself, supposing this to be early in the Fourth Glacial phase. Next came the primitive White element, down the Asiatic coast from North China, walking dry-shod like its predecessors onto what are now the Indonesian islands. This is the questionable element, since the one strongly indicated source of Australians is India, not north Asia. However, given the Ainus, there is nothing absolutely unlikely about it. Finally there came the Carpentarian strain, from India. Birdsell suggests that this lanky, primitive, straight-haired type could exist in south Asia, especially India, along with the Negritos, without the two mingling and blurring as they did in Melanesia, because they occupied different habitats: the Negritos, the rain forests; the Carpentarians the hot, dry plains of the Indian Peninsula. He believes the latter developed their hot country lankiness as an adaptation here, not in Australia itself.

This hypothesis has the virtue of being clear and straightforward. Birdsell presented it some time ago, and in the light of later information I would suggest an alternative. In the first place, the early skulls are of the Australoid type, not the Negrito. Secondly, I have already suggested that Solo Man may have had an influence on *Homo sapiens*, and one or two of the apparently old Australian skulls (not Keilor) are exceedingly heavy-browed and primitive.

Now the Solo skulls were found in Java, and we do not know whether the Australoid-looking people of India may represent his genetic influence, since we do not know how he was actually distributed. But Java is on the route to the Pacific, unavoidable for any late Pleistocene travelers with a primitive culture. If *Homo sapiens* came here in the form of the Niah Cave boy, this might have resulted in a variety of populations, some mixed with Solo, the whole lot ranging in nature from Negrito to Australoid. In such a case, for the Pacific itself it would make little sense to argue which arrived first. The situation would parallel that other hypothetical one in the west, in which an immigrant *Homo sapiens* might have mixed more with Neanderthals in the Near East than in Western Europe.

The Negro Puzzle Again

There is another problem of the dark-skinned races, one I consider the knottiest we face. Was there ever a Negro east of the Horn of Africa (before slave days), in all the tropics? Or have Negroes of the basic kind been confined, as the African evidence suggests, to the southern border of the Sahara in Africa, until their recent expansion east and south? The theory of Negritos grown up again to full size would allow for the "Negroes" of Melanesia. But that does not help us out of the hole. How do we get Negritos into the Pacific from Africa, or vice versa? For it is plain as the nose on your face that the Negritos are intimately related to fully developed Negroes—a specialized kind of man—in skin, hair form, nose shape, and so on. The Negritos are really all similar and must have had a common origin. And Negritos and Negroes cannot have appeared on separate continents; they too must have had a common origin. If Negritos developed as a diminished, forest form of the Negro, this must have been in a forest near which dwelt Negroes as we know them.

Was this in Africa? The ideal place, we have seen, is the forest border below the Sudan, the open belt running across Africa south of the Sahara. Border and belt may have shifted north or south with Pleistocene climates, of course. May we guess that the Negritos spread themselves right through the tropics, as a relatively heavy population, all the way to New Guinea and Australia; while the full-sized Negroes did *not* spread, for the reason that their old environment—open parklands—did *not* extend to the east? There are difficulties, right away. We need, at some time past, a wet forest right across the bottom of now-arid Arabia and the exceedingly barren, deserty shore of Baluchistan, to connect Africa and India, to let the Pygmies pass. And we learn only of dim suggestions of Negritos—no Negroes—in southeast Arabia. The only clear dark-skinned element not traceable to slaves is an Australian look in some of the people of the Hadramaut, southern Arabia, a look which Birdsell thinks represents a westward drift of Carpentarians from India.

Here the strait of Bab el Mandeb becomes important, where southern Arabia almost touches Africa. Though not wide, nor a formidable distance even for primitive man, the strait has probably not been dry land at any time during the Pleistocene, and the currents passing through it are strong. At any rate, the Arabian side, judging by archaeology, was no busy thoroughfare of early *Homo sapiens* or his predecessors. Miss Caton-Thompson found it, in fact, to be a dead end, a place where stonework stagnated in the later Paleolithic, in contrast to the liveliness and activity across the way in East Africa and the Horn. Only in the Mesolithic or Neolithic does this spot seem to have opened one eye, as a couple of African tool types make their appearance here. Therefore, this all-important part of Arabia, leading to the whole east, was in human terms much further away from Africa than it appears to be on a map. It does not seem to have been a bridge, thronged with Negroids and Negritos, in likely parts of the late Pleistocene. And we have already seen that by Upper Paleolithic times, at least, East Africa was in the hands of non-Negro people. This situation, at the Bab el Mandeb strait, is strange. The fact is that almost nothing is known about past climates and past habitation in this whole very suggestive zone, connecting India and Africa.

So we are left with a major dilemma. The Negroes themselves are bad enough: having to explain the connection between the African and Oceanic varieties. The worst part is getting the Negritos across a crucial crossing by any method but wishful thinking. I may have emphasized the difficulty of understanding the Negro stock, imitating the careless floor painter who paints himself into a corner of the room. We have painted the Negroes into West Africa, and then tried to connect them with Negritos on the other side of the world. But this is not dramatic effect; the puzzle is there. If we knew how the Negritos spread, and when, we might know the age of the whole Negro race stock; if we knew that in turn, we might begin to understand more about the age of *Homo sapiens* and the history of his other races.

23. LOOKING BACKWARD

In THIS BOOK we have looked at the record of our species. It is good to know as much as we know, but it is good to remember how much we do not know. How incomplete the fossils are is not always clear to us. For example, we know about living gibbons, lithe, long-armed and agile. We have fossil "gibbons," but their arms are not so long; we would be quite ignorant of an extraordinary ape if *Hylobates* had died out in the Pleistocene. As for the equally extraordinary orang, his only fossils are teeth. What would we know of that body, that skull, those arms and legs, if we could not see *Pongo* today? And the same applies to Negritos. Seen alive, they are important evidence of human history; without the living, we would have no clear evidence they had existed.

This is the lesson we have to apply. We do not even know what is missing. And so we will do well not to try filling blank spots with sheer guesswork. Already, I think, you will have seen that dating and understanding the more difficult fossils is something like lassoing an invisible calf with an imaginary lariat while riding an effort of will at a full gallop. In spite of all the evidence we have reviewed, we can move with but small confidence against the main problems of the human past.

We may, of course, begin in historic times, and work back along the lines traced in the last few chapters. We can with some assurance follow the Indians back to Asia, to become one with the earlier Mongoloids. We can move the later Mongoloids out of the southern parts of the Far East, toward the north, and push them back to a time when they become largely de-Mongolized; that is, they in turn become one with the American Indians. We can follow the Cro Magnons backward out of Europe, though unfortunately we do not know where to follow them to; perhaps into Siberia or the Far East, perhaps into India. And we can surely trace the natives of Australia back to Southeast Asia and India.

The Bushmen of South Africa backtrack to East Africa; that is to say, in the general direction of Asia. But the African Negroes, we have seen, backtrack to West Africa. Thus we might reconstruct a general spreading of the main racial types outward from Asia, except for the Negroes. I think it is better to confess ignorance rather than to argue and stretch points. However, there is this to be said. The Negritos of the Far East must have come out of Asia, probably from India. And they clearly represent a major spread, over land or narrow sea channels. Furthermore, they coincide too closely with the Negroes generally, in all their traits, to have developed by a kind of extreme parallel evolution. So there must be a connection, with Negritos apparently spreading all the way from Africa through a then-hospitable tropical forest belt, after the development of the Negro-Negrito stem from some earlier parent (perhaps in common with the Bushmen). Of course, it remains possible that both Negroes and Negritos entered Africa from Asia already developed.

Migrations and Changes

There is another thing to bear in mind. We need not imagine that all events happened at the same pace. Some racial distinctions came into being slowly: we can be sure that the Whites and American Indians existed long ago. But the strongly specialized (flat-faced) Mongoloids are very likely more recent (middle Würm?), and it is possible that the Negroes also are not of massive antiquity. (I am afraid I am being appropriately vague.)

Also, the spreads and movements of these people were not necessarily slow in the extreme. We think of the American Indians gradually penetrating throughout the Western Hemisphere, probably a fair view for Paleolithic hunters in a highly varied environment. But the Upper Paleolithic people seem to have taken command of Europe in the space of a few thousand years. And Dr. Birdsell did a careful pencil-and-paper analysis of his information on Australian tribes (rate of natural increase, tribal territories, and so forth) and concluded that the first invaders, even if of a most non-adventurous turn of mind, might have occupied that whole continent in about two thousand years. So the factor of spread is not much use in judging time.

We know already that the Bantu Negroes overran central and southern Africa in a few thousand years. And all the evidence suggests that the late, specialized Mongoloids had a similar explosion out of northern Asia, probably in the last few thousand years before the Christian era. So the picture of racial distribution at the time of Columbus may be viewed with suspicion, rather than used as a map of mankind's ancient racial homes.

We may be permitted to think of an early spread of certain general forms of *Homo sapiens:* the Whites, the American Indians, the Australians, and perhaps a parent Negro-Bush stock in Africa. Later there were radical shifts, as the Mongoloids expanded in Asia, the Negroes in Africa, the Polynesians in the Pacific and, finally, the Europeans all over the world. In such a light, a Negrito expansion through the tropical forests need not have been old or slow. All we need to explain it, and break the impasse, is more suitable connections between Africa and Asia.

The Trail is Lost

To resume our backward journey. Let us take the late Mongoloids as the most recent form of man. Rub them out. We are left with ancient American Indians (in Asia) and Whites, probably becoming more and more alike as we go back to 35,000 B.C. and beyond. We may guess that Negroes and Bushmen were doing the same in Africa. If I were to suggest that, still further back, the oldest White-Indian men (earlier than any we actually know) would begin to look more like the Australian aborigines, then I would be giving a fine example of how often hypothesis is used in place of fact in racial history. And yet the possibility of the Australians being an extremely archaic brand of "White" has been suggested by my colleagues often enough and with justice. I would like to go further and bring the already highly hypothetical Negro-Bush strain into the picture, but they are so different (even the heavy-browed Florisbad skull is not very Australian-like) from the others that this would really be stretching things. In addition we have no real idea how much we may allow for the picking up of genes from other kinds of man, such as Solo.

However, it seems fair to say from the evidence, until it is upset, that we can vaguely trace the ancestors of recent races moving outward from Asia. We can also see them going through late stages of specializing in some places: Mongoloids, Bushmen, Negroes, Negritos, White blonds and roundheads. And there were late movements: Negroes virtually blotting out Bushmen, and Mongoloids doing the same to Whites in eastern Asia.

But the backward journey is stopped abruptly at about 35,000 B.C. Just as we might actually be finding some of the connections to which the threads of evidence seem to be leading, we are frustrated. The evidence itself disappears. Back now in the first part of the Würm glaciation, we find ourselves without remains of *Homo sapiens* which can help us. Except for Rhodesian Man in the far south, and the Solo skulls in the far southeast, we have only Neanderthals. At this time they seem to be distributed throughout the northwest and into south central Asia. They appear to have covered, that is to say, the whole ice-free west, except where sapient man came pushing into Palestine, giving rise to the Skhūl people. The Neanderthals may even have cut Africa off from Asia, an important point.

Beyond and before this Neanderthal occupation we drop off to a still poorer level of information. The human remains are few and piecemeal, and therefore quite incompetent to answer most of the problems they raise. And the main one is still the birth of *Homo sapiens*. Now, we have seen that the argument is not as sharply drawn as once. Probably our modern species is neither tightly bound up with Neanderthals, nor so ancient as to let us expect that the Swanscombe Woman's forehead would have looked like one of ours. Obviously, sapient man developed from a more primitive ancestor, probably toward the middle of the Upper Pleistocene; that is to say, our forebears gradually became more "sapiens-like." And the evidence does seem to show that the Neanderthal line became more extreme, or more Neanderthal-like.

Now, the Neanderthal strain occupied a large territory in the Upper Pleistocene. If the sapiens line were to remain different from the Neanderthals and others, and especially if it were to become further differentiated into races, a similarly large tract is demanded for this line. On genetical grounds this is a requirement of the hypothesis. Otherwise the strain would have been swamped out, by contact with others over long periods of the Pleistocene; also, it could not have supplied representatives from time to time, like the people in the Fontéchevade cave, or the Kanjera men in East Africa.

But we do not know where this area was. The cupboard is bare of evidence. I will end here with a synopsis of man's history, as it seems to stand out from all we have reviewed. I wish I might see how such a history will be written a century from now.

Short History of Man

LATE TERTIARY From the middle of the Tertiary onward there existed small hominids, slender little ape-like creatures. They were almost certainly arboreal, skillful in the trees, and good brachiators; at the same time they did not become strongly specialized, top-heavy, and long in the arm. They always retained within the perimeter of their evolutionary possibilities that of standing erect and moving readily around in that posture. At the time of *Ramapithecus,* in the earlier Pliocene, these ancestors were short-faced, with short canine teeth. Though this might have been a disadvantage in ground life, in some suitable area or areas their ability to stand erect became so rewarding that strong adaptation for such a gait took place, probably rapidly. That is, the opposable toe was lost so that the muscles of the leg could work on a stiff arched foot, and effectively push the running animal forward. The gluteus muscle of the buttock was repositioned somewhat by changes in the pelvis, adding power to the leg at the hip joint. Holding the body erect was eased by a curving back of the lower spine and a broadening and strengthening of its vertebrae. The beginnings of such trends in the pelvis, spine, and trunk, however, were old, and had been a help in the original tendency to stand or walk erect.

LATE PLIOCENE, LOWER PLEISTOCENE   These transformed animals, now fully erect, were widespread in the Old World by the end of the Tertiary, appearing in the Lower Pleistocene as the australopithecines. Their brains were small and their jaws were powerful, but it was the molars, not the anterior teeth, which were large. There may have been minor imperfections in gait and use of hands compared to later man, but feet seem to have been fully hominid, and the basic hominid separation of function in arms and legs was clearly established. Two distinct lines of australopithecine already existed, and it is likely that at least one of them was using tools readily, in the form of animal bones and doubtless appropriately shaped random stones.

LATE LOWER AND MIDDLE PLEISTOCENE   The two australopithecine lines continued, with *Australopithecus* beginning actually to make patterned tools in stone. Involving a more highly controlled use of the hands, tool-making swung open the gate for brain growth and development. Both forms continued into the Middle Pleistocene: *Australopithecus* increased in body size and to some degree in brain size, undergoing a diminution of the jaw and molar teeth. *Paranthropus*, unmodified from the Lower Pleistocene, became extinct. *Australopithecus* reached the grade of *Homo erectus,* and was present in Africa and Asia, also apparently entering Europe for the first time.

LATE MIDDLE AND EARLY UPPER PLEISTOCENE   By the Second Interglacial a relatively modern brain case, of larger size and lighter construction compared to *Homo erectus,* existed in Europe, indicating steady evolution toward *Homo sapiens.* Otherwise these are the dark ages, yielding only the Kanjera fragments of Africa and the Fontéchevade skulls of Europe, as well as a very few early Neanderthals. Yet this period must have had in it the parents of the Neanderthals, of Rhodesian Man, of the Solo tribe, and probably of *Homo sapiens sapiens.* There was probably increasing diversity in human populations, at least to a small extent. The Solo men, remaining fairly close to *Homo erectus* of the Middle Pleistocene, must have coexisted with much more advanced forms of man in the west. Where Rhodesian Man fits in, we really cannot say today.

LATE UPPER PLEISTOCENE: THIRD INTERGLACIAL AND FOURTH GLACIAL Now the story becomes more familiar, with two clear populations, the Neanderthals and the sapiens men who succeeded them. The Neanderthal line, settling in Europe during the Third Interglacial, diverged toward an extreme form as time went on. In late times, at least, it also occupied Central Asia and North Africa. It did not, apparently, move down into the rest of Africa (though there is a Neanderthal-like jaw from Ethiopia); perhaps there was a Rhodesian population in possession.

Perhaps also there was a region of sapiens population in Asia, with a dark-skinned racial group in India, and another related group, north of the Himalayas, incipient for Whites and early Mongoloids. This is pure supposition; it is more or less what we are obliged to imagine. At any rate, after about 35,000 B.C. we begin to see *Homo sapiens* widely spread in the Old World, and entering the New World as well. Asia was the source of the men who went into the Americas and the Pacific. In the west the new men entered Europe; perhaps, in the early stages, the advance guard mingled with older types of man to produce what appear to be intermediate forms: mixing with the Neanderthals at Mount Carmel in Palestine, with the Rhodesians at Florisbad in South Africa, and with Solo Man in Southeast Asia or Indonesia. All this is less clear, and hypothetical in the extreme. But both Neanderthals and Rhodesians accepted their fate and vanished.

The formation of races of later times would not have been due to any single factor, but to a mingling of many. I believe *Homo sapiens* to be a generally unified and uniform stock of man, not the accidental result of parallel evolution everywhere, as Weidenreich held. But this does not mean his coming out of a single cave, forming several very distinct racial types in a small area, and then going out to conquer the earth. Rather, it implies a general revolution over a rather wide area, with no perfect homogeneity within the stock at any time. It implies physical traits evolving here and there, some of the new traits being passed around widely, some less widely. That is, some segments changed more radically from earlier types, some less so. It implies differentiation due partly to isolation, partly to climate, over the same wide area. Probably at certain times in the later Pleistocene, natural selection in north and south worked strongly in different directions. It suggests migrations outward from the main area, or even a change of the main area. Such migrations need not have been during any single period, and some might have been earlier than we know; perhaps the appearance given by 35,000 B.C. as a great turning point is exaggerated. It certainly implies considerable further differentiation and adaptation among racial groups, as they move into new places and climates, and also as they mix with one another, or with other sapiens men who went there earlier, or with men we would call non-sapiens.

These are all ideas which are sound in the light of what we know of the evolution of races and species in animals generally. They are also reasons why it would be infinitely difficult to judge what happened simply by looking into the faces of men now living in all the corners of the world. This will help, as will testing their blood and studying them in every possible way. So will an ever more precise knowledge of how evolution takes place, in man or any animal. But the story of what really happened lies in bones and fragments of bones still hidden in the ground. Year after year we must wait, look, and have luck.

24. HOW TO BE HUMAN

"WHEN I consider Thy heavens the work of Thy fingers," says the Eighth Psalm, "What is man, that Thou art mindful of him? . . . Thou hast put all things under his feet: All sheep and oxen . . . the fowl of the air, and the fish of the sea . . . O Lord our Lord, how excellent is Thy name in all the earth!"

How excellent! David, extolling the uniqueness of man, might have extended more appreciation to the rest of nature. We know now, better than the Psalmist knew, the meaning of the animals under man's feet. We know how slow was our coming, how long our preparation. We know, through millions of years, what powerful forces brought us out. We see what boons we had in skeletons, jaws, limbs, warm blood. Homely things, but with them any mammal is a testament of evolutionary creation. Add fingers and acute eyes, and you have something like a monkey. Add true hands and legs and you have the beginnings of a man. Then natural selection made our brains, and everything we do with them.

All this came gradually, in due course. Each patient step made possible the next. Each step gave rise to hundreds of kinds of successful animals, perfect in their own ways. Man himself could only appear when a very high organization had been attained. For hands and a big brain would not have made a fish human; they would only have made a fish impossible. Man's own trail, among the many trails in evolution, was well defined: he had to be a mammal and he had to be a primate.

Was he inevitable? Mankind long thought so, and Genesis entertains no doubt that the world was made for us. Being human, we find it hard to see things any other way. Not long ago it was shocking to ask whether man had evolved from other animals. It is doubtless equally shocking to ask whether man arrived simply as a matter of luck.

Actually it would be a futile question. One cannot pass judgment on such a thing without going straight on to the origins of the universe. It does not matter here what your religious views are, for man must be looked on as an extraordinary achievement of design and organization.

The universe itself is built on laws of matter. These are the foundation for laws of life; and on such a basis, we know, man at last came on the scene. He was not there to begin with, and he took a long time coming. But he came, and he expresses all the fullness of the possibilities of the organization of life as we understand it. How much of this is "chance"? There is no present answer.

I am not really trying to be profound, and I have only a few pages left in any case. Talking about chance, I am merely wondering if man was forced to take the shape he did. If we had it to do over again, would we choose all the same forks in the road, or would we turn out differently? Perhaps science fiction has the answer.

Doubtless there are other "men" in space. Led by the astronomers, we now face possibilities of life elsewhere at which the mind boggles. We know there are many billions of stars in our own particular galaxy, the Milky Way. Galaxies like ours are grouped in clusters, thousands to a cluster, and such clusters go on and on, out of reach of the telescopes, by the hundreds of millions. Planets to live on? Dr. Harlow Shapley has figured it out roughly.[1] Not many stars have planets around them, he thinks; perhaps one in a million. As in our own system, few planets are of the right kind, with water, days and nights, favorable temperature and chemicals, and so on. Perhaps one good place in about a trillion stars, all told. But these are really splendid odds, considering the number of stars; Dr. Shapley ends by guessing that there are about a hundred million worlds where higher life has actually been forged by evolution. "We are not alone." Intelligent beings abound in the universe, most of them far older than we ourselves.

We can try to imagine what such people are like. Here we get little help from the comic books, which only show us flying saucers, manned by flabby little web-footed goblins with knobs on their heads. We must be strictly scientific, starting from scratch and assuming nothing about the beings we are studying, except that they are "intelligent." But this at once means that they are "human," in the sense that they have culture, like ourselves: they communicate ideas to one another, and create things jointly. Otherwise intelligence means nothing. And we could never communicate with them, if they could not already communicate with each other.

Furthermore, we might just as well imagine them on a favorable world something like ours, in matters of temperature, gravity, some atmosphere and land surface, and so on, since it seems to be the kind most suitable for life. Very well. We have intelligent, communicating creatures, on a faraway Earth. Are they anything like us? I think they are.

[1] In *The Atlantic*, November 1953.

They might be considerably rearranged. They might "see" things we only "feel," like heat wave-lengths; or "feel" things we "hear," and so on. Their "bones," or whatever props them up, might be differently placed in relation to blood vessels and nerves. But they would have these things. Communicating, creating creatures must have motion—they could not be like trees, with little power to act and exert force. So they would have to be self-contained, moving about and getting their fuel like the animals of this world. They would need structure, and a nervous organization probably using electrical nerve impulses. They would need a liquid transportation system; we can hardly suppose that nourishment flows through their veins in the form of breakfast cereal. And so they must have begun their evolution, as we did ours, in a liquid medium, say water.

So much for raw material. What about design? Are the strangers round, or flat, or pointed? Do they smell through tail-fins and see through a radiator grill? The chances are excellent that they have a head end (which implies a tail end as well), because almost all the animals of this world which can move alertly and exert any real force are built on this same plan. It puts the senses where they will do the most good. And the main center of the nervous system is close by, so that sense impulses will not have to make a long journey aft to a brain in the rump. Therefore our men will have heads. And, like the more efficient of our own animals, they will doubtless do their eating at this end as well. So, if they are going to be intelligent, our distant cousins had better be plotted something like a vertebrate or an insect of our own vicinity.

But they will do well not to imitate insects, for many reasons. All the co-operation of insect life—warrior ants, worker bees—is printed on the nervous system of each single insect. They act without benefit of ideas, only from instinct. Their social "ideas" come from natural selection alone, not from thought. So intelligent creatures will have made a choice, early in evolution, of a nervous system which is more open to fresh impressions: a brain which can learn. Eventually such a brain will become large. Come to think, it will make quite a lump somewhere, probably in the head.

While we are roughing out shape, we might ask whether such a species will come in more than one form. Bees and ants do. And caterpillars turn into moths. Above all, the great majority of living things come in two sexes. It is one of nature's most popular ideas, and not for the first reason that will occur to you. Sex ensures a great plenitude of new gene combinations, different in each of the offspring, through the coming together of genes from two parents. This is one of the keystones of evolution, as you have seen. We on earth have long ago made all our arrangements on the basis of two sexes. Perhaps our extra-terrestrial equivalents have three sexes, like German nouns. Or more; who is to say? Certainly two is most likely. It is an almost universal rule here below, with no complaints.

We now have a Thing with one head and two sexes. (Two heads are *not* better than one; making up a single mind is more than most of us can do, as it is.) We had better assume that It goes on land. The water is far less promising as a medium for creation and communication, though perhaps not impossible. As for air, the birds have found that it does not work out well, if the goal is intelligence. Birds are beautiful but stupid, having been obliged to put their brain development largely in the service of co-ordination of movement, for flying.

Being on land, these men will have limbs as well as a head. They must have limbs, because they must have hands. If we can learn anything from our evolution, it is that we had to be able to *do* things to become human. And our whole struggle was the getting and freeing of hands to do them with. Surely, we would not have had large brains without them.

The hands will be better with fingers on them. There need not be five; perhaps a few more or less will serve. But you may have been struck by the fact that we have decidedly kept all five of the bunch handed down to us by *Seymouria* and his forefathers. So five seems like a good number, perhaps a minimum. Therefore look for plenty of fingers, on the ends of two arms. Two arms; not three, because the creatures should be symmetrical like us; and not four, because co-ordination would probably be too difficult for efficiency. Centipedes have to run their arms in teams.

Now for a big question. Will They be standing up and walking around like us? They would not look very human otherwise. But might they not have two hands and *four* legs, that is, three pairs of limbs? Insects have. Do we do anything well that a centaur could not do better? We are reasonably content with our own seating arrangements, but perhaps we are making the best of a bad job. You know already why we go around on only two legs: if we wanted hands to use, we had no choice.

The choice existed once, in the early fishes. But the lobe-fins and amphibians chose to keep only four limbs out of an original larger stock of fins. Unimaginative beasts, what was good enough for a bedstead was good enough for a labyrinthodont. And so these feckless ancestors nearly slammed the door on hands entirely, since later hand-users (or wing-users) among the vertebrates had to manage by balancing on the two remaining legs. Supposing that ancient vertebrates had found some simple use for an extra pair of forelimbs, like the insects, while they still had the chance. Then these forelimbs might have continued being sufficiently adaptive for evolution to hang onto, as their possessors came out on land. Had this happened, we might all have avoided the problems which turn up in the blueprints of bipeds. There might, in fact, have appeared on earth many intelligent, hand-using, four-footed animals. So I will lay a small bet that the first men from Outer Space will be neither bipeds nor quadrupeds, but bimanous quadrupedal hexapods. (I have just invented that last word, in the hope that it means "six limbs.")

Finally, will they be big or small? Who will make a nice pet for whom, when we finally meet? Here, of course, gravity would keep weight down. But, on this earth at least, an intelligent animal must not be too small. Its brain—or whatever it operates on—must be absolutely large. And there is no reason to suppose that the basic cells and fibers of the brain could be substantially smaller than the same things here, so there should be no saving of mass. Furthermore, small animals—the active, highly organized kind, like mammals—do not live as long as large ones, not long enough to afford them the luxury of behavior which is largely uninherited and must be learned very slowly. So other men should not be much less bulky than we are.

Perhaps they should be more so. We have not become bigger, ourselves, as we got brainier, and J. B. S. Haldane pointed out long ago the hazards of being too big. The giants in *Pilgrim's Progress*, or any story book giants, were amateurishly engineered. Being the same shape as ourselves, they would have collapsed in a heap, with broken thighs; their legs were not big enough to support their bulk. For, when an animal gets really large, its legs must become disproportionately thick and strong to keep up with its mass, its cubic content. This happens in elephants. Man, as a biped, is probably as big as is safe for him. Bipedal dinosaurs, it is true, got much larger, like *Tyrannosaurus*, but at the cost of being decidedly bottom-heavy, with great haunches and a fat tail. So the men of elsewhere, if bipeds, are probably no giants. But if they have four feet to hold them up, then they might well be as big as a horse, or larger, and still be both intelligent and maneuverable.

So, on the whole, perhaps mankind as represented by ourselves is a pretty good model for intelligent creatures. However, this does not tell us whether we had to happen at all. I have said what a "human" being might be like in other worlds than ours. But what about the chances of men coming into existence again, not elsewhere, but on this very planet? Supposing, in a moment of idiot progress, we really killed ourselves off. Would *Homo* rise again?

Man came from an australopithecine, which came in turn from some simpler hominid, perhaps like *Ramapithecus*. Those animals are gone;

man has competed them into the grave. There are still apes. They might do for a fresh start, but I strongly suspect they are too specialized, and too busy looking for fruit in the forest, to turn to freer use of hands. Monkeys? Just possibly, if something made it worth while for a species to stand up. The new men might then have tails. But, in fact, the monkeys have made no move to mimic the hominoids, or human ancestors, during about thirty-five million years.

No other higher mammals of this earth will serve. Horses, dogs, elephants, all are deeply committed to being what they are. The next try would have to come from a tree shrew, laboriously repeating all of primate history. And before little *Tupaia* could put forth progressive descendants now, the world would have to be swept clean of the kind of competition which might overwhelm them on the way up. This means: get rid of most higher mammals, above all, rats, cats, and monkeys.

If he fails us, we (or rather our carbon copies) are done for. The remaining links of progress are now missing links; the good chances are gone. The mammal-like reptiles gave out long ago; and getting something human from the specialized creatures in the next ranks is hopeless: birds, snakes, frogs. The fishes? Lobe-fins, with the makings of lungs and limbs, were put out of business eons ago by the ray-fins, who can never leave the sea. The main army of fishes has gone well past the fork that once led to the land. Only the lungfish remain, waiting in mud for the rain to come again, and the coelacanth, so deep in the ocean that he dies in shallow water.

We might need brand-new "vertebrates." Well, then, eradicate the fish, who rule the seas as we rule the land and who are not likely to stand aside while nature experiments with ridiculously crude forerunners of ostracoderms once more. Conceivably life would have to start afresh. In that case, wipe out everything that moves, to keep the necessary simple molecules from being eaten as they form. So all in all our hopes for repetition are not good, and we had better stay the hand that drops the bomb.

All this musing is not really science. I am taking it as a path to walk around our object, mankind, while we view his place in nature. We are inclined to swing back and forth between extremes in what we say about him. One moment he is a specklet in space and time, a nothing among millions of planets harboring life. The next, we are awed by his complexity of structure and his primacy on earth. The Psalmist, not too certain, seems to favor the second view, and I heartily agree, having no disposition to write about specklets. I hope this book does something toward putting man in perspective, for its moral is that our roots are long and deep.

Author's Note

I wrote an earlier book, *Mankind So Far,* with the same subject and a similar plan. A great deal has happened since. Important finds and facts have come to light: Piltdown Man and the australopithecines are only samples of the changes. Many things have been reconsidered, and opinions and understandings have shifted, certainly considerably in my own case. Accordingly, several years ago I asked my publishers to discontinue printing *Mankind So Far,* and I have written a new book to take its place. I have quoted a few adequate passages from the old one. But this is not a revised version; rather, it is a new book by a revised author.

In telling about the people who found fossil men, I have frequently been anecdotal but never inventive. I have made a particular effort to have these records as correct as I could make them, especially where the same episodes have been more romantically recounted in the past. In places I have used conversation as part of the narrative, but at the most this is reconstruction, never novelization. It represents what various people actually remember saying or hearing on these occasions. For example, I wrote in *Mankind So Far* that I had no idea what his mentors in Amsterdam said when Dubois threw up his job to go hunting missing links in the tropics. Eventually I was very kindly told what they said, by Dr. Antje Schreuder, who had herself for many years been Dubois' assistant and confidante.

My other debts are large. I have been learning from the writings and discussions of old friends and colleagues for years, and I trust them to recognize what I owe them. The following have given me direct help and advice at various points with the book itself: E. Mayr, H. L. Movius, Jr., and A. S. Romer, all of Harvard; R. A. Dart of Johannesburg; K. P. Oakley of the British Museum (Natural History); J. S. Weiner of Oxford; G. H. R. von Koenigswald of Utrecht; and D. A. Hooijer of Leiden. My appreciation for their kindness is great, for everything they did or said made the book better. Others have also been kind, in giving me important information or suggestions, or showing me material, while the book was under way; these were F. C. Howell of Chicago, F. Twiesselman of Brussels, W. Gieseler of

Tübingen, J. Hürzeler of Basel, and S. Sergi of Rome. Photographs for the plates were very kindly given me by Carleton Coon, Henry Field, Karl Heider, Laurence K. Marshall, and Douglas Oliver.

Two further people have my warm gratitude. The excellent drawings are by Janis Cirulis, an experienced illustrator lately come from Sweden. His endless patience and good humor in the face of my changes of mind and demands for the impossible were exemplary. Clara Claasen of Doubleday not only saw the book, like my previous books, through the press with skill and purposefulness but also helped at every turn with ideas and advance plans for many months while the book was being got ready.

February 1959

Note to the Revised Edition

Every author of a book on early man knows that a squadron of new fossils waits in hiding, to spring out when his work has appeared. I feel particularly victimized. The Leakeys, it is true, found "Zinjanthropus" while the original edition of this book was in proof, following it up with the really sensational series of recoveries at Olduvai in the next five or six years. They also brought "Kenyapithecus" to light, thus contributing, with Simons, to the recognition of *Ramapithecus* as a probable early hominid of the Pliocene. Simons also produced important new early "apes" from Egypt. The list of other new fossils is long and gratifying: at least four good Neanderthals; new Java skulls; from China, the Lantian, Mapa, and Liukiang men, and *Gigantopithecus'* jaws. The new information as to dates is so great as to defy specification. We still badly need fossils from the time between the Second (Mindel) and the Fourth (Würm) Glacial phases; we need more late fossils from Asia; we need Pliocene fossils from anywhere. If this revised edition has the proper effect, I shall have done my duty.

I wish to thank all my original helpers once again, and especially to mention thanks to Drs. von Koenigswald and Vértes for the use of photographs or information not yet published, and to Dr. Kurth of Braunschweig for comments made in connection with his excellent 1963 German translation of the original edition.

May 1966

Primates Among the Vertebrates

SUBPHYLUM *Vertebrata* (almost all of the Phylum *Chordata*)

SUPERCLASS *Pisces* (the fishes)
CLASS *Agnatha* (the jawless fishes: ostracoderms)
CLASS *Placodermi* (the armored fishes)
CLASS *Chondrichthyes* (the cartilaginous fishes, sharks and rays)
CLASS *Osteichthyes* (the bony fishes)
SUBCLASS *Actinopterygii* (the ray-finned fishes)
SUBCLASS *Choanichthyes* (fishes with internal nostrils)
ORDER *Dipnoi* (the lungfishes)
ORDER *Crossopterygii* (the lobe-fins)
SUBORDER *Coelacanthini* (the coelacanths)
SUBORDER *Rhipidistia* (fresh water ancestors of land animals)

SUPERCLASS *Tetrapoda* (the land animals, with four limbs)
CLASS *Amphibia* (the amphibians: 13 orders, living and extinct, including *Anura*, the frogs and toads; *Urodela*, newts and salamanders, and *Embolomeri*, labyrinthodont ancestors of reptiles)
CLASS *Reptilia* (the reptiles, with 5 subclasses, 16 orders, living and extinct, including the following)
SUBCLASS *Synapsida* (the mammal-like reptiles)
ORDER *Therapsida* (advanced mammal-like reptiles)
CLASS *Aves* (the birds)
CLASS *Mammalia* (some early mammals are of uncertain classification)
SUBCLASS *Prototheria* (the monotremes)
SUBCLASS *Allotheria* (the multituberculates, extinct)
SUBCLASS *Theria*
INFRACLASS *Pantotheria* (extinct ancestors of placentals?)
INFRACLASS *Metatheria* (the marsupials)
INFRACLASS *Eutheria* (the placental mammals, with 28 orders, living and extinct, including *Insectivora; Rodentia; Carnivora; Chiroptera* bats; *Perissodactyla* even-toed hoofed mammals; *Artiodactyla* (odd-toed hoofed mammals; and:)
ORDER **Primates**

Man Among the Primates

ORDER *Primates*

SUBORDER *Prosimii* (the prosimians or lower primates)
  FAMILIES: about 12. Six represent living forms (including some extinct members): tree shrews; lemurs; indris and woolly lemurs, aye-aye; lorises and galagos; Tarsius. Other families contain varied early Tertiary forms: plesiadapids (squirrel-like proto-lemurs); paromomyids (primitive and insectivore-like); carpolestids (specialized and unrelated to living forms); adapids (early lemurs); anaptomorphids (with resemblances to Tarsius); omomyids (the most likely general ancestors to higher primates).
SUBORDER *Anthropoidea* (the higher primates)
  SUPERFAMILY *Ceboidea* (primates of the New World)
    FAMILY   *Cebidae* (New World monkeys)
    FAMILY   *Callithricidae* (marmosets and tamarins)
  SUPERFAMILY *Cercopithecoidea*
    FAMILY   *Cercopithecidae* (Old World monkeys)
  SUPERFAMILY *Hominoidea*
    FAMILY   *Oreopithecidae* (Apidium, Oreopithecus)
    FAMILY   *Pongidae*
      SUBFAMILY *Hylobatinae* (gibbons and their ancestors)
      SUBFAMILY *Dryopithecinae* (Dryopithecus, Sivapithecus, Proconsul, Gigantopithecus)
      SUBFAMILY *Ponginae* (the living great apes)
    FAMILY   *Hominidae*
      GENUS   *Ramapithecus*
      GENUS   *Australopithecus*
      GENUS   *Paranthropus*
      GENUS   *Homo*
        SPECIES   *erectus*
        SPECIES   *sapiens*
          SUBSPECIES   *neanderthalensis*
          SUBSPECIES   *sapiens*

NOTE: especially for the Hominoidea, there is no "official" classification, but only a vague consensus with many individual disagreements. The above is a fairly economical and simple version. For example, Simons would put *Sivapithecus* and *Proconsul* into the genus *Dryopithecus;* Leakey would take *Proconsul* out of the subfamily Dryopithecinae entirely as something quite separate. Some would put *Australopithecus* and *Paranthropus* in a single genus; while both are usually put in a subfamily Australopithecinae as opposed to a second subfamily Homininae for *Homo.* The classification for *Homo* is not meant to accommodate Rhodesian Man; no classifications within *Homo* should be taken very seriously just now.

GLOSSARY

ADAPTATION, the fitness of an animal or plant species to its surroundings or way of life.

ADAPTIVE RADIATION, the evolutionary branching-out from a basic animal form, in following diverging lines of adaptation.

ALLEN'S RULE: other things being equal, warm-blooded animals of the same general kind in colder parts of the range will have shorter extremities (limbs, snout, tail), thus exposing less surface to heat loss.

AMNION, a fluid-filled sac surrounding the developing embryo in reptiles, birds, and mammals.

AMPHIPITHECUS, a problematical Eocene fossil jaw from Burma, possibly a hominoid.

ANTHROPOID, actually meaning "man-like," is ordinarily used only in connection with the "anthropoid apes" to distinguish these from monkeys.

ANTHROPOIDEA, suborder of Primates containing all the higher primates: New World and Old World monkeys, apes, and men, and their fossil relatives.

ANTIBODIES, protein substances in blood serum which exist, or form, reacting to various foreign substances, either diseases or antigens of blood cells foreign to the individual. The process of formation of antibodies is "immunization."

ASCENDING RAMUS, the vertical branch of the lower jaw.

ASSOCIATION AREAS, those parts of the neopallium, of the cerebral cortex of the brain, which are not distinctly connected with functioning of motor control or one of the senses, and are believed to be areas in which higher functions of association take place.

AUSTRALOPITHECINAE, a subfamily of the family Hominidae, containing the fossil "man-apes" (*Australopithecus* and *Paranthropus*) of the early Pleistocene but excluding all later or more advanced human forms.

AUSTRALOPITHECINE, pertaining to, or a member of, the subfamily Australopithecinae of the family Hominidae.

AUSTRALOPITHECUS, one genus of the proto-human australopithecines, known mainly from South Africa.

BERGMANN'S RULE: other things being equal, warm-blooded animals of the same general kind in colder parts of the range will be larger in general body size.

BILOPHODONT, or "two-crested," referring to the molar teeth of Old World monkeys, in which the cusps are arranged in pairs connected by transverse ridges. Other Anthropoidea lack this highly symmetrical cusp arrangement.

BRACHIATION, using the arms to swing through trees as a means of locomotion, as is characteristic of the anthropoid apes.

BRACHYCEPHALY: roundheadedness.

BRECCIA, a mass of material (e.g., earth, broken rocks, fossils, sand) which has become consolidated by some kind of cementing matrix, such as lime salts from water.

CALLITHRICIDAE, the family of the marmosets and tamarins of South America (tooth count 2-1-3-2), grouped with the Cebidae to form the Ceboidea, a superfamily of New World primates.

CANINE, the eye tooth, or dog tooth, lateral to the incisors, in mammals. Varyingly developed, but usually prominent and sometimes very large, in primates; relatively small in man.

CANINE FOSSA, or sub-orbital fossa, the hollow in the cheekbone over the sinus, on either side of the nose.

CARBON 14, a radioactive isotope of carbon, used in estimating dates from carbon preserved during the last 70,000 years.

CARTILAGE, "gristle," tough but resilient and translucent substance which lines skeletal joints and precedes most bone in the development of the skeleton.

CATARRHINE, "downward-nosed," a designation for the Old World higher primates (Old World monkeys, apes, man), to distinguish them from the Platyrrhines, or New World primates.

CEBIDAE, the family of the New World monkeys (tooth count 2-1-3-3), combined with the Callithricidae (marmosets) to form the superfamily Ceboidea.

CEBOIDEA, a superfamily of Anthropoidea or higher primates, containing the primates of the New World (families Cebidae and Callithricidae).

CENOZOIC (Recent Life), the Age of Mammals, beginning about 70 million years ago.

CERCOPITHECIDAE, the family of the Old World monkeys.

CERCOPITHECOIDEA, a superfamily of higher primates, containing only the family Cercopithecidae, Old World monkeys, to give these equal rank in classification with Hominoidea (apes and man) and Ceboidea (all the New World monkeys and marmosets together).

CEREBRAL CORTEX, the gray matter forming the outer layer of the cerebral hemispheres of the brain, especially developed in the mammals.

CHROMOSOMES, the carriers of inheritance, are thread-like structures in the nuclei of cells, on which genes are located. They are paired, one member of each pair being inherited from each parent. Man has an average of 23 pairs.

CINGULUM, when it occurs, is a shelving, or low collar ("girdle") around part or all of the base of the crown of a tooth, the cusps rising from within this girdle.

COCCYX, the tail vestige in man and apes, consisting of a few degenerate vertebrae generally fused together.

COELACANTHS, a marine branch of the Crossopterygii or lobe-finned fishes, related to the ancestry of land vertebrates but not on the direct line. At least two species survive in the Indian Ocean.

CONDYLE, a convex knob or joint surface of bone, to form a joint with a concave surface opposite. The condyle of the lower jaw is the hinder process on the ascending ramus. The occipital condyles of the skull, on either side of the *foramen magnum,* rest on the first vertebra, and form the joints of the skull with the spine.

CORONOID PROCESS of the jaw, the forward process of the ascending ramus, providing attachment for the large temporal muscle of the side of the skull.

CROSSOPTERYGII, a major Devonian group of the bony fishes, the lobe-fins, distantly related to the lungfishes, and containing the coelacanths and the ancestors of amphibians.

DENDROCHRONOLOGY, dating by counting tree rings.

DENTAL FORMULA, tooth count of different series of teeth. That of man and other catarrhines is 2-1-2-3, or two incisors, one canine, two premolars, and three molars, on either side of each jaw.

DIASTEMA, a gap, referring especially to a gap in either tooth row (particularly the upper) to receive the protruding canine of the opposite jaw.

DOLICHOCEPHALY: longheadedness.

DRYOPITHECINAE, a subfamily of the family Pongidae, containing a group of Miocene and Pliocene fossil apes related to the living great apes.

DRYOPITHECUS, an important genus of Miocene and Pliocene fossil apes, represented by several species, especially from Europe, foreshadowing the living apes.

ENVIRONMENTAL NICHES, special ways of life, or opportunities, within the whole environment, offering animals adapted to it a restricted degree of competition.

EOCENE, the second division of the Cenozoic or Tertiary era, lasting about from 55 million to 35 million B.C. This period probably saw the emergence of the first hominoids.

EOHIPPUS, a small, four-toed, primitive ancestor of later horses, whose proper name is *Hyracotherium.*

EPIPHYSIS, a joint surface or process of a bone which ossifies and grows separately, and unites with the body of the bone near the time of maturity; this is characteristic of mammals.

EVOLUTION, the fact of gradual change in species of animals or plants in succeeding generations, called by Darwin "descent with modification."

FLUORINE, an element occurring in ground water whose affinity for fossilizing bone allows estimates as to the correctness of assumed age.

FORAMEN MAGNUM, "large opening" in the base of the vertebrate skull, through which the spinal cord enters the skull.

FOSSIL, any evidence of an animal or plant preserved for a long period, but usually referring to a mineralized bone.

FRONTAL, the bone forming the forehead, and embracing the brow ridges and upper borders of the eye sockets.

GALAGOS, bush babies of Africa, members of the loris family (Lorisidae) of the prosimians, distinguished from the Asiatic lorises by a lengthened tarsus of the foot and active jumping habits.

GENERALIZED, the opposite of specialized, meaning an animal or organ not strikingly adapted to a given environment or way of life, generally closer to ancestral forms and probably more adaptable in different directions than corresponding specialized forms.

GENES, the units of inheritance, located on the chromosomes in the nuclei of cells. Since the chromosomes are paired, the genes occur in pairs, and the joint action of a pair modifies or controls the development of some characteristic of an individual.

GIGANTOPITHECUS, a fossil ape from the Middle (?) Pleistocene of China.

GLACIATION, the forming of ice sheets on land, either by extension of mountain glaciers in glaciated valleys or by the formation of continental glaciers during a glacial phase.

GORILLA, the genus name for *Gorilla gorilla,* the gorilla.

HETEROZYGOUS, having two different genes making up the gene pair under consideration. Often spoken of as the "single dose," with reference to a particular gene, as when one is "heterozygous" for the sickling gene, meaning that the subject has one sickling gene and one normal.

HOMINID, pertaining to the family Hominidae, of man, and thus relating to characteristics or members of this family; usually as distinguished from pongid, pertaining to members of the Pongidae, or apes. Distinct in meaning from "hominoid," which refers to both families together.

HOMINIDAE, the family of "man," including modern man and fossil man (in the subfamily of Homininae) and the man-apes (Australopithecinae) and probably the Pliocene form *Ramapithecus*. Characterized by upright bipedalism and traits of the dentition.

HOMININAE, a subfamily of the family Hominidae, containing the fossil men of the Pleistocene and living man (Java Man to *Homo sapiens*), but excluding the Australopithecinae.

HOMININE, referring to "men" within the family Hominidae; that is, to the subfamily Homininae in distinction to the subfamily Australopithecinae.

HOMINOID, pertaining to the superfamily Hominoidea, and thus relating to apes (pongids) and men (hominids) when considered together.

HOMINOIDEA, a superfamily of Anthropoidea or higher primates, containing and combining the families Pongidae (anthropoid apes) and Hominidae (man and australopithecines).

HOMOZYGOUS, having two genes which are identical (for the particular gene pair under consideration); often called the "double dose."

HYLOBATES, the genus name for the living gibbon.

HYLOBATINAE, a subfamily of the family Pongidae, to contain the gibbons, from the living form back to *Propliopithecus* of the Oligocene.

HYOMANDIBULAR, originally part of a gill arch, later taking part in attachment of the upper jaw to the skull in fishes, and eventually becoming the stapes of the middle ear in land vertebrates.

ICTHYOSAURUS, a water-living, shark-form reptile of the Mesozoic.

INCISOR, a tooth of the first series in mammals at the front of the mouth, usually somewhat chisel-shaped.

INSECTIVORE, an insect-eating mammal, member of the Insectivora, a group generally close to the early mammals of the Mesozoic.

ISCHIAL CALLOSITIES, bodies of tough fibrous tissue overlying the ischial bones (the "seat" area) of the pelvis. These are a particular specialization of the Old World monkeys, but occur also in gibbons and a high proportion of chimpanzees.

LABYRINTHODONTS, the major group of early amphibians, of the Paleozoic.

LIMNOPITHECUS, a fossil gibbon of the early Miocene of East Africa, known from two species, and relatively short-limbed compared to living gibbons.

LORISES, a family of prosimians (Lorisidae) akin to the lemurs, living in Africa and southern Asia.

LUMBAR, that part of the spinal column between the ribs and the pelvis; in man, it is strongly bent back in the "lumbar curve" to straighten the upper part of the body over the legs.

MARSUPIALS, the pouched mammals, which do not form a placenta in reproduction, but nourish the young from an early developmental stage in a marsupium, like the kangaroo. Once widespread, the group has only a few living representatives in the Americas (notably the opossum), and is the characteristic fauna only of Australia and New Guinea.

MESOLITHIC, "Middle Stone Age," but more correctly a group of hunting-gathering cultures in Europe between the end of the Pleistocene (about 8000 B.C.) and the appearance of Neolithic farming.

MESOZOIC (Middle Life), the Age of Reptiles, the geological period dominated by dinosaurs but containing the early development of mammals.

MIOCENE, the fourth division of the Cenozoic or Tertiary era, lasting from about 25 million to about 10 million B.C. Apes ancestral to modern forms were taking shape.

MODJOKERTO, a site in Central Java at which an infant skull was found with the Djetis fauna, evidently a child of Java Man.

MOLAR, teeth at the back of the mammal tooth row, usually more adapted for grinding or crushing than teeth of other series. Three are present in man as in original placental mammals. Commonly spoken of as "6-year," "12-year," and "wisdom" teeth.

MONOTREMES, egg-laying mammals of Australia and New Guinea, more primitive than marsupials and placentals. Represented only by the platypus and the spiny anteater, one form of the latter having a pouch like the marsupials.

MOUSTERIAN, a late, actually varied, complex of stone industries of the Lower Paleolithic, apparently exclusively associated with Neanderthal Man.

MULTITUBERCULATES, a group of early mammals, unrelated to the main marsupial-placental stock, which survived into the Eocene epoch.

MUTATION, refers mainly to a permanent change in some gene carried by an individual, producing a changed effect, in the trait to which the gene is related, in those of his descendants who receive the gene.

NATURAL SELECTION, the tendency for a population to change from generation to generation (to evolve) because some of its individuals are more adapted for a given situation, and therefore pass their inherited characteristics to the next generation in a greater proportion than the remainder.

NEOLITHIC, or "New Stone Age," more properly the period, anywhere, in which simple farming existed, without large communities or cities. It appeared perhaps as early as 10,000 years ago in the Near East and much later in Europe and other areas.

NEOPALLIUM, the "new cloak," or areas of the cerebral cortex of the brain devoted mainly to senses other than to smell, and to association. It forms the greater proportion of the cortex in mammals, especially in the Primates.

OCCIPITAL, pertaining to the back of the head: occipital bone, the back of the skull and hinder part of the base, including the *foramen magnum.*

OLIGOCENE, the third division of the Cenozoic or Tertiary era, lasting from about 35 million to about 25 million B.C. The first definite anthropoid ape dates from the early Oligocene.

OPPOSABLE, applied to the first digit (thumb and great toe) of typical primates, meaning a degree of rotation of this digit out of the plane of the others, allowing it to be opposed to them in grasping movements.

OREOPITHECIDAE, a family to contain the Pliocene fossil *Oreopithecus,* assigned to the Hominoidea, but not to either Pongidae or Hominidae.

OSTRACODERM, "shell-skinned," jawless fish, member of the Agnatha or earliest class of fishes, extinct except for lamprey eels and hagfishes.

PALEOCENE, the first division of the Cenozoic of Tertiary era, beginning about 70 million years ago. The period of early primate radiation.

PALEOLITHIC, the Old Stone Age, characterized by exclusive dependence on hunting, and by the use of stone tools. Divided into the Lower Paleolithic and Upper Paleolithic in Europe, the latter beginning about 35,000 B.C. and marked by varied utensils made on a flake-blade of flint.

PALEOZOIC, the Age of Fishes, the first geological period containing fossil remains of vertebrates.

PAN, the genus name for *Pan troglodytes,* the chimpanzee.

PANTOTHERES, a group of Mesozoic mammals, the Pantotheria. Although extinct themselves, they gave rise to the marsupials and the placentals.

PARANTHROPUS, one genus of the australopithecines of the early Pleistocene, known from South Africa and represented also by "Zinjanthropus" of East Africa and possibly *Meganthropus* of Java.

PARIETAL bones, the "walls" of the skull vault, forming the upper part of the sides of the skull on either side.

PEDOMORPHISM, change or evolution by retention of infantile characters into the adult stage.

PLACENTAL MAMMALS, those other than marsupials and monotremes. They form a placenta in reproduction, an organ in which the maternal and fetal blood streams come into close contact, attached to the fetus by the umbilical cord.

PLATYRRHINE, "flat-nosed," pertaining to the New World higher primates (families Cebidae and Callithricidae), whose nostrils are widely separated, to distinguish them as a group from the Catarrhines, or Old World higher primates.

PLEISTOCENE, the last division of geological time before the Recent: the Ice Age, lasting from perhaps 3,000,000 B.C. to about 10,000 B.C. All fossil human beings belong to this period.

PLIOCENE, the fifth division of the Cenozoic or Tertiary era, lasting from about 12 million to 3 million B.C. Ancestors of modern apes and of man were present; most *Dryopithecus* species, *Oreopithecus,* and *Ramapithecus,* are from this period.

PLIOPITHECUS, a fossil "gibbon" of the Miocene and Pliocene, relatively short-limbed compared to the modern gibbon, and having a tail.

PONGID, pertaining to Pongidae, generally as opposed to hominid (belonging to, or having characteristics of, man or the Australopithecinae) or cercopithecid (having the characteristics of Old World monkeys).

PONGIDAE, the family of the anthropoid apes, living and extinct, provisionally divided into the subfamilies Hylobatinae (gibbons), Dryopithecinae, and Ponginae (great apes). It is grouped with Hominidae, the family of man, in the superfamily Hominoidea.

PONGINAE, a subfamily of the family Pongidae, containing the living great apes.

PONGINE, pertaining to, or a member of, the Ponginae, the subfamily of the living great apes (orang, chimpanzee, gorilla) and their fossil relatives.

PONGO, the genus name for *Pongo pygmaeus,* the living orang utan.

PREADAPTATION, the accidental existence of some trait in an animal species which later proved to be adaptive or useful in a new situation.

PREHENSILE, applied to the digits of primates (and the tail of some New World monkeys), meaning their ability to enclose an object in grasping movements.

PREMOLAR, the teeth lying in front of the molars proper. "Bicuspid," or two-cusped, in man, but not in all mammals, nor strictly so in primates. Man has reduced the number in each side of each jaw from four, in original mammals, to two.

PRIMATES, an order of mammals, to which man, apes, monkeys, and lower primates belong. Divided into two suborders: Prosimii, the lower primates; Anthropoidea, monkeys, apes, and man.

PROCONSUL, a Miocene genus of ape, known from three species from East Africa.

PROSIMIANS, members of the Prosimii or lower primates, containing lemurs, lorises, tree shrews, and *Tarsius,* as well as many fossil forms.

RADIUS, the bone of the forearm, whose power end lies at the base of the thumb side of the wrist, which rotates on the ulna, the other forearm bone, to rotate the hand.

RAMAPITHECUS (including "Kenyapithecus"), a probable hominid, known from upper and lower jaws from India and Kenya, which manifest a short face and short canine teeth.

RODENT, a mammal with grinding molar teeth and continually growing, chisel-like incisors suited for gnawing bark and roots; a member of the Rodentia, which includes mice, squirrels, beavers, etc.

SACRUM, the fused vertebrae (usually five in man) which form the "keystone" of the pelvis, joined on either side (the sacro-iliac joints) to the two innominate, or hip, bones, and bearing the lumbar part of the spine above.

SCAPULA, the shoulder blade.

SEYMOURIA, a very early reptile, almost intermediate in its skeleton between amphibians and reptiles.

SIMIAN SHELF, a reinforcing shelf of bone lying across the inside of the arch of the chin region, in apes and Old World monkeys.

SIVAPITHECUS, an important genus of Miocene and Pliocene great apes, represented in India and Africa.

SPECIALIZED, an animal or an organ strongly adapted to a particular environment or way of life, carrying the connotation of tending to be limited as to other possibilities.

STEATOPYGIA, "fat on the buttocks," an emphasis of this region of fat deposition found especially among the women of the Hottentots, also of the Bushmen, and possibly rarely in some other peoples of the world.

STEREOSCOPIC VISION, the ability to merge impressions from both eyes in the brain in such a way as to allow good judgment of distance.

SYMPHALANGUS, the genus name for the siamang, the large member of the gibbon subfamily.

TARSIOID, resembling *Tarsius,* generally referring to a large group of extinct relatives of the living tarsier.

TARSUS, in man, the hinder part of the foot skeleton including the heel. In vertebrates generally, the part of the hind limb below the tibia.

TEMPORAL, the lateral part of the skull. Temporal bone, the part of the vault and base carrying the jaw joint, ear opening, and mastoid process. Temporal muscle, which raises the jaw, arises as a flat sheet from a large area of the side of the skull.

TETRAPODS, four-limbed vertebrates, i.e., the four classes of "land" vertebrates: amphibians, reptiles, birds, mammals, all built on an original four-footed plan, even though this has been changed or modified in whales, birds, man, etc.

THERAPSIDS, the advanced mammal-like reptiles of the late Paleozoic and early Mesozoic, from which the mammals arose directly.

TYRANNOSAURUS, a very large, bipedal carnivorous dinosaur of the Mesozoic.

ULNA, the forearm bone which forms the hinge joint at the elbow, and on which the radius twists to rotate the wrist and hand.

VERTEBRA, one of the parts of the spinal column. They are well differentiated in man and other mammals, but are increasingly similar in form along the spine as one goes down the scale to the fishes.

VERTEBRATES, the major group of animals to which man and all backboned animals belong. Strictly speaking, the Vertebrata are a subphylum of the phylum Chordata, all of which have a notochord or fibrous rod along the back, during life or preceding the spinal column in development; but the non-vertebrate members (lancelet, tunicates, etc.) are few and unimportant.

VILLAFRANCHIAN, an important fauna, or assemblage of animals, marking the beginning of the Pleistocene and constituting the appearance of the modern genera of horses, elephants, and cattle.

INDEX